Social Psychology in a Globalizing Era

Engaging with Disciplinary and Societal Challenges

Edited by Girishwar Misra and Purnima Singh

Routledge
Taylor & Francis Group
LONDON AND NEW YORK

First published 2025
by Routledge
4 Park Square, Milton Park, Abingdon, Oxon OX14 4RN

and by Routledge
605 Third Avenue, New York, NY 10158

Routledge is an imprint of the Taylor & Francis Group, an informa business

British Library Cataloguing-in-Publication Data
A catalogue record for this book is available from the British Library

ISBN: 978-1-032-57305-2 (hbk)
ISBN: 978-1-032-60964-5 (pbk)
ISBN: 978-1-003-46130-2 (ebk)

DOI: 10.4324/9781003461302

Typeset in Sabon
by Apex CoVantage, LLC

Social Psychology in a Globalizing Era

This volume locates social psychology in the context of contemporary societies in an increasingly globalizing world where time, space, and relationships are reshaped by powerful information, communication, and travel technologies.

The volume revisits the efforts thus far while commenting upon the treatment of pertinent issues in the emerging sociopolitical and academic climate of the globalized area. It discusses how globalization has led to multidimensional changes in the society, warranting newer ways of comprehending, conceptualizing, and navigating through the complexities of the emerging social world. While mapping the new changes shaping contemporary discourse, the book refers to the new emerging patterns of human relationships, which are acquiring different shapes and meanings, leading not just to restructuring but also to creating innovative ways of being and making sense of the world.

The volume would be useful to students and teachers of psychology, applied psychology, sociology, social work, public health, gender, and women studies. It would also be an invaluable companion to pediatrics, forensic medicine, psychiatry, and law enforcement authorities like police and judiciary.

Girishwar Misra was formerly a professor of psychology at the University of Delhi. Earlier, he taught at Gorakhpur University (1970–1079), Allahabad University (1979–1983), and Bhopal University (1983–1993), before joining as a professor at Delhi University in 1993, where he served for the rest of his career. He served as Vice Chancellor of Mahatma Gandhi Antarrashtriya Hindi Vishwavidyalaya in Wardha, Maharashtra (2014–2019). His teaching, research, and publications focus on cultural and indigenous psychology, human development, self and identity, and emotions. He was President of the National Academy of Psychology, India; Senior Fulbright Fellow at Swarthmore College, Philadelphia, and the University of Michigan, Ann Arbor; and Dean of Faculty of Arts, University of Delhi. He has been a visiting fellow at Ruhr University, Bochum, Germany; the University of Sussex, Britain; and the New School of Social Research, New York. He is a recipient of the National Fellowship of the National Academy of Psychology (NAOP), the National Fellowship of the Indian Council of Social Science Research (ICSSR), the S.C. Mitra Memorial Award of the Asiatic Society, and the Honorary Fellowship of the International Association of Cross-Cultural Psychology (IACCP).

Purnima Singh is Professor Emeritus at IIT Delhi, Delhi, India. Earlier, she was Institute Chair Professor at IIT Delhi and professor at the University of Allahabad. She is a past president and a fellow of the National Academy of Psychology. She is the editor of *Psychological Studies* (Springer). She is on the editorial board of the *International Journal of Psychology*. She is also in the Executive Committee of the IACCP and the President-Elect of Psychological and Societal Development (Division 3) of the International Association of Applied Psychology. Her research interests include justice, intergroup relations, structural variables, and education.

Contents

Illustrations

Figures

Tables

Contributors

John W. Berry is Professor Emeritus of Psychology at Queen's University, Canada, and a research professor at the National Research University Higher School of Economics, Moscow, Russia. He has published over 30 books in the areas of cross-cultural, intercultural, social, and cognitive psychology with various colleagues. He is a fellow of the Canadian Psychological Association, the Netherlands Institute for Advanced Study, the International Association for Cross-Cultural Psychology (IACCP), and the International Academy for Intercultural Research. He received the award for Contributions to the Advancement of International Psychology in 2012 (from CPA). He is also the winner of the 2024 Lifetime Career Award from the International Union for Psychological Science. His research interests include the role of ecology and culture in human development, acculturation, and intercultural relations.

Deborah L. Best, PhD, is William L. Poteat Professor of Psychology, Emerita at Wake Forest University, USA (previously Chair of the Psychology Department; Dean of the College of Arts and Sciences). She is Honorary Fellow (President: 2000–2002; Treasurer: 1988–1997) of the IACCP and is active in the Society for Cross-Cultural Research (President: 2011–2012). She is Special Issues Editor (2024—present; Editor-in-Chief—2012–2024; Associate Editor—1996–2012) of the *Journal of Cross-Cultural Psychology*. She has written and edited eight books, numerous book chapters, and research articles, including a 1990 landmark study of gender stereotypes in 30 nations that is currently being replicated in 60+ countries. Her research focuses on children's cognitive and social development and the role of culture.

Urmi Nanda Biswas is a professor in the Department of Psychology at Delhi University. She has been a visiting fellow at Roehampton University, London, and Gothenburg University, Sweden. She has completed over ten major research projects with funding from prestigious national and international agencies and produced 16 PhDs under her supervision. Her publications include *Social Psychology of Health: Issues and Concerns in India* and *Understanding Attractive Work in a Globalized Context*. Her upcoming book is titled *Building A Responsible and Resilient World: Perspectives from India* (Springer).

Ariel G. Gianukakis graduated from Wake Forest University, USA, where she was a member of a Developmental Psychology Lab (2019–2021). She was a research assistant at an infant neurocognitive development lab at New York University (2020). Additionally, she worked as a research assistant at Brown University, USA, where she focused on implementing measurement-based care in a child psychiatric hospital (2021–2023). She is now working toward her Master of Science in Nursing at Emory University, USA. She plans to work as a nurse practitioner specializing in child development and mental health.

Nick Hopkins is a professor at the University of Dundee. He is interested in group behavior and how identities are based upon our group memberships. He has been involved in a number of teaching and research skill training projects based at the University of Allahabad. One of his more recent projects is the ESRC-funded project looking at the social psychology of collective participation in the Magh Mela—a Hindu festival that takes place each year at Allahabad, North India. In addition to academic journals, his research concerning identity has featured in various governmental reports too, such as the UK Government's Foresight project "Future Identities: Changing Identities in the UK—the Next 10 Years." His research interests focus on the construction and implications of group-based social identities and minority group members' negotiation of their marginalization.

Nishtha Jain is a lecturer at the Jindal School of Psychology and Counselling, O. P. Jindal Global University, Sonepat. She is also a PhD candidate at the Indian Institute of Technology, Delhi. Her research focuses on exploring the kinds of critical decisions that arise in the treatment of cancer and how such decisions are taken within the Indian healthcare context. She recently won the Gary A. Klein Award for best paper contribution to Naturalistic Decision-Making (NDM) Theory at the 17th international conference of NDM, Auckland University of Technology, New Zealand, for her research. In her research journey, Nishtha aims to bridge the gap between psychological research and practical applications in healthcare, contributing to more effective decision-making processes and improved patient outcomes.

Preeti Kapur served as an associate professor of psychology at Daulat Ram College, University of Delhi, Delhi, for over four decades. She has taught undergraduate classes in social psychology, statistics, research methodology, and educational and community psychology. Her interest areas include cultural studies, religious studies, gender, health, and well-being. She has published papers in both national and international journals. Currently, she spends her time and energy on community outreach programs in the areas of primary education at NGOs and government school settings, mental health awareness, health and hygiene, and disability.

Arvind Kumar Mishra is a professor of psychology at Jawaharlal Nehru University (JNU), New Delhi. He has over 30 years of teaching experience. Before joining JNU, he taught at the University of Delhi and Jamia Millia Islamia, New Delhi. He is the coeditor of five books and numerous papers. His research interests focus on resistance to neoliberal modernity, the philosophy of social research, critical social psychology, the academic experiences of disadvantaged students, and self and identity processes among marginalized communities. He has been the principal investigator of a UK-India Education and Research Initiative (UKIERI) research project on *Social Identity, Well-Being, and Civic Participation among Social and Ethnic Groups in India*. He is on the Editorial Board of *Psychology and Developing Societies* (Sage).

Linda Escobar Olszewski is a clinical psychologist and the clinical director of Stuart House at UCLA Health. Dr. Escobar Olszewski also holds a faculty appointment in the Department of Psychiatry and Biobehavioral Sciences, David Geffen School of Medicine, UCLA. Dr. Escobar Olszewski has focused on working with children and adolescents from underserved and marginalized populations, treating complex trauma. She has diverse research interests, including trauma, parenting, and performance. Her current research focuses on the Latinx community and trauma correlates. Dr. Escobar Olszewski has presented her research at conferences and provides consultative services both nationally and internationally.

Pallavi Ramanathan is currently an assistant professor of psychology at FLAME University, Pune. She has recently completed her PhD in social psychology at IIT Delhi, and her thesis is titled "Understanding the Construction and Negotiation of Tibetan Refugee Identities in India." Her interests lie in the areas of social identity, the social and cultural context, and intergroup relations. She is keenly interested in the construction, negotiation, and contestation of identity at a group level, looking to understand the cross-section of identity and culture. Pallavi has presented her work at various international conferences and has been awarded various grants and honors, including the IACCP's SPARK Grant (2022). She also has several journal articles and book chapters to her credit.

Steve D. Reicher is Bishop Wardlaw Professor of Social Psychology at the University of St Andrews. Reicher completed his PhD at the University of Bristol, working closely with Henri Tajfel and John Turner. He is a fellow of the Royal Society of Edinburgh and a consultant editor for a number of journals, including *Scientific American Mind*. He is broadly interested in the issues of group behavior and the individual–social relationship. His research interests can be grouped into three areas. The first is an attempt to develop a model of crowd action that accounts for both social determination and social change. The second concerns the construction of social categories through language and action. The third concerns political rhetoric and mass mobilization—especially around the issue of national identity.

Richard Barry Ruback had a background in social psychology and law. Barry Ruback's interests were primarily in decision-making in criminal justice. He was particularly interested in the decision-making of crime victims and in the predictors and consequences of sentencing decisions, especially those concerning economic sanctions. In research funded by the National Science Foundation, the National Institute of Justice, and the Pennsylvania Commission on Sentencing, he examined the use and impact of economic sanctions (fines, fees, and restitution). He also had a long-standing interest in criminal victimization and crime victims' reporting to the police, which he is currently working on in connection with a BJS fellowship. Related to this interest is the work done with his graduate students regarding the occurrence and reporting of hate crimes in Pennsylvania.

Corinne R. Scannell, MS/SSP, recently graduated with a specialist degree in school psychology from Winthrop University, USA. She has presented at the National Association of School Psychology conference on the validity and utility of computer adaptive testing for elementary math (2024). She completed her undergraduate studies at Wake Forest University, USA. She was a member of a Developmental Psychology Lab at Wake Forest University (2017–2021). She was a research assistant in a Developmental Psychopathology Lab at Stony Brook University (2018) and in a Sports Psychology Lab at Universidad Pablo de Olavide, Spain (2019). She has volunteered at the National Eating Disorders Association Helpline (2019). She plans to pursue a career as a school psychologist in the K-12 setting.

Roomana N. Siddiqui is a professor of psychology at Aligarh Muslim University, Aligarh. She is a social psychologist interested in issues of social relevance. She earned her doctoral degree in the area of environmental psychology from the Centre of Advanced Study in Psychology, University of Allahabad. Her publications include *Dreams & Destinations: An Illustrated Publication of 100 Years of Women's Education*. She has worked with international collaborators on projects of significance. She has organized a number of training programs for research scholars and teachers. Her current research includes issues related to environment, identity, and intergroup relations.

Anup K. Singh has been Director General at Nirma University since 2013. He completed his doctoral studies at the University of Allahabad and postdoctoral fellowship at the University of Michigan, Ann Arbor. He was a visiting scholar at the JL Kellogg Graduate School of Business Administration,

Northwestern University, Evanston. He was a professor of organizational behavior at the Management Development Institute, Gurugram, and a professor and dean at the International Management Institute, New Delhi. He was also the director of the Jaipuria Institute of Management, Noida. Earlier, he was the director of the Nirma Institute of Management, Ahmedabad. He has many publications to his credit, comprising books, research papers in international and national journals, case studies, and book chapters, in addition to paper presentations at national and international levels.

Vanita Sondhi is a distinguished scholar and a professor in the Department of Applied Psychology at Vivekananda College, University of Delhi, with over 30 years of teaching and research experience. She earned her PhD from the University of Delhi, specializing in the area of eyewitness memory. Dr. Sondhi has made significant contributions to the field through her extensive research and publications in prominent national and international journals. Her work spans diverse topics, including resilience among orphaned adolescents, the psychosocial impact of globalization on young Indians, and mental health during crises such as the COVID-19 pandemic. She has also successfully developed courses for the University Grants Commission (UGC) e-pg Pathshala initiative.

Narayanan Srinivasan is currently a professor and the head of the Department of Cognitive Science at the Indian Institute of Technology Kanpur. He completed his undergraduate degree in physics at Madras University and master's degree in electrical engineering at the Indian Institute of Science, Bengaluru. His PhD is in psychology from the University of Georgia, Athens, USA. He uses multiple approaches to study mental processes. He has wide-ranging interests in cognitive science and is involved in projects in many different areas of cognitive science. His research interests focus on understanding consciousness, perception, attention, emotions, and decision-making.

Sonia Suchday is a professor and the chair of the Psychology Department and the interim university director of research at Pace University. She is the former chair of the U.S. National Committee on Psychological Sciences at the National Academy of Sciences and is a representative of the International Union of Psychological Sciences to the United Nations. She has extensive experience in building international educational and research programs and international partnerships. She has organized prestigious conferences, including one on diversity and disparity and the Israel–United States–India partnership. Her recent work includes the effects of spirituality on health and well-being. She is also the founder/director of Ashram On Park, a Workplace Wellness Consulting firm that she co-founded during the pandemic with three colleagues.

Jyoti Verma was awarded a PhD from Patna University and served as its faculty. She has been a consulting editor of the *Asian Journal of Social Psychology* and a member of the Editorial Board of the *Journal of Culture and Psychology*. Her expertise includes cross-cultural psychology and teaching organizational behavior in the MBA Program. Her extensive international experiences come from her research and professional visits to the United States, France, Italy, Germany, Finland, Poland, and so on, which have benefited her in interweaving psychology and Indian culture's understanding with cross-cultural experience in international business consultancy.

Colleen Ward is an American–New Zealand cross-cultural psychologist. She is a professor of psychology and the founder of the Centre for Applied Cross-cultural Research at Victoria University of Wellington. She obtained her PhD in social psychology from Durham University in 1977. She is interested in the experience and outcomes of cultures in contact, that is, acculturation. She is particularly concerned with the factors that facilitate or impede psychological ("feeling well") and sociocultural ("doing well") adaptation. As part of the acculturation process, she is also interested in how individuals negotiate their cultural identity, that is, heritage cultural identities and identity as a member of their new cultural group. As such, topics such as intercultural relations and multiculturalism form part of her research.

Preface

The Power of the Context

Professor Janak Pandey's Bequest to the Field of Social Psychology

Social Psychology in the Globalized Era is dedicated to Professor Janak Pandey, an incredibly influential figure in cross-cultural psychology and applied social psychology. Decades ahead of its time, he rooted his research in the understanding of social and cultural context, which influences our actions and emotions in his research on social influence processes, poverty and justice, and environmental issues. Trained at Patna University and Kansas State University, USA, he held faculty positions at the Indian Institute of Technology Kanpur and at Allahabad University, Allahabad. He also served as Director of G. B. Pant Institute of Social Sciences, Allahabad, and Founding Vice Chancellor of Bihar Central University, Patna. He had an international appointment at the East-West Centre, Honolulu, University of Manitoba, and Wake Forest University. As an author of more than 100 scientific papers and author/editor of more than 20 books in the field of cross-cultural psychology, attitude, environmental issues, and poverty, he has strengthened the teaching-learning of psychology within the spectrum of higher education in India. He also served as the associate/consulting editor of the *Journal of Cross-Cultural Psychology,* the *Asian Journal of Social Psychology, Psychology and Developing Societies*, and *Psychological Studies*. He also served as the convenor and president of the National Academy of Psychology (NAOP), India. He was also the National Fellow of the Indian Council of Social Science Research (ICSSR). His research, spanning over the last five decades, has shown how social development-related issues cannot be understood in a vacuum, the context determines the relevance of the issue, and how it is responded to, and this marks his pioneering contribution to the field of social psychology. The chapters in this volume have been authored by those who have collaborated with Professor Pandey in the past.

Psychology in India might not ever have been what it is today had it not been for some pioneers in the field, with Professor Pandey playing an important role in creating a niche for psychologists from India and also those from other majority world countries, the role that they have at present. In this brief commentary, we attempt to walk you through his contributions in an endeavor to understand the nature of social psychology through his works.

Though the canvas of his research interests is vast, social development-related issues have been at the core. Four broad areas are discernible, that is, challenges to social development—center-staging the issues of poverty, justice, prosocial behavior, environmental concerns in developing societies, social influence processes and their functionality in feudal hierarchical societies, and developmental trajectories of psychology in India. Of course, there are many other areas of research to which he has contributed and a large number of publications that do not find mention in this brief commentary; however, we attempt to give the reader a synoptic overview of his multidimensional contributions.

Challenges to Social Development

Social development is about bringing a change in the well-being of people. Crucial to the understanding of well-being is to have a perspective on the causes and consequences of poverty and injustice, which are major challenges for human development. In the context of the changing social-political and economic scenario of India's issues of poverty, its relative nature and the importance of subjective poverty and attribution of poverty attracted the attention of Professor Pandey. Examining issues like perceptions of poverty (Pandey et al., 1982a) and how political ideologies impact poverty explanation (Pandey et al., 1982b) and psychological factors in social mobility (Singh & Pandey, 1991), Pandey and his associates set the stage for understanding development in the Indian context (Pant & Pandey, 2004; Pandey, 2002), which culminated in an edited volume *Psychological Perspectives on Diversity and Social Development* (Pandey et al., 2019). Other social-development-related concerns focused on the conceptualization of fundamentalism (Pandey & Sinha, 1991), sex-trait stereotypes in India and Pakistan (Williams et al., 1982), helping behavior (Pandey & Griffit, 1977), and dependence proneness (Sinha & Pandey,1970a, 1971, 1972).

In a country like India in the 1960s, when national development was the major focus, the concern was to motivate people to excel and achieve. Pandey and Sinha (1968) examined the predicament of the need for achievement in a scarce resource context. His penchant for social issues can be seen in his work on justice perceptions and factors determining such perceptions (Pandey & Singh, 1989, 1997; Singh & Pandey, 1994), showing how justice evaluations and resource allocations are determined by characteristics of context and recipients.

Environmental Concerns in Developing Societies

Environmental issues have impacted flora, fauna, and human life worldwide. In developing societies, environmental issues are also social issues, as those most affected by environmental degradation are the poor and those on the periphery. This is a central theme in a number of his publications in the context of both India and countries in South Asia (which may be different due to political patterns but share rituals and social and religious practices). Population pressure on the environment and resources has created a vicious situation in this region. The experience of crowding and its impact on social behavior has been the focus of a large number of studies (Ruback & Pandey, 1991, 1992, 1996; Nagar et al., 1988; Ruback et al., 1997; Pandey & Jain, 2017), and his studies on urban stressors and their impact in South Asian countries, especially the impact on slum dwellers (Ruback & Pandey, 1996; Ruback et al., 2001; Pandey & Siddiqui, 2001; Pandey et al., 2000; Pandey, 1998), showcase his interest in poverty and environment as both interact and have a detrimental impact on the lives of slum dwellers. The numerous studies done by him and his associates extend his interest in poverty and justice to the environment and show their intricate connection in developing societies, which is a unique social milieu, hitherto neglected in Euro-American research.

Social Influence Processes in Context

Social influence has been a dominant research theme in social psychology and the central topic for Pandey. In the scarce resources and feudal hierarchical context of India, the nature of the social influence processes and the way they function is different. The volume titled *Nature and Dynamics of Social Influence: Interpersonal and Organizational Contexts* (2022) describes the research conducted by Pandey and his associates, showing ways in which forms of persuasion are used. The intricacies of social influence processes like self-presentation, impression management, ingratiation, persuasion, manipulative social behavior, and compliance as they are impacted by the cultural and social context in India are demonstrated through various studies. The tactics and strategies of social influence are impacted by social and cultural context. What makes certain tactics legitimate and acceptable varies from one context to another context. Interpersonal and organizational dynamics make certain tactics and strategies acceptable and others not that acceptable. The majority of studies (Pandey, 1981a, 1981b; Pandey & Kakkar, 1982; Pandey et al., 1983; Bohra & Pandey, 1984; Pandey & Bohra, 1984; Pandey & Singh, 1987) focus on other enhancement tactics and their functionality in the Indian scenario.

Trends in the Discipline of Social Psychology

As a psychologist known for the internationalization of psychology in the country and also a vociferous proponent of indigenous psychology, his contributions to the growth of the discipline of psychology in the country have been noteworthy. He had the honor to lead the third and the fourth rounds of a survey of psychology sponsored by the ICSSR, which led to the publication of a two-volume series of psychology titled *Psychology in India: The State-of-the-Art* published in 1988 (a three-volume set) and *Psychology in India Revisited: Developments in the Discipline* (Pandey, 2000, 2001, 2004). These volumes showcase critical developments in the discipline in India over two decades. How the discipline has moved from an era of replication to a focus on indigenization is very well captured in these volumes. There are significant resources in psychology.

His contributions to cross-cultural psychology are seen in edited volumes (Berry et al., 1996; Pandey et al., 1996). He also served as the president of the International Association of Cross-Cultural Psychology during 1994–1996, and in 2006, he was awarded an honorary fellowship. A seminal contribution has been the edited volume *Perspective on Experimental Social Psychology in India* (Pandey, 1981c), presenting contributions to experimental social psychologists. It is noteworthy to know that social psychology has been a key area of research in the country. A lucid depiction of the path traversed by social psychology in India with important milestones and trends of research can be seen (Pandey, 2019, 2022; Pandey & Singh, 2005), showing the connection between social context and research in social psychology. The way Professor Pandey could integrate both the internationalization of psychology and cultural and social inclusivity in his research shows the way forward for future researchers—to situate psychology research in a social-cultural context, and the dissemination of it in the global context is the way forward.

References

Berry, J. W., Poortinga, Y., & Pandey, J. (Eds.). (1996). *Handbook of cross-cultural psychology: Theory and method* (Vol. 1). Allyn & Bacon.

Bohra, K. A., & Pandey, J. (1984). Ingratiation toward strangers, friends, and bosses. *The Journal of Social Psychology*, *122*, 217–222.

Nagar, D., Pandey, J., & Paulus, P. B. (1988). The effects of residential crowding experience on reactivity to laboratory crowding and noise. *Journal of Applied Social Psychology*, *18*, 1423–1442.

Pandey, J. (1981a). A note about social power through ingratiation among workers. *Journal of Occupational Psychology*, *54*, 65–67.

Pandey, J. (1981b). Ingratiation tactics in India. *The Journal of Social Psychology*, *113*, 147–148.

Pandey, J. (Ed.). (1981c). *Perspective on experimental social psychology in India*. Concept Publishers.

Pandey, J. (1998). Environment in the Indian context: Socio-psychological issues and research. *Indian Psychological Abstracts and Reviews*, *5*(2), 205–234.

Pandey, J. (Ed.). (2000). *Psychology in India revisited: Developments in the discipline: Physiological foundation and human cognition* (Vol. 1). Sage Publishers.

Pandey, J. (Ed.). (2001). *Psychology in India revisited: Developments in the discipline: Personality and health psychology* (Vol. 2). Sage Publications.

Pandey, J. (Ed.). (2002). *Social development.* Ashish Publishing House.
Pandey, J. (Ed.). (2004). *Psychology in India revisited: Developments in the discipline: Applied social and organizational psychology* (Vol. 3). Sage Publication.
Pandey, J. (2019). Fifty years of Indian council social science research and development of psychology research in India. In B. B. Kumar (Ed.) *Understanding India and its problems* (Vol. 1). McMillan Publisher.
Pandey, J. (2022). *Nature and dynamics of social influence: Interpersonal and organizational contexts.* Springer.
Pandey, J., & Bohra, K. A. (1984). Ingratiation as a function of organizational characteristics and supervisory styles. *International Review of Applied Psychology, 33*, 381–394.
Pandey, J., & Griffitt, W. (1977). Benefactor's nurturance need, recipient's dependency and the effect of number of potential helpers on helping behavior. *Journal of Personality, 45*, 79–99.
Pandey, J., & Jain, U. (2017). Worldviews and perception of environmental problems. *Psychological Studies, 62*. https://doi.org/10.1007/s12646-017-0409-7
Pandey, J., & Kakkar, S. (1982). Supervisor's affect, attraction, and positive evaluation as a function of other enhancement. *Psychological Reports, 50*, 479–486.
Pandey, J., Kakkar, S., & Bohra, K. A. (1982a). The functional perception of poverty in India. *The Journal of Social Psychology, 117*, 149–150.
Pandey, J., Kumar, R., & Thapa, K. (Eds.). (2019). *Psychological perspectives on diversity and social development.* Springer Nature.
Pandey, J., Sharma, U., & Bohra, K. A. (1983). Perceived democracy in nomination, election and rotation methods of leader selection. *Indian Journal of Industrial Relations, 18*(4), 613–618.
Pandey, J., & Siddiqui, R. N. (2001). Perception of economic and environmental stressors by urban slum dwellers. *Psychology and Developing Societies, 13*(1), 93–103.
Pandey, J., & Singh, P. (1987). Effects of Machiavellianism, other enhancement and power position on affect, power feeling, and evaluation of ingratiator. *Journal of Psychology, 121*(3), 287–300.
Pandey, J., & Singh, P. (1989). Reward allocation as function of resources availability, recipients' needs and performance. *Psychology Monographs: Genetic, Social and General, 115*(4), 169–481.
Pandey, J., & Singh, P. (1997). Allocation criterion as a function of situational factors and caste. *Journal of Basic and Applied Social Psychology, 19*(1), 121–132.
Pandey, J., & Singh, P. (2005). Social psychology in India: Social roots and development. *International Journal of Psychology, 40*(4), 239–253.
Pandey, J., Sinha, D., & Bhawuk, D. P. S. (Eds.). (1996). *Asian contributions to cross-cultural psychology.* Sage Publications.
Pandey, J., & Sinha, J. B. P. (1968). Dependence proneness and perceived problems of adjustment. *Journal of Psychological Researches, 12*(3), 104–119.
Pandey, J., & Sinha, Y. (1991). Toward psychological conceptualization of fundamentalism. *Indian Journal of Social Science, 4*(3), 347–358.
Pandey, J., Sinha, Y., Prakash, A., & Tripathi, R. C. (1982b). Right-left political ideologies and attribution of causality to poverty. *European Journal of Social Psychology, 12*, 327–331.
Pandey, J., Varma, M., & R. Ruback. (2000). Perceived crowding in Indian classrooms: The effects of age, gender, and household density. *Psychology and Developing Societies, 12*(2), 139–154.
Pant, S. K., & Pandey, J. (2004). *Social development in rural India.* Rawat Publisher.

Ruback, R. B., & Pandey, J. (1991). Crowding, perceived control, and relative power: An analysis of households in India. *Journal of Applied Social Psychology*, *21*(4), 345–374.

Ruback, R. B., & Pandey, J. (1992). Very hot and really crowded: Quasi-experimental investigations of Indian "tempos". *Environment and Behavior*, *24*(4), 527–554.

Ruback, R. B., & Pandey, J. (1996). Gender differences in reaction to household crowding: Affiliation and stress in rural India. *Journal of Applied Social Psychology*, *26*(5), 417–436.

Ruback, R. B., Pandey, J., & Begum, H. (1997). Urban stressors in South Asia: Impact on male and female pedestrians in Delhi and Dhaka. *Journal of Cross-Cultural Psychology*, *28*(1), 23–43.

Ruback, R. B., Pandey, J., Begum, H., Tariq, N., & Kamal, A. (2001). Reactions to environmental stressors: Gender differences in the slums of Dhaka and Islamabad. *Journal of Cross-Cultural Psychology*, *33*(1), 100–119.

Singh, A. K., & Pandey, J. (1991). Psychological factors in social mobility. *The Indian Journal of Criminology & criminalistics*, *11*(1–2), 43–52.

Singh, P., & Pandey, J. (1994). Distributive decisions as a function of recipient's need performance variations and caste of allocator. In M. Bouvy, F. J. R. Vade Vijiver, P. Baski, & P. Schmitz (Eds.), *Journeys into cross-cultural psychology*. Swets & Zeitlinger.

Sinha, J. B. P., & Pandey, J. (1970a). Retention of experimentally induced changes in dependence proneness as a function of social support. *Indian Journal of Experimental Psychology*, *4*, 60–63.

Sinha, J. B. P., & Pandey, J. (1971). Dependence-prone persons under congruent and incongruent expectations. *Indian Journal of Psychology*, *46*(1), 13–29.

Sinha, J. B. P., & Pandey, J. (1972). Processes of decision making in dependence-prone persons. *Journal of Psychological Researches*, *16*(1), 35–37.

Williams, J. E., Best, D. L., Haque, A., Pandey, J., & Verma, R. K. (1982). Sex-trait stereotypes in India and Pakistan. *Journal of General Psychology*, *111*, 167–181.

Introduction

Social Psychology and Globalization: Some Trends

Girishwar Misra and Purnima Singh

The objective of this publication was to gather a range of social psychology perspectives from colleagues who work in many cultural contexts. The aim has been to examine social psychology within the framework of globalization, which includes both theoretical viewpoints and practical actions across many fields of study, cultures, and historical eras. This is a difficult undertaking. Social psychology primarily focuses on subjects such as identity, intergroup connections, affective processes, and social and societal transitions. Social psychology knowledge has developed over time in terms of understanding, explanation, and application. It has been influenced by a wide range of societal changes, encompassing both major and minor developments. Culture emerges as an entity that evolves in relation to other entities, mutually influencing each other.

The concept of "global" is thus characterized by the dual responsibility to take care of oneself in respect to others and as an individual. Indeed, the significance and influence of globalization depends on the balance of socioeconomic power. Take the case of India, which stands out as one of the most ancient civilizations that has managed to endure, boasting a documented history spanning 5,000 years. This example serves to demonstrate the topic at hand. The presence of continuity has been acknowledged within this cultural environment. Over the course of several millennia, the Indian viewpoint on social events and processes has experienced a significant metamorphosis. This evolution occurred simultaneously on the ecological, physical, and social levels. The process can be described as a co-evolutionary, where the mind, nature, and society all interacted in a way that strengthened each other.

Vedic literature provides numerous examples, illustrating the concept that undifferentiated existence comes before differentiated existence. The sages considered the social realm to be a developed condition with normative characteristics that enable both individual and collective actions. As a result, the person engaged in social activities and adopted collective intellectual frameworks that originated from those activities. It is crucial to emphasize that the scholastic discourses were highly varied, and the Indian thought traditions were marked by diversity rather than a sense of control or superiority. However, the ideological frameworks that governed social functioning were

DOI: 10.4324/9781003461302-1

inflexible and resistant to change, since they offered crucial support for individual and communal functioning while also maintaining stability in life. This is apparent in the enduring behavior patterns, attitudes, and rituals that have persisted for thousands of years. Furthermore, this also demonstrates the schema's versatility and usefulness.

The fundamental principles of this relational schema encompass Dharma (ethical behavior), Purushartha (life objectives), Ashram (stage in life), Sanskar (rituals and practices essential for community membership), Rina (a sense of obligation toward socially important individuals), Yajna (fulfilling duties and assigned tasks), charity (Dana), nonviolence (Ahimsa), and the quest for truth (Satya). These principles have been emphasized in Epics, Smriti, Puranas, and Dharma Shastra literature. In addition, they became an integral part of Loka Parampara, a form of indigenous customs and rituals that exhibit significant variations across various geographical areas. Together, they allowed a member of a group or community to participate in conscientious behaviors. It is important to mention that the written tradition (Shastra) and customs (Loka) have consistently and distinctly influenced one other in different places. The presence of foreign cultures have also exerted an influence. The Mughals and the British exerted substantial influence on various parts of life, although the extent of their impact varied. The British, who regarded India as a colony, imported modern Western norms of life and education by implementing colonial-oriented systems.

The study of some modern fields, such as social psychology, began during the period of British occupation. Hence, the Euro-American educational legacy had a profound influence on the conceptions, theories, and analyses. Researchers from Europe and America built and enforced the institutional structure of knowledge, including its content and methods, during British colonial control in India. This obscured the presence of indigenous knowledge traditions and cultural practices in the process of knowledge creation. The educational paradigm introduced by the British hindered the growth of scholarly Indian traditions. India maintained its commitment to Western-style education and research even after gaining independence in 1947. As a result, there was only a shallow understanding of the conditions, which therefore resulted in a weak development of theories. The primary focus of the research was on understanding Western conceptions and utilizing Indian civilization as evidence and examples to support and illustrate these Western perspectives and concepts.

The neglect of cultural foundations of theories, notions, categories, and subcategories of knowledge has resulted in substantial setbacks for the social sciences. As a result, our ability to make significant academic contributions to various disciplines of knowledge on a national or worldwide level was greatly reduced. The country's problem-solving efforts were only slightly influenced by the implementation of social sciences. Western knowledge remained the main source of reference. In recent past, the incorporation of indigenous social science into cross-cultural research has been undertaken to take into consideration cultural factors. However, these notions have not gained widespread acceptance or been extensively put into practice. The conventional scientific approach, rooted on positivism and highlighting objectivity and quantification to comprehend a static reality, is presently being questioned.

This volume is organized into four distinct sections: Part I focuses on the difficulties in comprehending the nature of social, Part II explores the impact of societal changes on social psychology, Part III delves into the topics of identity and intergroup relations, and Part IV examines the affective and cognitive processes involved in change. Each of these parts includes a wide range of social psychology studies.

Part I: Challenges in Understanding the Social Sphere

The chapters in this part focus on the difficulties related to understanding the social aspects. The social context is primarily characterized by human interactions, affinity, and dependency. For a significant period of time, experts have argued that social psychology research has neglected the importance of context, despite its crucial role in conducting effective social psychology studies.

Chapter 1 by Verma examines the contextualization and growth of social psychology in India. It focuses on the shift from Western-centric to indigenous knowledge, the importance of social relevance, and the adoption of postmodernist viewpoints. She begins her analysis of Western psychology. The roots of Indian psychology paralleled those of Western psychology, without a separate foundation, technique, or ideology. The recurrence continued until the late 1960s, when Indian intellectuals started questioning the relevance of Western concepts in the Indian sociocultural context. The study of psychology has seen a shift toward increased cultural awareness and social engagement in order to better align with the beliefs and needs of Indian culture. During the 1970s, Indian psychologists recognized that Western approaches were insufficient for addressing the social and psychological challenges specific to India. There was an increasing demand for intellectually and socially relevant Indian research, which in turn led to socioeconomic prosperity. In the 1980s, indigenization became prominent, as it entailed integrating culturally relevant knowledge and procedures into psychological research. This required the reevaluation of traditional notions and theories to match the sociocultural context of India. Verma illustrates that the theory of social representation emphasizes the importance of local interpretations and intuitive understanding in understanding social events, as well as the creation of knowledge through social processes. Verma's account emphasizes the importance of cultural sensitivity, social relevance, and indigenous knowledge in the advancement of Indian social psychology. Verma reflects on her work in social psychology, focusing on her efforts to understand and address global problems at the community level. She emphasizes the need of considering local viewpoints in global conversations and highlights the efforts of Indian social psychologists to promote culturally responsive approaches to understanding human behavior. The importance of "glocalization" has grown in the current interconnected world. Glocalization refers to the balance between global integration and local identity and traditions.

In Chapter 2, Berry discusses the topic of multilevel collaboration in various cultural situations. The Mutual Intercultural Relations in Plural Communities (MIRIPS) initiative, led by him, has been a substantial effort to define, measure, and understand the core difficulties in multicultural communities. The study examined the theories of diversity, contact, and integration in 17 civilizations with various cultural backgrounds. The multiculturalism theory suggests that individuals are more likely to exhibit tolerance toward others when they have a strong sense of personal, economic, and cultural security. When individuals view themselves as being threatened, they tend to reject others. The contact hypothesis suggests that intercultural contact might lead to increased mutual approval, but only under certain conditions. Finally, according to the integration hypothesis, persons who have a strong sense of identification with both their heritage culture and the larger community are more inclined to successfully adjust and adapt. MIRIPS utilizes a comprehensive methodology that incorporates several traits, methods, and cultural perspectives to examine these principles across different countries, while also considering cultural suitability. It explores both universal and specific cultural difficulties that arise in international relationships. The initiative is based on cross-cultural psychology, a field that focuses on uncovering universal psychological principles that govern human behavior. The chapter asserts that cross-cultural and intercultural psychology play a crucial role in understanding human behavior.

In Chapter 3, Ward has focused on utilizing psychological theory and research to tackle many significant societal concerns. She notes that the effectiveness of these projects depends on how they are spread and put into action, as well as the theoretical frameworks and research behind them. She claims that action-oriented, community-focused, and program-based research can have substantial influence. She notes that programmatic research consists of a series of interconnected studies that are supported by clear theoretical frameworks. She cites Herbert Kelman's research on conflict resolution, John W. Berry's research on acculturation, and Ed Diener's research on satisfaction. These comprehensive, enduring research endeavors help to the establishment of policies and practices that are supported by empirical data. Community-based research is used to create relationships with government agencies, organizations, and communities. Ward notes that applied research can be influenced by both inductive and deductive principles. Certain scholars commence their research by constructing theoretical frameworks to understand social phenomena, whereas others initiate their investigations by directly engaging with the subject matter and formulating hypotheses based on their empirical observations and personal encounters. Action research prioritizes the creation of theories while addressing social problems, as demonstrated by the study on cultural adaption among young Assyrian women. In order to develop a relationship between psychological theory and practice, it is imperative to engage in systematic research, include the community, and foster theoretical innovation. Ward believes that data-driven and problem-solving-oriented research is beneficial. She highlights the significance of sharing the findings of the study in order to accomplish the desired outcomes. Effective communication is essential for informing research, which in turn guides the development of policies and initiatives. It is important to consider political sensitivities, and the time required for study, as applied research has the capacity to impact policy. Ward has highlighted the significance of applied research by addressing practical problems and fostering engagement and cooperation with stakeholders to optimize the influence of research.

Part II: Societal Changes and Social Psychology

This section focuses on the field of social psychology and its relationship to changes in society. Most societies are experiencing rapid transformation. These alterations are causing a disturbance in the established social structure and introducing novel modifications that require individuals to adjust, resulting in social evolution. These changes have an impact on institutions, human behavior, and the environment. The modifications and their repercussions are the focal point of four chapters in this part.

In Chapter 4, Ruback examines research in environmental psychology, illustrating that the perception of control can ease congestion. However, the extent of this impact depends on the specific circumstances and the personal traits of the individual. Environmental psychology study has uncovered the way people perceive and experience crowding, as well as the resulting effects. This research has been conducted in the backdrop of the rapid urbanization and population growth in South Asia. Gender, culture, stress, and beliefs all contribute to the negative cognitive, social, and health effects of crowding. The results emphasize the importance of employing culturally sensitive research approaches and policy-relevant solutions to address environmental concerns in developing nations, where they are particularly severe. Through the implementation of a holistic strategy and cooperation with policy makers, social psychologists have the potential to improve the standard of living in South Asia and beyond. This will empower them to create efficient tactics for alleviating environmental stress. To do this, scholars must acknowledge the multitude of situations and experiences that vary across different areas and cultures. To address environmental concerns, it is imperative to do multidisciplinary research encompassing historical, cultural, and social aspects.

In Chapter 5, Siddiqui offers a thorough examination of environmental challenges. She begins her analysis by investigating the psychological and societal barriers that hinder effective action, as well as the unwillingness to recognize the seriousness of the issue. The chapter examines our environmental reaction, or absence thereof. She highlights that environmental deterioration has transformed into a worldwide issue that directly affects individuals, thereby heightening awareness but also fostering feelings of fear and uncertainty about the future. The importance of tackling these difficulties before they worsen is emphasized by comparing them to a pandemic. Psychological obstacles to effective action encompass the discrepancy between consciousness and behavior, as well as the physical and temporal distance from the issue, together with the diminishing of individual accountability. Trust in institutions and the media can either help or hinder collective action. For the well-being of future generations, it is essential to adopt sustainable lifestyles and effectively manage our resources. An examination of the environmental problems has revealed that denial and apathy can be related to cognitive fallacies, short-sighted thinking, and a lack of emotional involvement. Siddiqui examines the psychological obstacles that hinder successful action and emphasizes the importance of environmental education and unbiased media coverage in encouraging educated decision-making and group efforts. She proposes that the environmental catastrophe be addressed by engaging the international community, local communities, and people.

In Chapter 6, Misra examines the social and personal challenges that Mahatma Gandhi, the revered leader of India, encountered throughout his life and career. From the 1900s to the 1950s, Mahatma Gandhi, a dedicated practitioner of Karma Yoga, greatly influenced Indian society. He advocated for political and social reform, emphasizing the importance of human values and equality. Gandhi promoted the values of nonviolence, celibacy, and minimalism, emphasizing the significant influence of thoughts on one's life. To achieve inner tranquility and self-discovery, he advocated and implemented self-restraint, abstinence, and stillness. Gandhi's ideals were deeply rooted in his spiritual beliefs and values, and he emphasized the importance of incorporating indigenous knowledge and preserving culture in education. He strongly campaigned for a restoration of ancient values and self-governance, while expressing severe criticism toward Western civilization and its impact on Indian society. Gandhi's beliefs and acts still serve as a source of motivation and impact for the world today.

Chapter 7 delves into the impact of globalization on the identity, possibilities, and challenges faced by young individuals, as examined by Suchday. It compels individuals to harmonize their cultural identity with the pursuit of worldwide trends through exposure to novel concepts, beliefs, and customs from diverse cultures. Globalization impacts the decisions and possibilities available to young individuals by bringing about structural transformations, such as the movement of young people from rural areas to cities in pursuit of economic prospects. However, this mobility has the capacity to disturb family structures and support networks, leading to discontentment and marginalization. Globalization also brings about new health hazards, such as the rising incidence of chronic non-communicable diseases (NCDs) and mental health disorders like substance abuse, anxiety, and depression. Globalization offers both prospects and difficulties for the elderly, women, and teenagers in India. The enduring values of honoring and supporting older individuals persist, but the capabilities of women are limited by gender disparities. India's cultural heritage remains intact as it embraces globalization, whatever the challenges it encounters. This exemplifies its ability to withstand and adapt to swift transformations.

Part III: Identity and Intergroup Relations

Our interpersonal connections and the presence of both discord and agreement in social settings are shaped by our individual identities and affiliations with social collectives. To foster societies that value social welfare, it is imperative to comprehend the obstacles linked to collective social identity. The four chapters in this part focus on the process of identity building and negotiation among the main groups in society, along with their associated concerns.

Best and her colleagues provide useful insights on gender-trait stereotypes across multiple cultures in Chapter 8. Gender stereotypes were found to be present in both Western countries and Indian and Pakistani civilizations. Despite their variations, all countries displayed very similar qualities. Gender classification in Pakistan may have led to the early emergence of gender stereotypes. Intergenerational communication and age stereotypes displayed similarities. The younger generation in India and the United States are exhibiting a growing acceptance of older folks, a trend that can be related to the process of industrialization. In India, the practice of intergenerational living promotes favorable attitudes toward the old, with grandparents assuming a crucial role. The results illustrate the interconnectedness of familial relationships, culture, and attitudes toward aging. Developing positive interactions between generations depends on understanding changes in stereotypes.

To illustrate the impact of cultural environment on human behavior and its intricacies, Hopkins and his colleagues present a study on pilgrimage in India in Chapter 9. The examination of pilgrimage holds great importance in the realm of domestic travel in India, as the fields of psychology and culture intricately intertwine. However, the lack of material on this issue in textbooks highlights the need for psychological study in this sector. Psychology has faced challenges in incorporating culture, with some critics pointing out that the field's focus on behavior lacks consideration for cultural context. However, the Indo-British Hindu pilgrimage effort serves as an example of how identity theory may help bridge cultural gaps. Psychology must actively include and overcome Eurocentric biases, recognizing the importance of global, cultural, and psychological viewpoints. Undertaking a pilgrimage, whether it be physical or symbolic, motivates academics to explore unexplored areas in their quest for a psychology that is more accepting of many cultures. The examination of the Magh Mela highlights the complex interplay between memory, perception, and culture, as the participants' emotional encounters are linked to their capacity to form significant social bonds and convey religious and spiritual beliefs.

In Chapter 10, Biswas explores the correlation between gender and sustainable development and progress. She notes that the economic advancement, culture, and customs have an impact on the status and obligations of women. As specified in Sustainable Development Goal 5 (SDG 5), the achievement of gender equality and the empowerment of women are crucial for the promotion of sustainable and all-encompassing development. Indian women have challenges in achieving their goals and in maintaining a respectable and healthy lifestyle. Biswas highlights the importance of gender equality in sustainable development, emphasizing the impact of economic progress, culture, and traditions on the roles of women. She proposes a comprehensive plan that incorporates both professional and social contexts in order to achieve gender equality. Biswas also examines the impact of the decrease in the birth sex ratio on the personal and professional ambitions of Indian women.

Chapter 11 of the book examines how societal change affects interaction, as demonstrated by Singh, Misra, Kapur, Mishra, and Siddiqui. Global communities characterized by several ethnicities and diverse cultural traditions must strive to achieve reconciliation among different ethnic groupings. This undertaking is also difficult by globalization, dynamic social networks, and developing relationships. In India, governmental rulers may use identity politics for personal benefit or to foster cohesion, while conflicting identities can lead to marginalization and alienation. To attain peace, it is crucial to understand contrasting identities and create shared areas among varied groups. Social places that encourage interaction, learning, variety, and the interchange of viewpoints can cultivate interdependence and harmony. The conversation is primarily controlled by self-defined collective identities, while shared spaces and diversity are weakened by sociopolitical influences. Incorporating diversity into common spaces is crucial to improve their attractiveness without making them ethnocentric or elitist. An argument is made that a deeper and more subtle awareness of social reality, along with a concentration on interconnected groups, would enhance the understanding of social dynamics and the possibility of mutual understanding and coexistence.

Part IV: Affective and Cognitive Processes and Change

Change, whether occurring within a community or an organization, can elicit either support or criticism, which should then prompt the implementation of suitable measures. Cognitive and affective reactions do actually promote attitudes toward change. Various contextual and individual-level influences will shape these opinions. The three chapters in this part exemplify these shifts in diverse contexts.

Chapter 12 explores Sondhi's analysis of the scientific and artistic aspects of social influence, as well as the progress made in this subject. Social influence science encompasses a diverse range of theoretical frameworks and empirical studies, whereas social influence art refers to the ability to successfully apply these concepts in real-world scenarios. This chapter covers the issues of conformity, compliance, obedience, attitude change, persuasion, and self-presentation. Current research in the field of social influence highlights the importance of both interpersonal and group dynamics in shaping social actions, with an increasing focus on self-centered processes, including social categorization and social identification. Sondhi's research extensively illustrates the functioning of social influence in hierarchical and collectivist societies, such as India, where interpersonal dynamics are often impacted by ingratiation and other social techniques. Social influence techniques are not universally applicable, as demonstrated by the presence of cultural variations. Instead, they are inextricably interconnected with cultural values, social institutions, and group identities, which subsequently shape the impact individuals have on each other.

In Chapter 13, Singh discusses the complexities of leading institutions, highlighting the importance of being able to adjust to changing conditions, cultural differences, market trends, and the specific requirements of different tasks. Despite extensive research over several decades, no leadership theory has successfully comprehended all of its complexities. The theoretical foundations, wide range of approaches, and practical consequences of leadership training, mentorship, and advising have been extensively discussed. The need for leadership development arises from both personal goals and organizational necessities, while facing criticism. To successfully traverse the complexities of leadership in a rapidly changing society, it is crucial to carefully evaluate existing methods and understand the dynamics of leadership. Leaders, especially those in positions of authority, play a crucial role in facilitating organizational development. The charismatic and transformative leadership approaches offer attractive ideas, but they also bring about the possibility of risk diversion and only offer temporary advantages.

Jain and Singh examine the relationship between social complexity and decision-making in Chapter 14. The chapter argues that our decisions are influenced by cognitive and emotive variables. There are a multitude of options. Decisions are shaped by the surrounding circumstances, prevailing social standards, and the accessibility of resources. The Sanskrit phrases *Sankalp* and *Vikalpa* denote the cognitive process of decision-making. *Sankalp* denotes a definitive choice and the willingness to abide by it, while *Vikalpa* symbolizes an alternative possibility. Social cognition plays a role in shaping choices. Decisions are shaped by emotions, values, and social influence. Voting is impacted by social networks, party affiliations, and the stances of candidates. Research on decision-making is influenced by philosophical, statistical, and economic viewpoints. Decision-making models are present in cognitive psychology, medical informatics, commercial management, and political science. This is addressed by theories that are concerned with prescribing how things should be (normative theories) and theories that aim to describe how things actually are (descriptive theories). Normative theories promote the cultivation of optimal and rational decision-making processes. Descriptive theories analyze the cognitive process by which humans make decisions, as human judgment is complex. This chapter offers a comprehensive view of decision-making and its nuances.

The final chapter of the collection includes an epilogue written by Singh, Misra, and Ramanathan with an aim to discern patterns in the progress of social psychology in India. The development of social psychology in India has been shaped by philosophical traditions, research goals, contemporary events, and social and national difficulties, as observed. This review focuses on the most relevant findings from social psychology research, as well as previously overlooked phenomena. The intricacies of social reality have become more challenging to comprehend and elucidate due to experts' inclination to embrace a limited viewpoint. The intricate network of social reality is not sufficiently explored by the reductionist approaches of scientific social psychology, which often rely on unfamiliar cultural values. This leads to a condition known as "topic blindness" and the disregard of the normative aspects of the Indian context. Indian social psychologists have recently started exploring subjects such as identity, indigenization of psychological processes, health, and education. Programmatic research has not adequately adapted to the changes in the discipline, and the main driving force behind social psychology research is the observable nature of society problems. To enhance the impact of policy contributions, it is necessary to conduct a more thorough and nuanced analysis of data, taking into account its broader sociocultural context. Given the prevailing period of globalization, it is imperative for Indian social psychology to adapt and tackle the difficulties confronting the nation.

Concluding Remarks

The study of social psychology in the context of globalization is complex and varied. It is crucial to understand how cultural backgrounds and situations shape human behavior and how indigenous knowledge and cultural sensitivity can be incorporated into research. In India, the shift from Western-focused perspectives to indigenous understanding has led to more holistic methodologies for studying human behavior. The importance of working together with different stakeholders, promoting inclusivity, and considering cultural settings is emphasized in order to tackle social problems and promote beneficial social transformation. The authors propose a more inclusive and nuanced approach to social psychology research, which takes into account the varied viewpoints and experiences of people. They emphasize the importance of integrating cultural settings, promoting inclusive attitudes, and understanding cultural diversity in with a more inclusive approach to social psychology research, considering the diverse viewpoints and experiences of individuals and communities in an interconnected world.

Part I

Challenges in Understanding the Social

1 Making Sense of the 'Social,' Relevance of the 'Local,' and the Era of the 'Global'

Encounters of a Social Psychologist

Jyoti Verma

While interrogating the significance of 'social' in the discipline of social psychology, one would like to mention the happenings in France during early 1960s when voices started for 'de-individualizing' and 're-socializing' in this scholarly endeavor. The spirit behind such efforts was the belief that knowledge grounded in the inter-subjective world of a community made the real sense, and it cannot be reduced to individual-level discourse (Jovchelovitch, 2007). Inspired by the sociological orientation of considering 'social' more as an expression of 'collective representation,' it was realized that the integral 'social' component was neglected. A prominent reason for this was the dominance of Western-American empiricist tradition as the model for pursuing research and articulating its subject matter. However, the theory and approach of 'social representations' (SRs) led by Moscovici in 1960s strongly favored integration of the 'social' and the 'cultural' contexts. It ignited interest in addressing the 'social' part of social psychology with a fresh fervor.

Making Sense of 'Social' and the Significance of 'Local': Social Psychology in India

Social psychology in India showed inclination toward donning its 'social' face only later. The narrative begins with the state of 'felt discomfort' with the prevailing status of psychology in India after the country's independence. In this regard, some major events heightened the need for making the discipline socially more engaging and keener on recognizing the relevance of the local. These include (a) the 'felt discomfort' with the suitability of the Western empiricist tradition for doing research in India, (b) outgrowing the 'alien frame,' (c) need for becoming 'socially relevant,' (d) 'call for indigenization and making sense of the "local" or "native,"' and (e) the upcoming trends favoring 'postmodernist tradition' that believed in socially and culturally sensitive research, socially constructed reality and qualitative methodology. Let us examine these aspects in some detail.

DOI: 10.4324/9781003461302-3

The Felt Discomfort

The status of psychology after India's political independence remained a faint copy of the Western psychology or largely a Euro-American product. In fact, as the Indian psychologists engaged themselves in validating the work of Western researchers, the phase of expansion of the discipline remained primarily replicative in nature till 1960s (Sinha, 1986). That is, in the absence of serious objections against the imported modern scientific psychology rooted in experimental, mechanistic, materialistic, and positivistic tradition, 'the progress in social psychological research in India did not indicate any distinct mark in terms of context, method or ideological commitment' (Dalal & Misra, 2002, p. 17).

However, by the latter half of the 1960s, some Indian scholars (e.g., Sinha, 1968; Sinha & Pandey, 1970) questioned the relevance of Western theories (theory of n-Ach in this case) for the Indian sociocultural context. Similarly, referring to the Indian organizational context, J.B.P. Sinha (1984) reported that participative leader was perceived to be weak by majority of the Indian managers and many workers who preferred autocratic leaders. He remarked that these findings were suggesting about 'what was not working' rather than 'what does and can work' in the Indian setting. Apparently, the discomfort with the inconsistent and unexplained findings gave the required vigor to the mood of disenchantment from the Western frame of psychology.

Outgrowing the 'Alien Frame'

Call for outgrowing the 'alien' frame was meant to create awareness against the positivist/empiricist paradigm focusing on the patterns of cause and effect through empirical verification. The approach believed in experimental and manipulative methods (quantitative) and its data collection tools had to be valid and reliable. The effort was to obliterate the researcher's subjective biases, arrive at objective reality, and generalize the research findings. Under these parameters, social psychological research could not remain 'social': first, because the empirically derived individual data set was considered as the unit of analysis; and second, because the sociocultural context (an integral part of the discipline's domain) was either disregarded or treated very crudely. Within the field of social psychology, 'social' comes close to 'culture'; however, under the empiricist approach, the variables became 'stimuli' (as they could not be controlled) and were treated as 'source of error.' Under these circumstances, social psychological research in India did not show distinctive signs of breaking away from the alien frame.

Need for Social Relevance

By the 1970s, Indian psychologists became quite sure that their work was not addressing to the social psychological problems of the country and 'researches emanating from a genuine need, intellectual or social, from Indian soil were very limited' (Dalal & Misra, 2002, p. 17). Similarly, there was increasing evidence to suggest that Western social psychological theories could not offer solution to the complex problems of social change and development faced in India. On the other hand, the west-oriented training was unlikely to encourage enthusiasm for studying Indian context and concepts of Indian origin (Ganguli, 1971; Krishnan, 1961; Parmeshwaran, 1978). Apparently, Indian social psychology had not yet arrived at an identity of its own.

It became progressively clear that social psychology should be working toward becoming a proactive discipline committed to social reality, societal values, sociocultural development, and the country's needs and concerns and should be offering better insights into the society's problems and their solution (Pareek, 1981). Accordingly, the demand for utility of psychological research started gaining ground around late 1960s (see Tripathi, 1988; Muthayya, 1988). This progression may be seen as the effort toward making psychology a socially relevant discipline and social psychologists as socially responsible people, working toward their country's socioeconomic change and development.

Socially Relevant Research: Illustrations From the Work of Professor Janak Pandey

One of the most prominent Indian social psychologists, Professor Janak Pandey, has widely addressed to the country's contemporary economic and environmental issues and development processes with an unfaltering interest in the social and cultural perspective for understanding social behavior. He is well known for his research on social influence process and for showcasing the status of psychology in India through the numerous publications. A few titles will make the point: *Perspective on Experimental Social Psychology in India* (Ed.) (1981), *Psychology in India: The State-of-the-Art* (1988, 3 Volumes), and *Psychology in India Revisited* (2000b, 2001, 2004b, 3 volumes).

It is beyond the scope of this chapter to refer to the voluminous research publications by Professor Pandey. Nevertheless, a few examples will illustrate his concern for the country's problems and socially relevant research. He has worked extensively on poverty (Pandey, 2000a; Pandey & Singh, 1985; Singh & Pandey, 1990; Siddiqui & Pandey, 2003), crowding (Pandey, 1978, 1999; Pandey & Nagar, 1987; Ruback & Pandey, 1992), and environment (Pandey, 1998). Professor Pandey has contributed in the area of indigenous psychology significantly (Adair et al., 1995; Pandey, 2004a) while his contributions in the field of cross-cultural psychology and lately on the advances of cognitive sciences are noteworthy too (not being mentioned here).

Call for Indigenization for Making Sense of the 'Native'

Mainstream psychology received a major jolt in the 1980s with the popular preference for including culturally appropriate 'local' or 'native' knowledge and the gradual awakening of social psychology against the imposition of positivist frame. Additionally, another development took place at the plane of cross-cultural psychology. Both these event gave impetus to the process of making the discipline suitable to the sociocultural soil of the country or the progression of 'indigenous psychology.' The indigenization movement was pioneered in India by Professor Durganand Sinha (1990, 1993, 1994, 1997, 1998). The interest in reinterpreting the categories of observation and looking for indigenous concepts and theories drew several Indian scholars (see Misra & Mohanty, 2002). As stated by Kim (1990), indigenous psychology emerged as psychological knowledge that is (a) native, (b) not transported from another region, (c) is designed for its people, and (d) is about understanding how the local context affects, shapes, and guides psychological description, explanation, and application.

Coming to the developments in cross-cultural psychology, the discipline during its formative years aimed at discovering the cultural universals (etics) and differences (emics) (Pike, 1967). However, its claims of 'mono-cultural' nature of modern psychology and 'universality' were challenged, and it was argued that psychologists cannot remain 'culture blind' or 'culture bound.' 'Emic' was the localized culture-specific dimension of human psychology applicable to only one culture and not to the others (Triandis, 1994). Notably, as the indigenous approach does not assume existence of universals on a priori basis, its acceptance was conditional to empirical verification.

Sinha (2000, 2002, 2003) wrote on indigenization of psychology in India and argued in favor of indigenization of psychological research in theory and methodology. Moreover, he suggested multi-method approach for understanding Indian culture and preferred integration of etics and emics (Sinha, 2004). Others too (e.g., Mukherjee, 1980; Nandy, 1974; Pareek, 1981) supported the idea that scientific understanding of Indian social reality would benefit from indigenous psychological knowledge. Though set in motion, looking for new concepts and theories leading to the phase of indigenization of Indian psychology took time.

Understandably, the source of indigenous psychological understanding is embedded in belief systems, metaphysical and religious concepts, basic theories about human nature and behavior, and relationship with their surroundings. However, this is often disregarded in psychological research. India's ancient wisdom too, based on experiences, intuitions, and insights of the seers secured in the secret and mystical elements, is the source of indigenous psychological information and folk wisdom. Misra (2011) contended that one reason why the values of historical conversation and tradition were ignored has been the contemporary trend of doing psychological investigation with strict adherence to psychological constructs. Ironically, this situation created hindrance in the understanding located in and transmitted from collective past while the 'richness, depth and continuity of the Indian tradition made it even more difficult' (p. 63). Fortunately, with the call for indigenization, traditional psychological knowledge and its sources started making real sense and so did the idea of common sense understanding of knowledge grounded in the history and culture of people.

Having said this, it may be added that by the end of 1970s, Indian and Asian social psychologists felt convinced that it made sense to study psychology of a group or a culture in terms of culturally provided (indigenous) native categories instead of taking recourse to interpolated foreign concepts (see Misra & Gergen, 1993). Apparently, the course of indigenizing psychology in India progressed in stages and was only articulated by 1980s.

The Postmodernist Trend

The postmodernist approach presented a bold perspective against the positivist-empiricist premise which believed that objective reality existed somewhere outside waiting to be perfectly mapped and neglected the social and cultural dimensions of reality. However, the postmodernist trend was sensitive toward the cultural aspect and understood that concepts behave differently in different cultural contexts and certain concepts are differently viewed from the culture's point of view. Back in 1993, Misra and Gergen had expressed their concern for 'reorienting the human scientific enterprise in a culturally sensitive fashion' and observed that 'so far psychological discourse and culture had remained intimate strangers' (p. 238). In view of the fact, that culture and social psychology are mutually associated, recent years have seen scholars 'moving towards, reorienting psychological discourse by locating it in culturally rooted conceptual space' (Misra & Mohanty, 2002, p. 15). Misra (2000) talked about implications of culture for psychological knowledge; similarly, social constructionist, cross-cultural and cultural approaches have been the major forces behind prominently recognizing the role of cultural variables for the understanding of psychological phenomenon.

Misra and Kumar (2010) quote Gergen (1996) who observes that 'Post-modern contour for psychology can be drawn only if it is willing to accommodate multiple realities, shared meanings of symbols, "folk" psychologies, culture and local idioms, which contribute to individual and social behavior' (p. 354). Interestingly, Gergen talked about 'local' truths, 'established within various scientific fields, within the various communities of humankind and these must surely be honored from within the traditions of these communities.' According to him, the 'future well-being of the world community depends on facilitating dialogue among these local traditions' and 'Declarations of truth beyond tradition are a step toward tyranny and, ultimately, the end of communication' (Kenneth Gergen in Conversation with Peter Mattes and Ernst Schraube, 2004).

Moreover, the postmodernist approach gives immense importance to the communication and practices of the real people in actual transactions of real life. It values knowing how people understand, analyze, and socially construct a phenomenon which gains legitimacy through discussion and sharing made during social meetings. The tag line is 'knowledge is socially constructed,' and hence, reality is relative. Tripathi (2011) observed:

> [V]arious cultural concepts that are used to understand and give meaning to our experiences may gather new meanings in the face of exchanges and interactions that are taking place among the people around the world based on interactions brought about by new information and communication technologies.
>
> (p. 372)

The observation seems very apt in reference to the globalized world we live in today.

Apparently, the postmodernist trend contends that knowledge cannot be value free, and therefore, subjectivity exists and understanding of human phenomenon requires an understanding of the 'human made world.' In sum, constructionist and cultural psychologists take the position that culture is not 'given' but individuals construct it. 'In cultural psychology, culture and behavior are not separable. Cultural psychology studies psychological processes associated with culture. Culture is within the individual and it is a way of knowing, experiencing, and interacting in the world' (Pandey, 1996, p. 358).

SRs and Move Toward 'Social' and the 'Locally Embedded Meaning': Lay Explanations, Common Sense, and Folk Wisdom

One of the well-known postmodernist theories is that of SRs articulated by Moscovici (1961, 1984, 1988). It endorses the idea of 'socially elaborated and collectively shared' knowledge by focusing on the 'locally embedded meanings and functions of a phenomenon.' The theory underlines that the process of socially constructing a phenomenon and the resulting product (representation) is inseparable from the process which creates it. Apparently, the purpose is to understand how people use their 'common sense' thinking or practical knowledge to orient themselves to their social world and put it into practice in their everyday life. It is suggested that the world of common sense is 'consensual' born out of 'shared traditions' enriched by many 'experiments' and 'observations' unlike the 'reified' world of the research scientist (see Moscovici, 1984; Moscovici & Hewstone, 1983).

The core proposition of the SRs theory is that socially relevant knowledge has social genesis, and there is meaningful link between the 'local' and the 'social.' For instance, when an affair eludes direct experience, perception, and simple causal explanation, effort is needed to capture and analyze the information, making rounds at the local levels regarding the issue's lay version, and try to reach people's perception of that object (Farr, 1993). Lay explanations can be reached from where they originate, that is, at the public, social or group medium of communication (i.e., talk, discourse, and interactions).

People from different nationalities (i.e., China, Japan, and Australia) are found to endorse different lay theories about the route of globalization and views on how the specific circumstances of cultures entering the global market can result in notable differences in making sense of globalization and social change (Kashima et al., 2011; Yang et al., 2011). Indeed, the manner in which globalization is experienced varies considerably within a particular society (Norasakkunkit & Uchida, 2011; Gelfand et al., 2011).

The Methodology of Postmodernist Tradition

The post-modern approaches do not endorse the idea of universally applicable absolute laws and principles and care for methodologies that are comfortable with the definition that knowledge was continually constructed, negotiated, revised, and assumed subjectivity of meaning and centrality of setting in meaning making. If it is believed that individual principles emanate from social processes, and knowledge doesn't exist independently of the knower and the process of knowing, the implication is that meaning takes shape in the 'discourse' and not by 'labeling' of the objective reality. Therefore, for the qualitative methods, the source of data and the unit of analysis, lie the descriptive content located in talks, texts, social interactions, discursive acts, etc. (see Prakash, 2011).

However, the researcher must keep looking for the shared pattern in the live actions and words of the people in a particular social setting, empathize with their values, and assure in-depth participation in research. Let us appreciate that the postmodernist trend has taught us to give value to knowledge grounded in the inter-subjective world of a community instead of considering it as an individual property. It is a matter of concern that there is widespread unawareness concerning appreciation and analysis of local truths, contents of everyday thinking, folk wisdom, and common sense for understanding socially contextualized knowledge.

Relevance of the 'Local' in the Era of Globalization

One hears about 'turning inward' in recent times whose undertone seems analogous to 'turning to local.' Sharma (2020) refers to the magnifying 'inward tendencies' observed during the economic crisis of 2008 and compares it with the globally rampant Corona virus Pandemic of 2020. He writes:

> Populist leaders more emboldened to bash foreigners; nations less willing to expose themselves to world trade, global banks and international migration; national economies more reliant on local industries; people everywhere retreating to corona virus free safety of home to pursue employment, education and entertainment in the immersive world of the online economy.
>
> (p. 12)

He observes further that the growing anti-China rhetoric in a number of nations (including India) and anti-trade expression has come even from the French President, one of the last high-profile champions of globalization who feels that 'Delegating our food supply to others is madness' and, hence, control has to be reinstated.

In other words, the economically devastating COVID-19 pandemic has inspired many nations to rethink about going back to all their 'local' assets. Indian Prime Minister's address to the nation before the fourth lockdown in May 2020 emphasized the urgency for a self-reliant India. He pleaded for utilizing India's local resources, skills and capabilities, indigenous forms of art and handicraft, youth power and the brilliant Indian minds in science, pharmaceuticals, medical science and technology, etc. The call for 'make in India' is the call for turning to the 'local' but with an eye on the 'global' quality and market.

The marketing world has cleverly demonstrated that for globally endorsed preferences and products, the relevance of 'local' depends much upon how to market the desired global preferences into a local avatar. There is no dearth of material showing that consideration for local culture, norms, and practices can save millions for a company while insensitive marketing messages can lead to costly re-positioning. Even use of a number, name, or symbol in a culturally inappropriate way can derail product sales. Hence, companies have proactively adapted their products and marketing strategies to entice their international customers. The product-driven 'glocal' strategy adopted by the popular international brand McDonald's is pretty obvious as it sells the local forms of McSpaghetti in Philippines, the McAloo Tikki Burger in India, and the McArabia wrap in the Middle East. Similarly, technology- and hospitality-based businesses have opted for product-driven localization. For instance, mobile phone brands offer flashlights and anti-dust keypads for Asian and African markets, and hotel chains operating in the Middle East and North African region provide facilities keeping in view the religious values of their local clientele. The present author was told that all the international flights originating from Europe and heading to India, or vice versa, do not serve beef or pork. Apparently, companies' distribution, logistics, retailing infrastructure, and even merchandising are largely based on the preferences of the local consumer. The distribution methods dealing with retailing in India have incorporated cycles, rickshaws, bullock carts, trucks, and even boats to ensure connectivity with the Kirana shops in rural communities. Occasionally, even price and product size are adjusted to suit the rural population of non-affluent countries.

The crucial concerns are (a) not underestimating the value of localization and (b) striking a balance between the 'local' and the global attributes which should not be limited to international brands entering local markets but also for the regional brands with global aspirations. In the latter case, taking cognizance of the social and cultural norms is equally vital and is exemplified in fashion accessories and dresses bearing Indian motifs and material that are especially created to meet the taste and utility of the European customers.

However, when envisioning the complex challenges of development and sustainable development goals (SDGs) for a highly diversified country like India, the need is to align around a common agenda, choosing strategy driven by local voices and considering the proposed solution befitting to the local context (see, Singh, 2012, and Gagan Bhalla www.brandz.com/articlenew/global-strategy-local-relevance-1714). In general, and in reference to the macro-scenario, it appears that local and global are entwined, and people's actions are regionally and locally contextualized.

Globalization and the Moves Made by Psychologists

Globalization is perceived as a process which stamps everyday life experiences and standardizes ideas globally due to movement of merchandise. The process includes far-reaching and inescapable contact among people of different cultures and territories and is bound to leave social, cultural, economic, and political interdependencies and consequences. Simply said, 'globalization is the process through which products, services, cultural influences and so on, move across national boundaries' (Sinha, 2008, p. 358). Contributing factors of globalization include sophisticated communication and transportation technologies and services, mass migration, travel and economic activities expanding beyond the national markets through industrial combinations and commercial groupings, etc. Globalization offers huge potential profits to business houses and countries through international agreements but not without complications due to widely different local and contextual expectations, standards of living, values, cultures, and the legal systems.

Talking of psychologists, as knowledge moves around globally, sensitive psychologists get an opportunity to look for the relevance of the 'local' knowledge besides the globalization enthused thoughts on society and its system, on the political, economic, and social values, plus the native identities of people, communities, and nations. Moreover, they may also be interested in identifying local solutions for neutralizing some unsettling impact of globalization. However, a seemingly apathetic stance has been observed toward the phenomenon of globalization in psychology although, the discipline has the potential for offering new conceptual and empirical perspectives on matters related to social and cultural implications of globalization (see Arnett, 2002; Chiu & Cheng, 2007; Gelfand et al., 2011; Ghosh, 2011; Gogineni et al., 2018).

Hermans and Dimaggio (2007) and Marsella (2012) observe that globalization is a 'trans-disciplinary macro-social concept' not conceptually connected with the psychosocial and bio-psychological levels of functioning with which psychology prefers to work with. Not that psychologist have ignored this pervasive phenomenon totally; however, their contribution has been largely indirect. The question before psychologists is this:

> How people make sense of and respond to globalization and its socio cultural ramifications; how people defend the integrity of their heritage

> cultural identities against the 'culturally erosive' effects of globalization, and how individuals harness creative insights from their interactions with global cultures.
>
> (Chi-yue Chiu et al., 2011, p. 663)

There is need for interdisciplinary inquiry into the psychology of globalization. Peoples' understanding of globalization, including its determinants and implications, is warranted. Understanding of social psychological factors that can help mitigating negative effects and exploring the factors that can enhance these positive effects would be very pertinent.

Psychologists have also touched upon 'values' while discussing consumerism, upsurge of market-driven economy, changing family structure and individualism, etc., that are linked to globalization. Marsella (2012) observed that globalization could threaten traditional sources of meaning and values. The connections between global and local do need serious attention. As Tripathi (2011) has put:

> We wait for the emergence of a new kind of psychology, which is global as it seeks and believes in essential unity of the psychic minds yet allows itself to be influenced by cultures and minds that may have emerged in different contexts. For want of a better name let us call it 'glocal psychology'.
>
> (p. 372)

Having touched upon the endeavors of psychologists in addressing globalization, and having mentioned that knowledge travels globally offering opportunity to recognize the importance of the local, a valid question would be, 'how has social psychology in India moved back and forth globally to realize the salience of the local?' The author would choose to respond to this question first, by asking to recall the social psychology narrative from the post-independent India, and the pioneer role played by Indian social psychologists toward indigenization of psychology. Second, she would like to take note of Indian social psychologists who looked for the relevance of the 'local' and tried for the contextual understanding in construction, representation, and use of knowledge. J.B.P. Sinha's autographical essay (1997) provides an account of his transformation that led to evolution of the sensitivity to realize the salience of the local and culturally rooted psychology. A number of Indian psychologists, including Professors D. Sinha, Janak Pandey, Girishwar Misra, R.C. Tripathi, Ajit Dalal, T.S. Saraswati, Lilavati Krishnan, and Purnima Singh, had acquired psychological knowledge generated and shared globally but converged in favor of the culture-specific local concerns.

Author's Encounters as a Social Psychologist

The purpose of this reflective account is to give a glance at the author's encounters as a social psychologist and ask whether she tried making sense of the 'social' in her discipline, thought of the relevance of the 'local,' and addressed to global issues? Talking of her career, she had the good fortune of having Professor J.B.P. Sinha as her teacher at Patna University and later as her PhD supervisor. J.B.P. Sinha is among the front line Indian social psychologists who questioned the applicability of western theories for the Indian circumstances. On her part, as a young researcher, the author was too naïve to ask whether social psychology was truly representing the 'social' component of its subject matter on the basis of individual data.

Her long-pursued interest in the area of collectivism and individualism almost for a decade was inspired by J.B.P. Sinha and Professor Harry Triandis. During her Fulbright Postdoctoral Fellowship at the University of Illinois (Urban-Champaign) in 1984, the author got opportunity to work with Professor Triandis. During the latter part of 1980s and further in the 1990s, she worked in the area of Indian collectivism and published several papers independently (Verma, 1885, 1986, 1988, 1999, 2003) and in collaboration with J.B.P. Sinha and others (Sinha & Verma, 1987, 1994; Sinha et al., 1994, 2001; Triandis et al., 1986; Verma & Triandis, 1999). Notably, for a long period of time, she chose quantitative methods for conducting research, and her focus remained unraveling the Indian idea of collectivism and its measurement.

While looking back, the author realizes that for some years, she was not quite certain about what interested her most. For instance, she found the 'women studies' area interesting but did not pursue it for long. Nevertheless, she might mention her chapter titled 'Transformation of women's role in India,' published in a volume edited by Jaan Valsiner (1995) and recall an early interview-based paper on the 'Life Patterns and Thinking of Three Generations of Middle Class Bihari Women' (1985). She also supervised a doctoral study at on 'Sources of Power and Influence of Middle Class Bihari Women' at Patna University (1992).

Similarly, she found the study of 'values' engaging and wrote a chapter on 'Social Values' in the fourth Indian Council of Social Science Research's (ICSSR's) Survey of Psychology (Verma, 2004a), while one of her joint papers empirically examined the structure of 'Indian Value Types' in the backdrop of Shalom Schwartz's universal value structure (Sinha & Verma, 2006; Verma, 2011a). During 1980s and 1990s, she participated in several national and international conferences and learnt about indigenous psychology and the process of indigenization.

An important turning point in her career came in 1994 when she visited Paris under the Indo-French exchange program. This visit was a rare opportunity where she had the privilege of being in contact with Professor Moscovici, who extended the SRs theory and approach in different cultural contexts. The author also had advantage of meeting other scholars from this area and one of them Wolfgang Wagner subsequently visited Patna with his student. Wagner was studying representations of 'madness' in a relatively traditional society. My collaboration with him yielded a couple of publications (Wagner et al., 1999, 2000).

In the beginning of 2001, the author was invited to join a major project on 'Representations of Food, Body and Health' sponsored by Observatoire Cidil de L' Harmonie Paris, France. Part of the study was done at Patna with the help of focus group discussions. The findings from Patna were published in 2004 and later utilized in a chapter introducing the SRs approach in the 'Handbook of Psychology in India' (2011b). The author's last comprehensive research in the tradition of SRs was completed in 2008–2009 in connection with a study of 'Trust in Organizations' (schools) in Finland, India, and Cameroon supported by the University of Helsinki, Finland. The aim was to understand cultural differences in representations of trust between superior and subordinates in the school setting.

At the University of Helsinki, the author had a firsthand experience of qualitative data analysis. First, the massive descriptive data from the focus group discussions and interviews were translated from Hindi to English by her, and later minutely transcribed by a small team of Finnish colleagues with the help of software (Atlas). Project Director Professor Pirttila Backman, some colleagues, and the present author struggled with analysis and interpretation of the data. This led to a joint publication (Pirttila Backman et al., 2017). In subsequent work, the present author often used both qualitative and quantitative methods, including her ICSSR project on '*Deteriorating Relationships of Bihari Migrants with Local Population in Mumbai*' in 2011.

The author also ventured to study issues related to Indian immigrants, acculturation concerns, and perhaps the process of identity in general (Arnett, 2002). She did undertake a study of acculturation experiences and adaptive strategies of Indian immigrants leading to the notion of bicultural identity. The author also had opportunity to work as intercultural communication consultant for a small Warsaw-based Polish consultancy, where her responsibility was to help resolve communication-related misunderstandings between the Indians and the Poles. She has recently completed a narrative-based paper on 'culture shock' (In press) which connects with globalization and emerging cultural issues.

Concluding Comments

In case of India, a primary feeling of uneasiness with the purely positivist-empiricist tradition helped creating the temper for doing socially relevant research and placing faith in indigenous concepts, methods, and tools. Moreover, the voices favoring 'de-individuation' and 're-socialization' of social psychology that emanated from France in 1960s were an inspiration for studying the social genesis of knowledge and the locally ongoing interactive processes that created it. Gradually, this trend facilitated the postmodernist approach and the belief that social and cultural dimensions were important for understanding and interpreting behavior. However, the academic engagements in social psychology in India are yet not at par with the international developments in the field. Coming to the 'global' part, it appears that despite the pervasive global values of consumerism and individualism, 'local' is still relevant, and it is worthwhile to 'turn inward' and build on a society's local human and material resources. Finally, taken that knowledge travels back and forth globally, Indian social psychologists too obtained, produced, and shared their knowledge globally and realized the relevance of the 'local.'

References

Adair, J., Pandey, J., Begum, H., & Puhan, B. N., & Vohra, N. (1995). Indigenization and development of the discipline: Perceptions and opinions of Indian and Bangladeshi psychologists. *Journal of Cross-Cultural Psychology*, *26*, 392–407.

Arnett, J. J. (2002). The psychology of globalization. *American Psychologist*, *57*(10), 774–783.

Bhalla, G., *Global strategy, local relevance*. www.brandz.com/articlenew/global-strategy-local-relevance-1714

Chiu, C. Y., & Cheng, S. Y. Y. (2007). Toward a social psychology of culture and globalization: Some social cognitive consequences of activating two cultures simultaneously. *Social and Personality Psychology Compass*, *1*, 84–100.

Chiu, C. Y., Torelli, C. J., & Cheng, S. Y. Y. (2011). Toward a social psychology of globalization. *Journal of Social Issues*, *67*(4), 663–676.

Dalal, A. K., & Misra, G. (2002). Social psychology in India: Evolution and emerging trends. In A. K. Dalal & G. Misra (Eds.), *New directions in Indian psychology*, Vol. 1, *Social psychology* (pp. 1–26). Sage.

Farr, R. (1993). Theory and method in the study of social representations. In D. Canter & G. Breakwell (Eds.), *Empirical approaches to social representations* (pp. 15–38). Clarendon Press.

Ganguli, H. C. (1971). Psychological research in India; 1920–1967. *International Journal of Psychology*, *6*, 165–177.

Gelfand, M. J., Lyons, S. L., & Lun, J. (2011). Toward a psychological science of globalization. *Journal of Social Issues*, *67*(4), 841–853.

Gergen, K. J. (1996). *Realities and relationships: Soundings in social construction*. Harvard University Press.

Gergen, K. J. (2004). Kenneth Gergen in conversation with Peter Mattes and Ernst Schraube. *Forum: Qualitative Research*, *5*(3), Art. 27.

Ghosh, B. (2011). Cultural changes and challenges in the era of globalization: The case of India. *Journal of Developing Societies*, *27*(2), 153–175.

Gogineni, R. R., Kallivayalil, R. A., Sharma, S., Rataemane, S., & Akhtar, S. (2018). Globalization of culture: Impact on Indian psyche. *Indian Journal of Social Psychiatry*, *34*(4), 303–312.

Hermans, H. J. M., & Dimaggio, G. (2007). Self, identity, and globalization in times of uncertainty: A dialogical analysis. *Review of General Psychology*, *11*, 31–61.

Jovchelovitch, S. (2007). *Knowledge in context: Representations, community and culture*. Routledge.

Kashima, Y., Shi, J., Tsuchiya, K., Cheng, S. Y. Y., Chao, M. M.-M., Kashima, E., & Shin, S. H. (2011). Globalization and folk theory of social change: How globalization relates to societal perceptions about the past and future. *Journal of Social Issues*, *67*, 696–715.

Kim, U. (1990). Indigenous psychology: Science and applications. In R. W. Brislin (Ed.), *Applied cross-cultural psychology* (pp. 142–160). Sage.

Krishnan, B. (1961). A review of the contributions of Indian psychologists (1950–1960). In T. K. N. Menon (Ed.), *Recent trends in psychology* (pp. 119–41). Orient Longman.

Marsella, A. J. (2012). Psychology and globalization: Understanding a complex relationship. *Journal of Social Issues*, *68*(3), 453–471.

Misra, G. (2000). Implications of culture for psychological knowledge. In J. W. Berry, R. C. Mishra, & R. C. Tripathi (Eds.), *Psychology in human and social development* (pp. 31–67). Sage.
Misra, G. (2011). Psychology through the works of professor Jai. B. P. Sinha: Some reflections. In J. Pandey, T. N. Sinha, & A. K. Sinha (Eds.), *Dialogue for development* (pp. 58–66). Concept.
Misra, G., & Gergen, K. (1993). On the place of culture in psychological science. *International Journal of Psychology*, *28*(2), 225–243.
Misra, G., & Kumar, M. (2010). Psychology in India: Retrospect and prospect. In G. Misra (Ed.), *Psychology in India* (Vol. 4, pp. 340–376). Pearson.
Misra, G., & Mohanty, A. K. (2002). *Perspectives on indigenous psychology*. Concept.
Moscovici, S. (1961). *La Psychanalyse: Son image et son public*. Presses Universitaires de France.
Moscovici, S. (1984). The phenomenon of social representations. In R. M. Farr & S. Moscovici (Eds.), *Social representations* (pp. 3–68). Cambridge University Press.
Moscovici, S. (1988). Notes towards a description of social representations. *European Journal of Social Psychology*, *18*, 211–250.
Moscovici, S., & Hewstone, M. (1983). Social representations and social explanation: From the naïve to the amateur scientist. In M. Hewstone (Ed.), *Attribution theory*. Blackwell.
Mukherjee, B. N. (1980). Psychological theory and research method. In Udai Pareek (Ed.), *A survey of research in psychology, 1971–76*, Part I (pp. 91–135). Popular Prakashan.
Muthayya, B. C. (1988). Dynamics of rural development. In Pandey, J. (Ed.), *Psychology in India: The state-of-the-art*. Vol. 2, *Organizational behavior and mental health* (pp. 225–278). Sage.
Nandy, A. (1974). The non-paradigmatic crisis in India psychology: Reflections on a recipient culture of science. *Indian Journal of Psychology*, *49*, 1–20.
Norasakkunkit, V., & Uchida, Y. (2011). Psychological consequences of post-industrial anomie on self and motivation among Japanese youth. *Journal of Social Issues*, *67*, 774–786.
Pandey, J. (1978). Effects of crowding on human social behavior. *Journal of Social and Economic Studies*, *5*(1), 37–41.
Pandey, J. (Ed.). (1981). *Perspective on experimental social psychology in India*. Concept Publishers.
Pandey, J. (Ed.). (1988). *Psychology in India: The state-of-the-art. Vol. 1 Personality, and mental processes. Vol. 2. Basic and applied social psychology. Vol. 3 Organizational behavior and mental health*. Sage.
Pandey, J. (1996). Coda. In J. Pandey, D. Sinha, & D. P. S. Bhawuk (Eds.), *Asian contributions to cross-cultural psychology* (pp. 357–361). Sage.
Pandey, J. (1998). Environment in the Indian context: Socio-psychological issues and research. *Indian Psychological Abstracts and Reviews*, *5*(2), 205–234.
Pandey, J. (1999). Socio-cultural dimensions of experience and consequences of crowding. In J. C. Lasry, J. Adair, & K. Dion (Eds.), *Latest contributions to cross-cultural psychology* (pp. 11–22). Swets and Zeitlinger.
Pandey, J. (2000a). Perception of poverty: Socio-psychological dimensions. In A. K. Mohanty & G. Misra (Eds.), *Psychology of poverty and disadvantage* (pp. 72–88). Concept.
Pandey, J. (Ed.). (2000b). *Psychology in India revisited: Developments in the discipline: Physiological foundation and human cognition* (Vol. 1). Sage.
Pandey, J. (Ed.). (2001). *Psychology in India revisited: Developments in the discipline: Personality and health psychology* (Vol. 2). Sage.

Pandey, J. (2004a). Psychology in India enters the twenty-first century: Movement toward an indigenous discipline. In J. Pandey (Ed.), *Psychology in India revisited: Developments in the discipline* (pp. 342–370). Sage.
Pandey, J. (Ed.). (2004b). *Psychology in India revisited: Developments in the discipline: Applied social and organizational psychology* (Vol. 3). Sage.
Pandey, J., & Nagar, D. (1987). Experience of indwelling and out dwelling crowding and social psychological consequence. *Social Science International*, *3*(1), 1–9.
Pandey, J., & Singh A. K. (1985). Social psychological responses to perceived and objective indicators of poverty in India. In I. R. Lagunes, & Y. H. Poortinga (Eds.), *From a different perspective: Studies of behavior across cultures* (pp. 148–156). Swets & Zeitlinger.
Pandey, M. (1992). *Women's source of power and influence* [Unpublished doctoral dissertation in psychology]. Patna University.
Pareek, U. (1981). *A survey of research in psychology: 1971–1976, part 2*. Popular Prakashan.
Parmeshwaran, E. G. (1978). Psychology in Indian universities. *Manas*, *25*, 69–79.
Pike, K. L. (1967). *Language in relation to a unified theory of the structure of human behavior*. Mouton.
Pirttila Backman, A.-M., Menard, A., Verma, J., & Kassea, R. (2017). Trust among teachers and principals in Cameroonian, Indian and Finnish schools. *Journal of Social and Political Psychology*, *5*(1), 29–57.
Prakash, A. (2011). Qualitative methods in psychology. In G. Misra (Ed.), *Psychology in India*. Vol. 4 *Theoretical and methodological developments* (pp. 227–71). Pearson.
Ruback, R. B., & Pandey, J. (1992). Very hot and really crowded: Quasi-experimental investigations of Indian "tempos". *Environment and Behavior*, *24*(4), 527–554.
Sharma, R. (2020, Tuesday, May 5). The pandemic isn't changing everything. *The Times of India (Patna Daily)*, 12.
Siddiqui, R. N., & Pandey, J. (2003). Coping with poverty by an urban poor minority group. *Psychological Studies*, *48*(3), 66–71.
Singh, A. K., & Pandey, J. (1990). Psychology of poverty. *The Indian Journal of Social Work*, *51*(4), 624–632.
Singh, N. (2012). Adapted and excerpted from: *Localization strategies for global e-Business*. Cambridge University Press.
Sinha, A., & Verma, J. (2006, October). Indian value types: An empirical study. *Psychological Studies*, *51*(4), 235–244.
Sinha, D. (1986). *Psychology in a third world country: The Indian experience*. Sage.
Sinha, D. (1990). Indigenization of psychology. *Bulletin of the National Academy of Psychology* (India), *1*, 3–5.
Sinha, D. (1993). Indigenization of psychology in India and its relevance. In U. Kim & J. W. Berry (Eds.), *Indigenous psychologies: Research and experience in cultural context* (pp. 3–43). Sage.
Sinha, D. (1994). Indigenization of psychology in India. *Indian Psychological Abstracts and Reviews*, *1*, 179–215.
Sinha, D. (1997). Indigenizing psychology. In J. W. Berry, Y. Poortinga, & J. Pandey (Eds.), *Handbook of cross-cultural psychology: Theoretical and methodological perspectives* (Vol. 1, pp. 129–169). Allyn & Bacon.
Sinha, D. (1998). Changing perspectives in social psychology in India: A journey towards indigenization. *Asian Journal of Social Psychology*, *1*(1), 17–31.
Sinha, J. B. P. (1968). The nAch/nCooperation under limited/unlimited resource conditions. *Journal of Experimental Social Psychology*, *4*, 233–248.
Sinha, J. B. P. (1984). Towards partnership for relevant research in the third world. *International Journal of Psychology*, *19*, 169–178.

Sinha, J. B. P. (1997). In search of my Brahman. In M. H. Bond (Ed.), *Working at the interface of cultures: Eighteen lives in social science* (pp. 77–84). Routledge.
Sinha, J. B. P. (2000). Integrative indigenization of management in India: Practices and prospects. *Indian Journal of Industrial Relations*, *35*(4), 439–460.
Sinha, J. B. P. (2002). Towards indigenization of psychology in India. In G. Misra & A. K. Mohanty (Eds.), *Perspectives of indigenous psychology* (pp. 440–457). Concept.
Sinha, J. B. P. (2003). Trends toward indigenization of psychology in India. In K. S. Yang, K. K. Hwang, P. B. Pedersen, & I. Daibo (Eds.), *Progress in Asian social psychology: Conceptual and empirical contributions* (pp. 11–27). Praeger.
Sinha, J. B. P. (2004). *Multinationals in India: Managing the interface of cultures*. Sage.
Sinha, J. B. P. (2008). *Culture and organizational behavior*. Sage.
Sinha, J. B. P., Daftuar, C. N., Gupta, R. K., Mishra, R. C., Jayseetha, R., Jha, S. S., Verma, J., & Viayakumar, V. S. R. (1994). Regional similarities and differences in people's beliefs, practices, and preferences. *Psychology and Developing Societies*, 6(2), 131–150.
Sinha, J. B. P., & Pandey, J. (1970). Strategies of high n-Ach persons. *Psychologia*, 210–213.
Sinha, J. B. P., Sinha, T. N., Verma, J., & Sinha, R. B. N. (2001). Collectivism coexisting with individualism: An Indian scenario. *Asian Journal of Social Psychology*, *4*, 133–145.
Sinha, J. B. P., & Verma, J. (1987). Structure of collectivism. In C. Kagitcibasi (Ed.), *Growth and progress in cross-cultural psychology* (pp. 123–129). Swets & Zeitlinger.
Sinha, J. B. P., & Verma, J. (1994). Social support as a moderator of the relationship between allocentrism and psychological-well-being. In U. Kim, H. C. Triandis, C. Kagitcibasi, S. C. Choi, & G. Yoon (Eds.), *Individualism and collectivism: Theory, method and applications* (pp. 267–275). Sage.
Triandis, H. C. (1994). *Culture and social behavior*. Mc Graw-Hill.
Triandis, H. C., Bontempo, R., Betancourt, H., Bond, M., Leung, K., Brenes, A., Georgas, J., Hui, H. C., Marin, G., Setiadi, B., Sinha, J. B. P., Verma, J., Spengenberg, J., Touzard, H., & de Montomollin, G., (1986). The measurement of the etic aspects of individualism and collectivism across cultures. *Australian Journal of Psychology*, *38*(3), 257–267.
Tripathi, R. C. (1988). Applied social psychology. In Pandey, J. (Ed.), *Psychology in India: The state-of-the-art*. (Vol. 2.), *Organizational behavior and mental health* (pp. 95–157). Sage.
Tripathi, R. C. (2011). In search of a global psychology. In G. Misra (Ed.), *Handbook of psychology in India* (370–373). Oxford University Press.
Verma, J. (1985). Life patterns and thinking of three generations of middle class Bihari women. *Social Change*, *15*(2), 25–28.
Verma, J. (1986). Perceived causes of norm violation as a function of individualism and collectivism. *Psychological Studies*, *31*(2), 169–176.
Verma, J. (1988). Allocentrism, collectivism, in-group influence and some background variables. *Psychological Studies*, *3*(1), 20–23.
Verma, J. (1995). Transformation of women's social roles in India. In J. Valsiner (Ed.), *Child development within culturally structured environments: Comparative-cultural and constructivist perspectives* (Vol. 3, pp. 138–163). Ablex Publishing.
Verma, J. (1999). Collectivism in the cultural perspective: The Indian scene. In J. Lasry, J. Adair, & K. Dion (Eds.), *Latest contributions to cross-cultural psychology* (pp. 228–241). Swets & Zeitlinger.
Verma, J. (2003). Situational preferences for different types of individualism-collectivism. In U. Vindhya (Ed.), *Psychology in India: Intersecting crossroads* (pp. 54–77). Concept.

Verma, J. (2004a). Social values. In J. Pandey (Ed.), *Psychology in India revisited* (Vol. 3, pp. 69–117). Sage.
Verma, J. (2004b). Relationship among food, body and health: Some representations from Bihar. *Psychological Studies*, *49*(4), 227–237.
Verma, J. (2011a). Values as force behind development. In J. Pandey, T. N. Sinha, & A. K. Sinha (Eds.), *Dialogue for development* (pp. 252–274). Concept.
Verma, J. (2011b). Representations of food, body and health. In G. Misra (Ed.), *Handbook of psychology in India* (pp. 239–253). Oxford University Press.
Verma, J., & Triandis, H. C. (1999). Measurement of collectivism in India. In W. J. Lonner, D. L. Dinnel, D. K. Forgys, & S. A. Hayes (Eds.), *Merging past, present, and future in cross-cultural psychology* (pp. 256–265). Swets & Zeitlinger.
Wagner, W., Duveen, G., Themel, M., & Verma, J. (1999). The modification of tradition: Thinking about madness in Patna, India. *Culture and Psychology*, *5*, 413–46.
Wagner, W., Duveen, G., Themel, M., & Verma, J. (2000). "I have some faith and at the same time I don't believe"-cognitive polyphasia and culture change. *Journal of Community & Applied Social Psychology*, *10*(4), 301–314.
Yang, D., Chen, X., Cheng, S. Y. Y., Kwan, L., Tam, K.-P., & Yeh, K. H. (2011). Lay psychology and its social impact. *Journal of Social Issues*, *67*, 677–695.

2 Living Together in Culturally Diverse Societies

John W. Berry

Introduction

In all culturally diverse societies, such as India and Canada, achieving social stability, cohesion, and mutual accommodation are goals that citizens and policy makers in most culturally diverse societies are now seeking (Banting & Kymlicka, 2003; Berry, 2013; Berry & Sam, 2013). This chapter outlines a program of research that seeks to conceptualize, measure, and interpret some fundamental issues in a number of plural societies. It reports on a project "Mutual Intercultural Relations in Plural Societies" (MIRIPS; see Berry, 2017).[1] It was carried out as a basis for attaining the goals of social cohesion and mutual acceptance among all groups that co-inhabit diverse societies in many parts of the world. We do this by proposing and then empirically examining three core psychological principles of intercultural relations: multiculturalism, contact, and integration (Berry, 1984). This research was carried out across 17 culturally plural societies: Australia, Azerbaijan, Canada, Estonia, Finland, Germany, Greece, Hong Kong, India, Italy, Latvia, Malta, Norway, Portugal, Russia, Spain, and Switzerland. The first goal of the project is to evaluate these three hypotheses of intercultural relations across these 17 societies. The second goal is to examine the findings to see whether they constitute some "universal" principles of intercultural relations that may be applied in many societies. If they are, it may be possible to propose some policies and programs to improve the quality of intercultural relationship globally (Berry et al., 2022; Berry, 2023).

The design of the project is an exercise in replication across contexts in order to discern what may be culturally universal and what may be culturally specific in how diverse groups of peoples engage in their intercultural relations. Across the whole project, these replications were carried out with a shared conceptualization and research instrument. However, the project employed culturally appropriate operationalizations of the concepts and methods with highly varied samples. It thus represents a multi-trait/multi-method/multi-cultural approach, providing a robust examination of the three principles and hypotheses.

DOI: 10.4324/9781003461302-4

The three principles that are evaluated in the MIRIPS project are as follows:

(i) Multiculturalism hypothesis: When individuals feel secure in their cultural, economic, and personal place in a society, they will be able to better accept those who are different from themselves; conversely when individuals feel threatened, they will reject those who are different.
(ii) Contact hypothesis: When individuals have contact with and engage with those who are culturally different from themselves, under certain conditions, they will achieve greater mutual acceptance.
(iii) Integration hypothesis: When individuals identify with, and are socially connected to, both their heritage culture and to the larger society in which they live, they will achieve higher levels of adaptation (psychological well-being, sociocultural competence and intercultural tolerance) than if they relate to only one or the other culture or to neither.

Psychological Approaches to Intercultural Relations

The MIRIPS project focuses on the psychological aspects of intercultural relations but takes into account some of the social and political contextual features of the larger societies and of the interacting groups within them. The study is situated within the broad field of cross-cultural psychology (Berry et al., 1997, 2011), which seeks answers to the question: are individual human behaviors shaped by the cultural context in which they develop? The eventual goal is to achieve a set of universal psychological principles that underlie human behavior globally. By universal, we mean: (i) a phenomenon that shares a common, species-wide substrate of psychological processes and functioning, and (ii) a phenomenon that also exhibits behavioral variations across cultures as this substrate is differentially developed and expressed in daily life. Much research in cross-cultural psychology has been carried out within the "ecocultural framework" (Berry, 2018), including studies with Adivasi peoples in India examining their ecological and intercultural adaptations (Mishra et al., 1995; Mishra & Berry, 2017).

The project is also situated in the field of intercultural psychology (Sam & Berry, 2016). This field deals with the question: "If individual behaviours are shaped in particular cultural contexts, what happens when individuals who have developed in different cultural contexts meet and interact within another society?" There are two domains of psychological interest here: (i) *ethnocultural group relations* and (ii) *acculturation*. The study of ethnocultural group relations has usually examined the views and behaviors of the dominant group(s) toward the non-dominant ones, using concepts such as ethnic stereotypes, attitudes, prejudice, and discrimination. These views are often assessed with regard to a number of non-dominant groups, such as specific ethnocultural groups and immigrants. This "one-way" view of examining ethnocultural relations misses understanding the important reciprocal or mutual views held by non-dominant groups toward dominant group(s). The MIRIPS study has examined the intercultural views of both kinds of groups in contact, using the same concepts and measures with both dominant and non-dominant groups.

The second domain of psychological interest in intercultural psychology is that of acculturation, defined as "the process of cultural and psychological change that takes place as a result of contact between cultural groups and their individual members" (Berry, 2005). Four kinds of changes have been identified: changes in the *customs and repertoire* of groups and individuals that can be relatively easy to accomplish (such as the food, dress, and language); more problematic and challenging changes leading to the phenomenon of *acculturative stress*; the development of a set of *strategies and expectations* about how to deal with living interculturally; and some long-term *adaptations* as people settle into their intercultural lives.

As in the case of research on ethnocultural group relations, research on acculturation has also typically been a "one-way" approach. When examining the changes, stress, strategies, and adaptations of non-dominant peoples, research has usually missed examining those of members of the dominant group(s) regarding how they think that non-dominant groups and individuals *should* acculturate and live in the plural society. These views of dominant groups (their attitudes) and of the larger society in general (public policies) have come to be known as *acculturation expectations* (Berry, 2003). In addition, the acculturative changes of the dominant group are also examined.

General Framework for the MIRIPS Project

The MIRIPS project is guided by a framework that identifies the main concepts and variables and suggests their interrelationships (see Figure 2.1). This figure shows five kinds of acculturation and intercultural relations phenomena: (i) the characteristics of the two or more cultural groups (A and B) prior to contact; (ii) the nature of the contact between them; (iii) the cultural changes that are taking place in both groups; (iv) the psychological changes experienced by individuals in both groups in contact; and (v) the long-term adaptations that may be achieved.

At the cultural group level (on the left of Figure 2.1), we seek to understand key features of the two (or more) original cultural groups prior to their major contact, the nature of their initial and continuing contact relationships, and the resulting dynamic cultural changes in the groups as they emerge as ethnocultural groups during the process of acculturation. Such changes may occur due to invasion and domination, colonization, migration, or globalization. These cultural changes can range from being rather easily accomplished (such as evolving a new economic base) through to being a source of major cultural disruption (as a result of becoming colonized or enslaved).

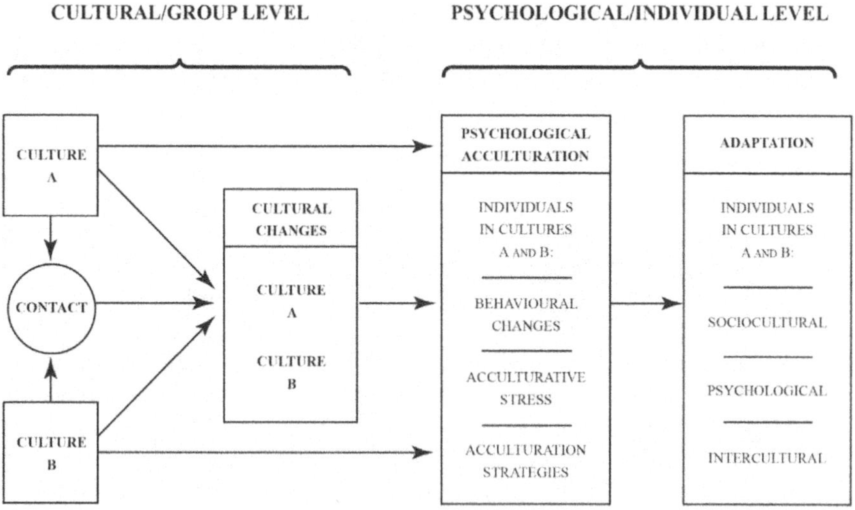

Figure 2.1 General Framework for MIRIPS Project

At the individual level (in the middle), we consider the psychological acculturation that individuals in all groups in contact undergo. Identifying these changes requires sampling a population and studying individuals who are variably involved in the process of acculturation. These changes have been examined extensively by psychologists and psychiatrists over many decades (e.g., Berry, 1997; Bhugra, 2020), with a complex set of findings that need to be considered critically. The figure shows three kinds of psychological changes resulting from contact: behavioral; stress; and strategies. Behavioral changes can be a set of rather easily accomplished changes (e.g., in ways of speaking, dressing, and eating), or they can be more difficult to accomplish (e.g., changes in identities, self-concept, and values). Second are changes that are due to acculturation experiences that are challenging, even problematic, in which *acculturative stress* becomes manifest. Third, individuals also develop and engage in *acculturation strategies* and *expectations* (Berry, 1980) as their preferred way to acculturate and relate to each other.

Following from these three kinds of psychological changes are some long-term outcomes, referred to as *adaptations* (on the right). Three kinds of adaptations have been discerned: psychological, sociocultural, and intercultural. Ward (1996) distinguished between *psychological adaptation* and *sociocultural adaptation*. The first refers to adaptations that are primarily internal or psychological (e.g., sense of personal well-being and self-esteem, sometimes referred to as "feeling well"). The second refers to adaptations that are sociocultural and are sometimes called "doing well." This form of adaptation is manifested by competence in carrying out the activities of daily intercultural living (such as in the community, at work, and in school).

A third is *intercultural adaptation* (Berry, 2005), which refers to the extent to which individuals are able to establish harmonious intercultural relations, with low levels of prejudice and discrimination ("relating well").

Intercultural Strategies and Expectations

One concept that is central to and underlies all aspects of acculturation and intercultural relations phenomena is the way in which people seek to relate to each other in culturally plural societies. As noted above, these are the *strategies* and *expectations* that all groups and their individual members have, whether acknowledged explicitly or just implicitly, when they acculturate and engage in intercultural relations. These strategies and expectations can be held by both the dominant and non-dominant individuals and groups that are in contact.

They are based on three underlying issues: (i) the degree to which there is a desire to maintain the group's culture and identity; (ii) the degree to which there is a desire to engage in daily interactions with other groups in the larger society, including both dominant and non-dominant one(s); and (iii) the relative power of the groups in contact to choose their preferred way of engaging each other (Berry, 1980).

Four strategies have been derived from the first two issues facing all acculturating peoples (see Figure 2.2). There are two sets of concepts, one for the *strategies* of non-dominant groups and their individual members; how do they wish to live interculturally? The other are the *expectations* of dominant

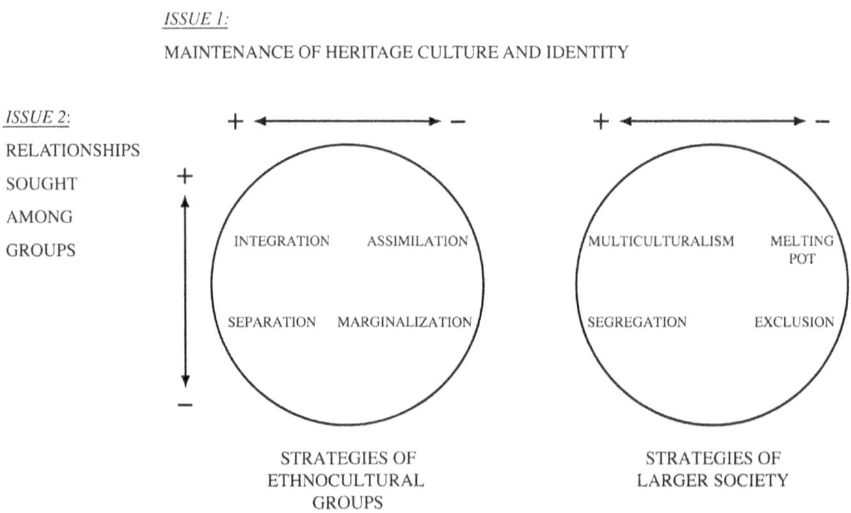

Figure 2.2 Society 2: Acculturation Strategies and Expectations Among Ethnocultural Groups and the Larger

groups in the larger society and of their individual members; how do they think that non-dominant groups and individuals should live interculturally? The power relations between these two sectors of the population in a plural society are present in the differences between these strategies and expectations. Typically, the dominant group has more power than the non-dominant group to decide on the policies and practices that are operating in the plural society.

These issues can be responded to on attitudinal dimensions, on which generally positive or negative orientations to these issues intersect to define four ways of acculturating. Preferences for these ways carry different names, depending on which groups (the non-dominant or dominant) are being considered. From the point of view of non-dominant ethnocultural groups (on the left of Figure 2.2), when individuals do not wish to maintain their cultural identity and seek daily interaction with other cultures, the *Assimilation* strategy is defined. In contrast, when individuals place a value on holding on to their original culture and at the same time wish to avoid interaction with others, then the *Separation* alternative is defined. When there is an interest in both maintaining one's original culture and having daily interactions with other groups, *Integration* is the option. In this case, there is some degree of cultural integrity maintained while at the same time seeking, as a member of an ethnocultural group, to participate as an integral part of the larger society. Finally, when there is little possibility or interest in cultural maintenance (often for reasons of enforced cultural loss) and little interest in having relations with others (often for reasons of exclusion or discrimination), then *Marginalization* is defined.

Different terms (but parallel terms) are used to refer to the four expectations held by members of the larger society (on the right of Figure 2.2). Assimilation when sought by the non-dominant acculturating group is termed the *Melting Pot*. When separation is forced by the dominant group, it is *Segregation*. Marginalization, when imposed by the dominant group, is *Exclusion*. Finally, for integration, when cultural diversity is a feature of the society as a whole, including all the various ethnocultural groups, it is called *Multiculturalism*. With the use of this framework, comparisons can be made between individuals and their ethnocultural groups and between non-dominant peoples and the larger society within which they are acculturating.

Of course, non-dominant individuals and groups do not have the freedom to choose how they want to live interculturally. When the dominant group enforces certain forms of acculturation or intercultural relations or constrains the choices of non-dominant groups or individuals, then the third element of the framework becomes necessary: the power of the dominant group to influence the strategies available to, and used by, the non-dominant groups (Berry, 1980). As a result, there is a mutual, reciprocal process through which both groups arrive at strategies that will work in a particular society and in a particular setting. For example, integration can only be chosen and successfully pursued by non-dominant groups when the dominant society is open and inclusive in its orientation toward cultural diversity (i.e., a form of multiculturalism). Thus, a mutual accommodation is required for integration to be attained, involving the acceptance by both groups of the right of all groups to live together as culturally different peoples. This strategy requires non-dominant groups to adopt the basic values of the larger society, while at the same time, the dominant group must be prepared to adapt national institutions (e.g., education, health, labor) to better meet the needs of all groups now living together in the plural society.

MIRIPS Project

Three hypotheses are evaluated in the MIRIPS project: the *multiculturalism hypothesis;* the *contact hypothesis;* and the *integration hypothesis.* These hypotheses have been derived from the multiculturalism policy advanced by the Federal Government of Canada (1971). This policy promotes the maintenance of groups' cultural heritages as well as social interaction and sharing among groups.

The *multiculturalism hypothesis* is expressed in the policy statement that confidence in one's identity will lead to sharing, respect for others, and to the reduction of discriminatory attitudes. That is, confidence rooted in the cultural maintenance component of the policy will lead to the mutual acceptance goal. We have considered this confidence to involve a sense of security (or conversely, a sense of threat) to one's person or ethnocultural group. The multiculturalism hypothesis (first advanced by Berry et al., 1977, p. 192) is that such a sense of security in one's identity is a psychological precondition for the acceptance of those who are culturally different. Conversely, when one's identity is threatened, people will reject others.

Three kinds of security have been conceptualized by Berry et al. (1977): *cultural, economic,* and *personal.* Cultural security refers to a sense that aspects of one's culture (such as identity and language) have a secure status in the society. Economic security refers to the sense that one's economic status (such as job security and house prices) are not going to be diminished in culturally diverse settings. Personal security refers to the sense that one is free to move around without being accosted or attacked. The MIRIPS project assess all three forms of security.

In sum, the multiculturalism hypothesis proposes that a high sense of security will predict a preference for the strategies that engage in contact and participation in the larger society: integration and assimilation. In addition, this hypothesis proposes that secure individuals will achieve a higher level of intercultural adaptation, including higher scores on multicultural ideology and tolerance. Conversely, when individuals are threatened, especially by acts of discrimination, they will prefer the separation and marginalization strategies and exhibit low levels on the multicultural ideology and tolerance scales.

The *contact hypothesis* derives from the second link in the policy framework, which proposes that intercultural contact and sharing will promote mutual acceptance. The contact hypothesis asserts that "Prejudice . . . may be reduced by equal status contact between majority and minority groups in the pursuit of common goals" (Allport, 1954). Allport proposed that the hypothesis is more likely to be supported when certain conditions are present in the intercultural encounter. The effect of contact is predicted to be stronger when there is contact between groups of roughly equal social and economic status; however, in most intercultural situations, equal status is rare. A second condition is that the contact should be voluntary (sought by both groups, rather than imposed). A third condition is that contact should be supported by society, through norms and policies promoting contact and laws prohibiting discrimination.

In sum, the contact hypothesis proposes that under certain conditions, more intercultural contact will be associated with more mutual acceptance. Specifically, more contact will predict higher intercultural adaptation (both Multicultural Ideology and Tolerance) and should also predict a preference for the two strategies of integration and assimilation.

The *integration hypothesis* proposes that when individuals and groups seek integration (by being doubly or multiply engaged in both their heritage cultures and with other groups in the larger society), they will be more successful in achieving a higher level of adaptation than if they engage only one or the other of the cultural groups. Much research has demonstrated that the integration strategy is usually associated with better psychological well-being (e.g., Berry et al. 2006; Berry & Hou, 2016). Based on a review of numerous studies, Berry (1997) made the generalization that integration was the most successful strategy for both psychological well-being and sociocultural adaptation. This generalization has been examined in a meta-analysis by Nguyen and Benet-Martinez (2103), who concluded that integration ("biculturalism" in their terms) was associated with the most positive outcomes for migrants' well-being.

In sum, the integration hypothesis proposes that when individuals prefer the integration strategy or have the multiculturalism expectation (i.e., when they are doubly or multiply engaged), they will achieve higher scores on psychological, sociocultural, and intercultural adaptation than when they prefer any of the other three strategies. Conversely, especially when individuals are marginalized (when they have no or few engagements), they will achieve lower adaptations. Preference for the assimilation and separation strategies should result in mid-levels of adaptation being expected.

Method

Samples

The project sought to include a wide range of culturally plural societies. These included those that are "settler societies," with both new migrants and settled ethnocultural groups; those that are experiencing migration relatively recently; those with return migrant flows of "co-nationals"; and those that have residual populations of non-dominant groups following political realignment. The samples are also diverse, including adults and school children, community groups, online forums, and both snowball and random samples. The total numbers of participants were 7,485 members of the dominant group in a society and 5,888 members of the various non-dominant groups.

Variables

There are three categories of variables assessed in the study:

1. Socio-demographic variables: Age, Gender, Education, Religion, Socioeconomic Status, Languages known and used, and Ethnic Origin.
2. Intercultural variables: Social contacts; Cultural identities (*ethnic/national*): Security (*cultural, economic, personal*); Acculturation Strategies/Expectations (*Integration/Multiculturalism; Assimilation/Melting Pot; Separation/Segregation; Marginalization/Exclusion*).
3. Adaptation variables: Psychological (*Self-esteem; Life satisfaction; Psychological problems)*; Sociocultural; Intercultural (Multicultural Ideology; Tolerance; Attitudes toward immigrants).

Data Collection and Analysis

Each country research team employed the MIRIPS instrument in a way that met their research needs and their social conditions. Thus, the findings are not strictly comparable across countries. Nevertheless, the core concepts and the three hypotheses remain common, even if they were operationalized somewhat differently. Because of these variations, the goal of the MIRIPS project has *not* been to place all the data collected in all the societies into one data base and thereby to carry out pan-cultural analyses (as was done, e.g., in the study of immigrant youth; Berry et al., 2006).

Each MIRIPS team chose to analyze their data in a way that met their particular requirements, taking into account their selecting and operationalizing the variables, their local research issues, and the requirements of their funding sources. In some cases, simple mean differences and bivariate correlations were used to evaluate the three hypotheses. In other cases, multivariate statistics, such as factor analysis, profile analysis, and path analysis, were carried out. And in some cases, a combination of these methods was used to gain multiple perspectives on the validity of the three hypotheses.

Results

In the 17-country studies, based on all the samples, there was a maximum of 44 possible evaluations of the three hypotheses (making a total of 132 evaluations overall). These studies included samples of both dominant national and non-dominant ethnic groups in most of the countries; in some countries, there was more than one study—and more than one dominant and non-dominant sample. In some studies, not all hypotheses were evaluated, reducing the total number of possible evaluations to 112 across the three hypotheses.

Despite the lack of strict comparability in the operationalization of the variables across the 17 societies, when examining the findings across the three hypotheses, a fairly clear pattern emerges. First for the multiculturalism hypothesis, in 36 of the 39 possible evaluations, there was support for the hypothesis; in three cases, there was no support (in two cases, there was no relationship between security and acceptance of others, and in the other case, there was a contrary finding). There were five cases where this hypothesis was not evaluated.

Second, for the contact hypothesis, in 28 of the 35 possible evaluations, there was support for the hypothesis. In the seven cases of no support, there were six cases of no relationship between intercultural contact and the acceptance of others, and one case of a contrary finding. There were nine cases where the hypothesis was not evaluated.

Third, for the integration hypothesis, in 29 of the 37 possible evaluations, there was support for the hypothesis; there were eight cases of no support (six cases of no relationship between preferring integration/multiculturalism and well-being, and two cases of contrary findings). There were seven cases where the hypothesis was not evaluated.

This general picture shows that these three hypotheses are supported much more often than not; 92%, 80%, and 78% of the evaluations are positive for the multiculturalism, contact, and integration hypotheses, respectively. Of particular importance is that there are very few contrary findings; there are only one, one, and two such negative findings for the three hypotheses.

Discussion

A summary of evaluations according to the type of sample (dominant or non-dominant) shows that there is a generally common level of support in these two types of samples across the countries in the study. That is, there is little variation in the level of support between dominant national and non-dominant ethnic samples. This may be taken as evidence for the presence of *commonality* in intercultural relations in most of these societies.

We are interested not only in evidence of shared support but also in the degree to which there is *agreement* about these issues between dominant and non-dominant people living in the same society. This is the core of the question of *mutual* intercultural relations; is there support (or not) for the hypotheses in *both* dominant and non-dominant groups within a society? We found a level of mutuality that varied across the three hypotheses. For the multiculturalism hypothesis, there was agreement in the findings between the two kinds of samples in each country in 15 of the 17 societies. For the contact hypothesis, there was agreement in 11 of the 17 societies, and for the integration hypothesis, in 9 of the 17 samples, there was agreement. Overall, we found agreement in 35 of the possible 51 society evaluations (69% of cases).

On this basis, there is some possibility of developing policies and programs to improve intercultural relations in those societies. This is most likely to be successful where there is both support for the hypotheses and mutual agreement between groups in their support. However, in those societies where there is limited support for a hypothesis, there is still a possibility of developing policies and programs by working with that sector of the society, where such limited support was found.

Implications

Universals

The evidence produced by the MIRIPS research teams in these societies on the validity of these three hypotheses, while variable, has provided a large degree of general support for them. Do they qualify as universals of intercultural relations? Second, does this level of support provide a basis for claiming that these three hypotheses are likely to be global in their validity? And third, if so, can they provide a basis for advancing policies and programs that will improve the quality of intercultural relations elsewhere in the world? In my view, the empirical findings do allow us to promote them as candidates for being universal psychological principles of intercultural relations.

Policy and Program Implications

If the claim for some universality is accepted, we can ask the fundamental question: is such universality sufficient to serve as a basis for promoting these three principles as a valid basis for developing intercultural policy and program in many societies? Although the three principles were drawn from extant intercultural policy (in Canada, Australia, and the European Union) and have been largely supported by empirical research in WASP psychology (Western Academic, Scientific Psychology) as well as in the present study in a variety of societies, do they provide a relevant basis for policy development in other plural societies?

In some of the societies just mentioned, there has been a policy transition over the past decades from attempts to assimilate non-dominant (indigenous, ethnocultural, and migrant) peoples into a homogeneous society, to one that is more integrationist and multicultural (Berry & Kalin, 2000). Is it possible to emulate this transition in other plural societies? The lesson here is that change in intercultural policy is possible; if this has been the case in these societies, what conditions may be required in other societies in order to move toward this more pluralist vision?

In contrast, some societies appear to have transitioned away from the multiculturalism vision, preferring to seek a more uniform society in terms of culture, language, and religion. These transitions are usually contentious and, in some cases (e.g., in India), lead to political polarization and community conflicts.

One possible answer to the question of how to live together in culturally plural societies is that the kind of evidence provided by the MIRIPS project may be useful to persuade these societies to move away from both the emerging assimilation policies that are designed to achieve a culturally homogeneous society and the policies that exclude those that are different (by way of segregation or exclusion) toward a more multicultural one. In my view, policies that are evidence-based are more likely to be successful than those based only on preconceptions or political expediency. However, evidence alone (such as that provided in this project) is unlikely to shift public policy toward more pluralist ways of living together. Other factors are also important, particularly public opinion, political ideology, and the availability of resources.

Widespread public education, both in schools and in the society at large, is required in order to bring about any policy change from assimilation toward a multicultural way of living together. The benefits of the multicultural vision need to be articulated and advocated widely in ways that the general public can understand and accept this vision. Particularly important is the claim that life for everyone is enriched culturally, psychologically, and economically in multicultural societies (Berry, 1998; Berry & Sam, 2014).

These three principles of intercultural relations (of providing a secure and non-discriminatory social and cultural environment, of opportunities for equitable intercultural contact and participation, and of ways to be engaged in and identify with more than one culture) offer a clear basis for moving toward achieving a more harmonious plural society. If this goal of attaining more positive intercultural relations is valued by the general population of the larger society and by policy makers and leaders, then the path forward should be clear to them. Despite the obvious difficulties in many contemporary societies, the three psychological principles of intercultural relations examined in the MIRIPS project and articulated in this chapter would be a good place to start.

Conclusions

The ideas and research findings reported in this chapter are situated in the disciplines of cross-cultural and intercultural psychology. The first main feature of these approaches is that cultural experiences shape the development and expression of human behavior. The second is that these behaviors are brought to the intercultural arena by both (all) groups and individuals that are in contact. The third main feature is that in order to discern which features of cultural experience shape behaviors in which way, the comparative method is required. And, finally, by examining the evidence obtained by empirical research across cultures to identify any general patterns, there is the possibility of discovering some basic pan-cultural (universal or global) psychological principles of intercultural relations. In the MIRIPS project, we have followed the steps on this path, using the *emic/etic* strategy. We have sought to articulate these principles, first by conceptually defining some psychological processes that may be theoretically related to intercultural behaviors and then by empirically examining them across societies.

In a sense, the project is an example of extended replication. Current controversies about the reproducibility of psychological findings, even within the same society, suggest that our knowledge base is not as secure as previously thought. So, it will be useful to attempt to repeat the empirical examination of the same three hypotheses in a number of different societies in order to broaden our knowledge base. In this project, despite highly variable conditions (demographic, cultural, historical, and policy), there has been a modest degree of replication of psychological findings across contexts. However, more needs to be done to expand the conceptual and empirical basis for appropriate policy development.

Note

1 This chapter stems from an international collaborative project "Mutual Intercultural Relations in Plural Societies" (MIRIPS; www.victoria.ac.nz/cacr/research/mirips). I thank all my colleagues for their contributions to this research: Nadezhda Lebedeva, Victoria Galyapina, Zarina Lepshokova, Tatiana Ryabichenko, Alexander Tatarko, Raivo Vetik, Maaris Raudsepp, Jüri Kruusvall, Larissa Kus-Harbord, Marianna Makarova, Aune Valk, Asteria Brylka, Inga Jasinskaja-Lahti, Tuuli Anna Mähönen, David L. Sam, Katja Hanke, Marieke C. van Egmond, Anette Rohmann, Klaus Boehnke, Andrea U. Haenni Hoti, S. Heinzmann, M. Müller, A. Buholzer, R. Künzle, Vassilis Pavlopoulos, Frosso Motti-Stefanidi, Cristiano Inguglia, Pasquale Musso, Alida Lo Coco, Gordon Sammut, Maryanne Lauri, Felix Neto, Joana Neto, Hector Grad, R. C. Mishra, S. Bano, R. C. Tripathi, Algae Kit Yee Au, Bryant Pui Hung Hui, Sylvia Xiaohua Chen, Justine Dandy, Kevin Dunn, Jolanda Jetten, Yin Paradies, Lena Robinson, Tahereh Ziaian, Saba Safdar, Gui Yongxia, R. C. Annis, and R. Gibson.

References

Allport, G. W. (1954). The nature of prejudice. Addison-Wesley.

Banting, K., & Kymlicka, W. (2013). Is there really a retreat from multiculturalism policies? New evidence from the multiculturalism policy index. *Comparative European Politics*, *11*(5), 577–598.

Berry, J. W. (1980). Acculturation as varieties of adaptation. In A. Padilla (Ed.), Acculturation: Theory, models and some new findings (pp. 9–25). Westview Press.

Berry, J. W. (1984). Multicultural policy in Canada: A social psychological analysis. *Canadian Journal of Behavioural Science*, *16*, 353370.

Berry, J. W. (1997). Immigration, acculturation and adaptation. *Applied Psychology: An International Review*, *46*, 5–68.

Berry, J. W. (1998). Social psychological costs and benefits of multiculturalism. *Trames: Estonian Journal of Social Sciences*, *2*, 209–233.

Berry, J. W. (2003). Conceptual approaches to acculturation. In K. Chung, P. Balls-Organista, & G. Marin (Eds.), *Acculturation: Advances in theory, measurement, and applied research* (pp. 17–37). APA.

Berry, J. W. (2005). Acculturation: Living successfully in two cultures. *International Journal of Intercultural Relations*, *29*, 697–712.

Berry, J. W. (2013). Achieving a global psychology. *Canadian Psychology*, *54*, 55–61.
Berry, J. W. (2017). *Mutual intercultural relations*. Cambridge University Press.
Berry, J. W. (2018). Ecological perspective on human behaviour. In A. Uskul & Oishi, S. (Eds.), *Socio-economic environment and human psychology* (pp. 3–32). Oxford University Press.
Berry, J. W. (2023). The search for some general psychological principles for improving intercultural living in plural societies. *Psychology and Developing Societies*, *35*.
Berry, J. W., & Hou, F. (2016). Acculturation and wellbeing among immigrants to Canada. *Canadian Psychology*, *57*, 254–264.
Berry, J. W., & Kalin, R. (2000). Multicultural policy and social psychology: The Canadian experience. In S. Renshon & Duckitt (Eds.), *Political psychology: Cultural and cross-cultural foundations* (pp. 263–284). MacMillan.
Berry, J. W., Kalin, R., & Taylor, D. (1977). *Multiculturalism and ethnic attitudes in Canada*. Ministry of Supply and Services.
Berry, J. W., Lepshokova, Z., MIRIPS Collaboration, & Gorigoryev, D. (2022). How shall we all live together?: Meta-analytical review of the mutual intercultural relations in plural societies project. *Applied Psychology: An International Review*, *71*(3), 1014–1041.
Berry, J. W. Phinney, J. S., Sam, D. L., & Vedder, P. (Eds.). (2006). Immigrant youth: Acculturation, identity and adaptation. *Applied Psychology: An International Review*, *55*, 303–332.
Berry, J. W., Poortinga, Y. H., Breugelmans, S. M., Chasiotis, A., & Sam, D. L. (2011). *Cross-cultural psychology: Research and applications* (3rd ed.). Cambridge University Press.
Berry, J. W., Poortinga, Y. H., & Pandey, J. (Eds.). (1997). *Handbook of cross-cultural psychology, Vol. 1, Theory and method*. Allyn & Bacon.
Berry, J. W., & Sam, D. L. (2013). Accommodating cultural diversity and achieving equity: Psychological dimensions of multiculturalism. *European Psychologist*, *18*(3), 151–157.
Berry, J. W., & Sam, D. L. (2014). Multicultural societies. In V. Benet-Martínez & Y.-Y. Hong (Eds.), *Handbook of multicultural identity: Basic and applied perspectives* (pp. 97–117). Oxford University Press.
Bhugra, D. (Ed.). (2020). *Migrant psychiatry*. Oxford University Press.
Government of Canada. (1971). *Multicultural policy: Statement to house of commons*. Ottawa.
Mishra, R. C., Bano, S., & Tripathi, R. C. (2017). Intercultural relations in India. In J. W. Berry (Ed.), *Mutual intercultural relations* (pp. 291–310). Cambridge University Press.
Mishra, R. C., & Berry, J. W. (2017). *Ecology, culture and human development: Lessons for Adivasi Education*. Sage.
Mishra, R. C., Sinha, D., & Berry, J. W. (1995). *Ecology, acculturation and psychological adaptation: A study of Adivasi in Bihar*. Sage.
Sam, D. L., & Berry, J. W. (Eds.). (2016). *Cambridge handbook of acculturation psychology* (2nd ed). Cambridge University Press.
Ward, C. (1996). Acculturation. In D. Landis & R. Bhagat (Eds.), *Handbook of intercultural training* (2nd ed., pp. 124–147). Sage.

3 The Highs and Lows of Taking Psychology Out Into the Real World

Colleen Ward

> Social psychology has the potential to make critical and distinctive contributions to public policy and toward the resolution of pressing world problems.
>
> —Pettigrew (1988, p. 206)

> A longstanding and fundamental interest of cross-cultural psychology has been the application of the findings of the field to the improvement of both the life circumstances and the quality of life of people everywhere.
>
> —Berry et al. (2011, p. 305)

> The most critical objective of indigenous research is to interpret and discuss results in terms of cultural considerations and application of the results in policy formulation and amelioration of local social problems.
>
> —Pandey (2004, p. 350)

In many ways, social and cross-cultural psychology are well-positioned for application in the real world. Both of these fields operate across multiple levels of analysis and are oriented toward linking individual experiences to broader contextual factors. For social psychology, the context may be defined by situational factors, such as the presence of intergroup tensions or the features of an educational environment. For cross-cultural psychology, connections are made between individual behaviors and experiences and culture-level factors, such as values, norms, and beliefs. As social issues such as deprivation and racism cut across all of these levels, the micro-individual, meso-situational, and macro-societal multilevel solutions are required (Esses & Dovidio, 2011; Pettigrew, 1988, 1998). Indigenous psychology can ensure culturally appropriate interpretation of theory and data across all of these levels. In principle, then, social and cross-cultural psychology, imbued with indigenous perspectives, are at an advantage compared to social sciences like sociology, political science, or economics that operate almost exclusively on the macrolevel. "In principle" is one thing, however, and "in practice" is something else.

Despite this disciplinary advantage, few social and cross-cultural psychologists have the inclination or skills to embark upon explicitly applied

DOI: 10.4324/9781003461302-5

research. Overall, the interest in pursuing applied research has been low largely because it is not encouraged or rewarded in our institutions. Dovidio and Esses (2007) maintain that universities—at least universities in WEIRD (Western, Educated, Industrial, Rich, and Democratic) countries—prioritize and reward basic research and rapid publications. In contrast, applied research conducted in the field generally takes much longer to produce and is often dependent upon the cultivation of partnerships and relationships within communities, which are time-consuming endeavors. Even with strong interests in research applications, psychologists, compared to other social scientists, are less likely to make significant impact in the real world. Indeed, we appear in the media, influence public opinion, and act as consultants for public policy less frequently (Dovidio & Esses, 2007; Pettigrew, 1998). Why? A simple reason is that we have largely failed to make ourselves visible. Perhaps this is because it is too troublesome to do so as it takes time away from our basic science pursuits, but it is also the case that we have limited experience and few skills for operating in this arena.

With the exceptions of professional programs (e.g., counseling, clinical, and community qualifications), psychologists are rarely trained to make a "real-world difference," and we generally have poor insights into the process of policy-making. We often lack appropriate networks for accessing applied research opportunities via government departments or voluntary organizations, and we are not generally adept at dissemination of our findings in popular media (Pettigrew, 1988). Moreover, most of us are unable to communicate well with either the general public or professional audiences such as law-makers or policy analysts who do not have a background in psychology. This is a question of using not only an abundance of psychological jargon but also other annoying disciplinary idiosyncrasies that stymie our communication effectiveness. Because our theories in social and cross-cultural psychology are "messy" and complex, we tend to be overly cautious when discussing the implications of our research (Pettigrew, 1988). We are prone to insert too many "it depends" in our explanations, and we call for more research with such alarming frequency that potential stakeholders, both public and professional, are unlikely to find us convincing (Dovidio & Esses, 2007). We may be very adept in communicating with our scholarly peers, but we are generally very poor at translating our theories and research to other groups of information consumers.

Bridging the Divide: Applying Psychological Research to Social Problems

Dovidio and Esses (2007, p. 10) note that in order for psychological research "to be valuable in addressing real world social problems," it should be: 1) programmatic; 2) conducted in the real world; 3) grounded in theory; and 4) communicated beyond our scholarly peers. I suggest making real-world impact is also dependent upon cultivating networks and partnerships as these provide the avenues for supporting applied research and disseminating its findings.

Programmatic Research

Programmatic research is defined by an overarching research theme (e.g., improving educational outcomes or reducing poverty) supported by coherent theoretical frameworks. It involves a series of inter-related, multifaceted, and multi-method studies. Programmatic research is often multidisciplinary and generally provides a strong base for translational science. Programmatic research may be more easily developed in research teams or in established research centers and institutes than by individuals; however, there are notable individuals in social and cross-cultural psychology who have used their programmatic research to affect policies and practices.

Ed Diener's decades of systematic research on happiness has supported the development of a national happiness index and moved countries beyond economic and political concerns in policy-making to psychological ones (Diener, 2000; Diener et al., 2009; Diener & Suh, 1997). Oishi and Diener (2014) have clearly described ways in which self-reported happiness can be used to evaluate public policy. John W. Berry's programmatic research on acculturation and intercultural relations has provided evidence-based support for Canada's Multiculturalism Policy and has been used to inform the development of policies and practices in Estonia and other former Soviet states (Berry et al., 1977; Berry, 2013; Kruusval et al., 2009).

Herbert Kelman's programmatic work focused less on national policies and more on the application of research for program development to foster peace and conflict resolution in the Middle East (Kelman, 1998). This involved the development and delivery of interactive problem-solving workshops based on theory and research on international conflict, social influence, and intergroup interactions (Kelman, 1972, 1979). Bringing together highly respected and influential members of Arab and Israeli political parties, the workshops encouraged perspective-taking to generate novel approaches to managing conflict. According to Kelman (1998), the long-term objective of the workshops, launched in 1971, was to introduce interactive problem-solving perspectives into subsequent political debate and decision-making in communities. Overall, the workshops were very successful as Kelman (1995) described three ways in which they contributed to the mutual recognition between Israel and the Palestinian Liberation Organization in 1993: 1) by establishing groups on both sides who were willing to engage in productive negotiations; 2) by sharing of novel workshop-generated ideas to shape the content and outcomes of the negotiations; and 3) by fostering a positive political atmosphere.

As can be seen from these examples, programmatic research takes time. Serpell (2011) has described his programmatic research on child development in Africa that spanned more than a quarter of a century and its implications and applications for indigenous education. Combining two threads of research on children's everyday experiences and skills acquisition and adults' conceptualizations of the processes and outcomes of child development, he began with foundational quasi-experimental, cross-cultural comparative studies of children's perceptual skills and quasi-ethnographic studies of adults' estimates of children's intelligence. This was followed by deepening and refining his insights and exploring the external validity of his theory and research. Over the course of more than 25 years, Serpell set out to investigate the broader implications of his research findings, specifically the discrepancies between indigenous perspectives and experiences and the assumptions underlying the formal education system in Zambia. This led on to implementing and evaluating culturally appropriate interventions to address the social and educational challenges, culminating in the delivery of the Child-to-Child program, designed to promote social responsibility in pre-adolescent children. Subsequent evaluations showed that those who completed the Child-to-Child program were better prepared for the practical challenges of life in rural villages, and their parents were positive about the promotion of the indigenous tradition of social responsibility. Beyond demonstrating the benefits of educational practices consonant with indigenous perspectives and experiences, Serpell then stepped back to reflect on the methodological strategies used in cultural psychological research, providing a meta-theoretical contribution to our field.

Community-Based Research and Relationships

Programmatic research is ambitious and bold, and although it may not require an entire academic career to make impact, it does ultimately require research in the real world. Studies may start in a lab, but research needs to be taken into communities to test its external validity. This is one reason why it is so important to establish relationships and networks, whether with community members, professional associations, voluntary organizations, or government departments. At Centre for Applied Cross-Cultural Research (CACR), we have pursued multi-purpose partnerships with a wide range of individuals and organizations. This may be primarily for data collection, which could involve employing field assistants from various ethnic communities as was done in our recent research with New Zealand Koreans (Ward et al., 2020) or by working with organizations, such as the Hellenic New Zealand Congress, which involved the co-design of a survey on cultural identity and a formal presentation to the organization at the conclusion of the research (Ward, Ng Tseung-Wong, et al., 2018). Sometimes, the impetus for research comes from the communities themselves. For example, the New Zealand Federation of Multicultural Councils (NZFMC) approached our Centre to initiate research on the dynamics of acculturation and adaptation of recently immigrated parents and children. We worked together to obtain funding from the

New Zealand Families Commission and to plan the study's design. NZFMC provided an avenue for accessing research participants while we collected and analyzed the data in consultation with NZFMC and ultimately co-authored a paper by CACR Fellows and the NZFMC President (Stuart et al., 2010). This project was only possible because of the long-standing relationship between our Centre and NZFMC, including our continuous support as contributors to many of their community forums.

Relationships with government can also be beneficial, particularly in cases of data sharing or when partnerships bring mutual benefits. At the most basic level, just keeping the lines of communication open between academics and government departments can be useful. This permits you to call on these departments to endorse your research, which is helpful when seeking funding. Beyond that, researchers can collaborate with government in a range of ways. This could involve acting in an advisory capacity, which might allow an academic to recommend items to be included in a national survey. It might also involve multi-purpose collaborations. To these ends, we were offered the opportunity to merge our national survey data on attitudes toward immigrants with Immigration New Zealand's Longitudinal Immigration Survey on immigrant experiences. This permitted us to examine questions such as do attitudes toward immigrants vary as a function of immigrant density across regions, and how do attitudes toward immigrants relate to immigrants' experiences? Among our key findings was a curvi-linear effect on attitudes toward immigrants with negative attitudes found in the low- and high-density areas. Immigrants were less likely to report discrimination in regions with higher proportions of overseas-born residents. In addition, immigrants were viewed as less threatening in regions with higher incomes, and immigrants themselves felt safer in those regions (Ward et al., 2011).

Despite the benefits research partnerships offer, establishing and maintaining these types of relationships are challenging for academics due to our many responsibilities and time constraints. Not only are there efforts involved in maintaining relationships in the face of staff turnovers, but collaborations typically involve time-consuming obligations, such as the return of the findings to organizations, departments, and communities. While it is not impossible for individuals, it is certainly easier when the commitments are shared among academics with overlapping interests—even better if the relationships are supported by professional staff in a research center.

Theory and Applied Research

Beyond programmatic and community-based research, Dovidio and Esses (2007) argue that impactful applied research should also have a solid theoretical base. This is not to suggest that the research is designed with the expressed purpose of testing a particular theory. Rather, as Buschini et al. (2010) argue, there are two approaches that address pressing social issues with theory. The most common way is to analyze a problem or propose an evidence-based intervention in light of one's preferred theories. For example, Stephan and Stephan (2000) have applied Integrated Threat Theory to understanding the nature of prejudice. They identified four major threats to positive intergroup relations: realistic threat, symbolic threat, intergroup anxiety, and negative stereotypes, and they demonstrated how each of these operate in intergroup settings. Their early research examined Americans' attitudes toward immigrants and mutual perceptions of Blacks and Whites, Mexicans and Americans, and natives and Whites, supporting the external validity of their theory and demonstrating somewhat different magnitudes in the relationships among these threats and attitudes across different ethnic groups (Corenblum & Stephan, 2001; Stephan et al., 1999, 2000, 2002; Stephan & Stephan, 2000). Subsequent meta-analyses have shown that each of these threats is significantly associated with negative outgroup attitudes (Riek et al., 2006). Over the last two decades, Integrated Threat Theory has occupied a central position in studies of intergroup dynamics, and independent groups of researchers have set about exploring ways in which threats can be reduced to improve intergroup perceptions and relations. Intergroup contact (Berry, 2017; Pettigrew & Tropp, 2006; Ward & Masgoret, 2006), intragroup support (Stevenson et al., 2020), and enhancing a common group identity (Riek et al., 2010) have been shown to provide routes to threat reduction and more positive outgroup attitudes.

A second approach is to start with the problem, which requires the researcher to be theoretically eclectic. Put in other terms, "the problem is no longer at the service of the researcher, but the researcher begins to serve the problem" (Buschini et al., 2010, p. 7). Much of my own research falls into this category. Many of my studies of acculturation start with the question: Which factors facilitate or impede the adaptation of sojourners, immigrants, and minority groups? This is a complex question that crosses different aspects of adaptation, originally discussed in terms of psychological and sociocultural adaptation (Searle & Ward, 1990) and more recently extended to intercultural adaptation (Berry & Sam, 2016). The theoretical frameworks required to span Affect, Behaviors and Cognitions (i.e., the ABCs of acculturation) include Stress and Coping, Culture Learning, Social Identity, and Intergroup theories (Ward, 2001; Ward et al., 2001). More recently, we have added to the "alphabet of acculturation and adaptation" in reviewing acculturation theory and research by applying a developmental perspective, particularly to issues of cultural identity and well-being (Ward & Szabó, 2019). These diverse and comprehensive theoretical frameworks permit us to incorporate micro-individual and meso-situational factors as predictors of adaptation, but because we operate from a cross-cultural perspective, we also include macro-societal level factors in our research. For example, the International Comparative Study of Ethno-Cultural Youth, which spanned 13 countries, examined diversity and diversity policies as macrolevel factors and their impact on the psychological and sociocultural adaptation of young immigrants (Berry et al., 2006). The findings revealed that cultural diversity per se was associated with lower levels of psychological adaptation, but stronger diversity policies predicted better sociocultural outcomes (i.e., better school adjustment and fewer behavioral problems) for immigrant youth. Clearly, these findings have relevance for the formulation of diversity policies.

Putting the problem first is also a characteristic of action research, which can be more about generating new theory rather than integrating eclectic conceptual frameworks to interpret social problems. While Buschini et al. (2010) described the most common ways to address pressing social issues with theory, they neglected the discussion of action research, which adopts a bottom-up action-oriented approach that generates theory while confronting social dilemmas. Along these lines, Dick et al. (2009, p. 8) point out that theory is "emergent from and grounded in experience and action." Indeed, action research is undertaken with the expressed purpose of understanding and collectively resolving social problems that affect groups and communities (Kindon et al., 2007). Its dynamics involve a spiral process of planning for social change; acting and observing; and reflecting. Put in other words, action research unfolds with action (i.e., social change) and research (i.e., understanding, explaining, generating theory) achieved at the same time.

Our post-graduate student Philippa Collie along with CACR Fellows undertook a form of culturally sensitive participatory action research with young Assyrian women in New Zealand (Collie et al., 2010a, 2010b). Their project had both community and academic goals. The community goals were described in terms of facilitating a research process where participants' views were heard and respected, and there was an opportunity to initiate a project that addressed participants' concerns. The academic goal, which emerged and was refined over the course of the study, related to understanding how young women managed expectations about how they should maintain their heritage culture and how they should adapt to life in New Zealand. Adopting an ethnographic approach, the researchers observed how the young women positioned and repositioned themselves in relation to these cultural ballasts. They resolved tensions between ethnic and national identities by both fusing and alternating identities; however, their choices were shaped by the situation at hand rather than a general preference for one strategy or the other. The findings by Collie et al. (2010a) challenged the dominant paradigm in studies of acculturation that reflects a categorical approach (integration, separation, assimilation, or marginalization) and a rather static snapshot in time (Berry, 1997; Berry et al., 2006, 2011; Berry & Sam, 2016). Rather, as the researchers argued, acculturation theory must address the dynamic processes that unfold in the everyday lives of immigrants and former refugees. At the same time, the community goals were met in a culturally appropriate way by the production of a jointly authored (but anonymous) document generated by the research participants. The document was presented to community leaders by Philippa who acted as a liaison between the young women and Assyrian elders. This process permitted the participants to "negotiate a collective opinion on the topic of cultural maintenance and adaptation" (Collie et al.,

2010b, p. 143). Moreover, this oblique approach to parents and community elders was viewed by the participants as offering the opportunity to convey their complex views without appearing disrespectful or disloyal.

As can be seen from the above example, the degree to which the development of problem-led research is guided by theory or fosters theory development varies significantly across projects. In contrast to the description of the eclectic theoretical bases that have guided our evolving program of research on acculturation and adaptation and unlike the participatory action research with the Assyrian community, there are also simple but influential studies, such as needs analyses, that are best described as data-led "fact-finding missions." Needs analyses refer to formal, systematic research processes that identify gaps in the resources required to achieve specific goals. Such analyses are used in a variety of contexts, often to gain insights into the comprehensiveness of various programs or services. The applications of this approach, however, are wide ranging and include the investigation of broad-based community needs and challenges. As an example, our Centre was contracted by a regional Multicultural Council to conduct a series of workshops with the objectives of identifying the needs faced by new immigrants and former refugees and to probe potential solutions as to how their needs could best be met. Working with our post-graduate students, we designed workshops that posed two key questions for small group discussions: *What are the major challenges faced by migrants and former refugees in your region? What is required to settle successfully and make New Zealand your home?* Second, the identified needs and challenges were subjected to SWOT analyses, where participants assessed strengths, weaknesses, opportunities, and threats associated with meeting their prioritized needs. Finally, on the basis of the SWOT analyses, participants generated recommendations about how best to move forward in addressing the needs and challenges for immigrants and former refugees in their region.

Although some may describe this type of research as atheoretical, our report drew on related studies to situate and interpret the findings. We used theory and research on cross-cultural adaptation to demonstrate a convergence of the participants' identified needs and to provide evidence for the merit of their recommendations. Figure 3.1 presents a simplified representation of the needs identified in the workshops and reflects the key factors that are known to be associated with cross-cultural adaptation (Masgoret & Ward, 2006). It not only illustrates the core importance of language proficiency, which is necessary to operate effectively in a new cultural context, but also shows that culture-specific skills are required. Linguistic and cultural competence contribute to establishing and maintaining social relations, which, in turn, broadly affect health and well-being (Ward, Lescelius, et al., 2018). Although this project did not result in an academic publication, it was a worthwhile endeavor. It gave our students the opportunity to engage in intercultural interactions and conduct meaningful research in the real world. More importantly, the project made a difference. On the basis of the report,

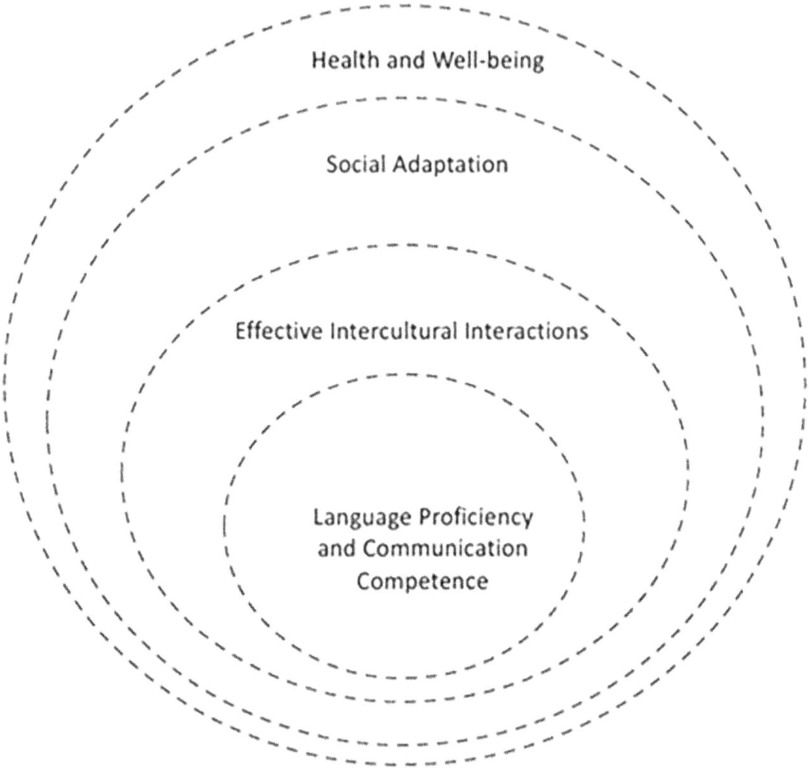

Figure 3.1 Cross-Cultural Adaptation

Source: Modified from Masgoret & Ward (2006)

regional public service directors made a commitment to provide resources for interpreters, cross-cultural workers, and intercultural trainers, addressing the needs relating to language proficiency and cultural competence.

Communicating Our Research Findings

Dovidio and Esses (2007) identify the ability to communicate our research findings beyond our scholarly peers as the final step in making real-world impact. This is particularly challenging for most of us as it fundamentally requires translating our findings into everyday language. Effective communication typically requires succinct summaries of key points without an overelaboration of conditional outcomes. It may also necessitate the use of "spin" to make your findings appear more interesting and relevant to specific stakeholders. In many cases, communication specialists and related services in your university can assist in preparing and releasing press statements about important research findings. You may also have access to university workshops on how to be effective science communicators. All of these channels can increase the profile of your research for external stakeholders. In the end, however, it is up to the scientist to take initiative.

As academics, many of us find it easier to communicate our findings in writing as this allows us more time to consider how best to convey our research results or offer a professional commentary. Even something as simple as a letter to the editor can be used effectively for public education under the right conditions. For example, my colleague, CACR Co-Director James Liu, and I wrote to the *Auckland Herald* in response to their piece "Council Divisive Survey Slammed." The survey, which used the common convention of the "feelings thermometer" to gauge warmth toward various ethnic groups in the region, was described as "racist." We briefly explained the history of the feelings thermometer in social science research, including its widespread use in New Zealand. We argued that "surveys such as this are not racist though responses to the questions may be" and "if the responses are racist, it is important for us to know." We then went on to explain that findings from studies like these can inform policy and planning across a range of areas, including health, education, and employment, for the betterment of the city as a whole. At the same time, our colleague and CACR Fellow Ron Fischer (2014) blogged on "Political correctness gone mad: The issue of the 'racist' survey in Auckland." In a similar vein, he asked: "How are you going to plan policies and make decisions about ethnic relations, if you have no understanding of the intergroup relations in your community?"

Political op-eds also offer an opportunity to showcase your research and provide insights into social issues and political events. Our CACR Fellow Jaimee Stuart (2019) produced a piece for CNN on "How Hate came to my Hometown" in response to the tragic attacks on the Christchurch mosques. Why did this happen? Jaimee set out by describing the sociopolitical context in New Zealand, summarizing our attitudes toward diversity and multiculturalism in general (very positive), describing our perceptions of Muslims (less favorable compared to other groups) in particular, and referring to programs for promoting diversity and social inclusion both within and across ethnic and religious groups. She also described the experiences of our Muslim community members, highlighting incidents of racism and discrimination, based on her long-term research with young Muslims. In the end, she argued that understanding what happened in the Christchurch terror attacks requires us to view New Zealand in the wider global context and to regard violent extremism "as the global problem that it truly is, rather than simply as another local tragedy." Indeed, an earlier study in New Zealand showed that the extent of exposure to news, which in New Zealand comes largely from international sources, is associated with more negative attitudes toward Muslims (Shaver et al., 2017). Embedded in Jaimee's emotionally moving piece written in everyday language are links to studies that have formed part of our programmatic research on acculturation and intercultural relations (e.g., Stuart, 2014; Stuart & Ward, 2018; Ward & Masgoret, 2008), illustrating the relationship between applied research and everyday experiences.

Making your research accessible and communicating in a way that engages other social scientists and the public more broadly can certainly be challenging. These were the goals of our Centre's book *New Zealand Identities: Departures and Destinations* (Liu et al., 2005). James Liu brought together CACR Fellows and associates to engage academics, government, and community organizations in productive dialogues that could contribute to building a more inclusive society. Combining editors from different ethnic backgrounds (New Zealand European, Māori, Pacific, and Asian) and contributors from diverse disciplinary (psychology, sociology, political science, and religious and cultural studies) backgrounds, the book presents interconnected conversations. James described the book as an "academic town hall," arising from "the conversations that New Zealanders have at the dinner table and in front of the evening news," that is, their everyday experiences. For many of us who contributed to the book, multiple drafts and revisions were required; learning to minimize disciplinary jargon and to communicate in a way that resonates with friends, neighbors, and community members was a learning process. I remember my own journey in the production of our chapter "Immigration, Acculturation and National Identity in New Zealand." In the end, I became comfortable citing Tana Umaga, the then captain of the All Blacks, New Zealand's national rugby team, alongside John W. Berry while describing integration. In Umaga's words:

> I am a New Zealander with Samoan parents. . . . I will never forget my culture and I am proud of that. . . . I'll never forget the Samoan part of me, but I was born in New Zealand and I am a New Zealander first.
>
> (Ward & Lin, 2005)

Along similar lines and in an effort to communicate our research in plain language, our Centre now produces one-page, simple to read, summaries of our research and publications. In essence, these summaries translate our findings for the general public as well as relevant government and non-government stakeholders. The summaries follow a template: a simplified title, research citation, background, main findings, relevance of findings to New Zealand, and contact person. We typically involve our post-graduate students in generating these summaries, selecting the research, interviewing the researcher(s), and drafting the one-pagers. We have received highly positive feedback on these summaries both nationally and internationally, including requests from other universities to teach students how to translate their own research for community members and policy makers. An example of a CACR one pager can be found in Figure 3.2 (Centre for Applied Cross-Cultural Research, 2016). More examples of the research summaries can be found on our center's website at: www.wgtn.ac.nz/cacr/research/1-page-research-summaries.

RESEARCH SUMMARY

Social influences on the adaptation to a new cultural environment

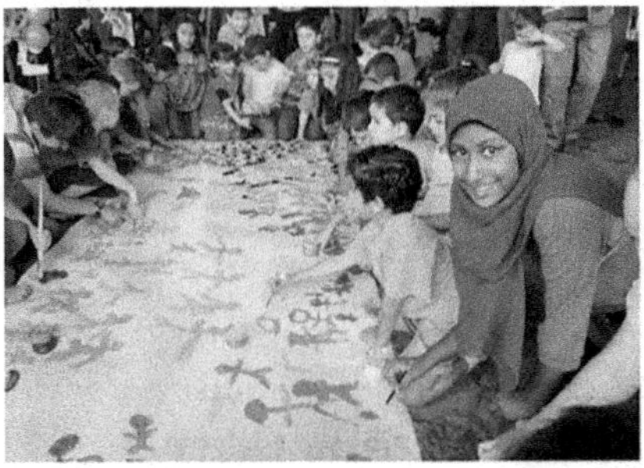

RESEARCH

'Advancing acculturation theory and research: The acculturation process in its ecological context'

by Professor Colleen Ward and Dr. Nicolas Geeraert (2016)

Published in *Current Opinion in Psychology 8*, 98-104.

Background

In a highly globalised world travellers, migrants, and those living in multicultural countries must confront different values and practices in their adaptation to the new host country.

The adaptation process often involves a re-evaluation and change in one's beliefs, behaviours, and identities. This change can be stressful and people often cope with it in different ways, which can affect how well they adjust.

What distinguishes those who adapt well from those who don't?

The Centre for Applied Cross-cultural Research, part of Victoria University of Wellington, re-evaluated the current psychological frameworks we use to understand acculturation research in order to consider the many different factors that influences a person's successful adaptation into a new culture.

Main research findings

Researchers are more often finding that most immigrants and short-term travellers are coping with their new environment by adopting features of their new host culture.

Although there are individual differences associated with cross-cultural adaptation, such as emotional stability and personality characteristics, many researchers forget to take into account the social contexts such as the influence of family, institutions, and society.

It has been found that family dynamics are also an important part of the adaptation process with a more cohesive family unit leading to better adjustment.

In schools, pressures from peers and teachers to conform to the traditions of the host culture can lead immigrants to feel separated. In contrast, giving more social support can lead to more positive attitudes toward the settlement country and as a result lead to better adaptation. This extends to the business and policy environments, where more inclusive policies help minority groups become more engaged.

Relevance of findings to New Zealand

With immigrants making up a large portion of the New Zealand population, it is important for skilled migrants to feel well adjusted in their new environment. In order to achieve this we need to have a complete conceptualisation of how the acculturation process works so successful adaptation can be facilitated.

New Zealand schools systems can contribute by showing support to immigrant students. Businesses should embrace diversity in the workplace by showing it is valued. Finally, policies should reflect the appreciation of diversity.

Social service professionals and counsellors should consider how all of these social contexts might affect students. Employers, team leaders, and advisors should also consider how policies and the social work environment might facilitate or hinder the successful adaptation of migrants and workers.

VICTORIA UNIVERSITY OF WELLINGTON TE HERENGA WAKA

Centre for Applied Cross-cultural Research
Te Pae Rangahau Tauhōkai Ahurea

PO Box 600, Wellington 6140, New Zealand
Phone +64-4-463-5311
Email cacr@vuw.ac.nz
Website www.wgtn.ac.nz/cacr

Figure 3.2 One-Page Research Summary From the Centre for Applied Cross-Cultural Research

Source: Photo "Harmony Day" (5475651018) from Wikimedia Commons. Permission granted to share and distribute under Creative Commons Attribution 2.0 Generic License. https://commons.wikimedia.org/wiki/File:Harmony_Day_(5475651018).jpg.

Notes: Text by author and CACR students.

Beyond the written word, opportunities for communicating research findings also come from invitations to speak or give interviews. If you want your research to "get out there" into the real world, it is important to be available. This is not to suggest that you must accept all offers, rather choose what you see as the best opportunities to make the points you believe should be heard, to reach your target audience, and/or to pick what you think you would most enjoy. While I occasionally invest time with radio or newspapers, I am more likely to prioritize engagement with government bodies and voluntary organizations as I see these at the coalface of working for social change, whether this involves policies and practices or grassroots social movements. Our Centre has widely shared our research findings in on-site presentations to government agencies such as the Office of Ethnic Communities, Ministry of Business, Innovation and Employment, and Ministry of Social Development on topics such as multiculturalism and social inclusion, attitudes toward ethnic and immigrant minorities, and the experiences of Muslims in New Zealand. We also participate in government-organized summits and conferences, for example, the inaugural *Settlement Summit: Collaborating for Outcomes*, which brought together government and service providers to enhance settlement outcomes for immigrants and the 2016 Pathways, Circuits and Crossroads Conference, *From Global to Local: Impacts of Migration, Mobility and Diversity*, targeted at government and voluntary organization stakeholders. Not only do these initiatives reach the people who can take concrete actions to precipitate social change and make a difference, but our messages are often disseminated more widely than we would normally achieve. As an example, my presentation on "A Multicultural Nation in a Bicultural Context" delivered at the Human Rights Commission's annual Diversity Forum not only reached government and voluntary organization stakeholders at the time but later attracted 4,900 viewers on YouTube, far more than could be reached by my course lectures and post-graduate seminars at the university.

One critically important aspect of communicating our findings to external stakeholders is the issue of "spin." It is crucial to know your target audience and have a strategy for communicating your ideas in an appropriate way. Regrettably, what is appropriate is not always obvious. On one occasion, I was invited by a friend and colleague at Immigration New Zealand to share some of my research with her department. I suggested a presentation on new series of studies on multiculturalism (e.g., Stuart & Ward, 2019; Watters et al., 2020; Ward, Gale, et al., 2018). A few days later and after discussion with her section head, she came back to me, having been told that it was an election year and that their department "had no business" discussing multiculturalism. A few years later, however, and after the tragedy of the Christchurch mosque attacks, I was invited to share my research at another government department. I was able to present the key findings about the benefits of a "diversity-receptive environment," one that was characterized by diverse groups in contact with one another, a widespread appreciation of diversity, and policies and practices to support diversity (i.e., multiculturalism); however, on this occasion, I delivered the well-received presentation under the topic of fostering social inclusion without referencing "the M word." Frankly, I am still learning how to spin, but if you want your findings to reach those who can apply your research in the real world, this is an essential skill to develop.

Making Impact in the Real World: From Individuals to Communities

Although few of us will make large-scale national impact with our applied research, it is important to recognize that even the modest impacts are noteworthy, whether targeting individuals, public sectors or communities. Beyond the role that academics play in public education, we can also apply our knowledge of theory and research to program development. The ExceLL (Excellence in Cultural and Experiential Learning and Leadership) program is an outstanding example of this, combining theory and research on acculturation with the principles of social learning. The program has five stages: alliance building; development of cultural maps; demonstration, feedback, practice, and coaching; goal setting and contracting; and transfer of learning to achieve educational, social or employment goals (Westwood et al., 2000). The use of co-facilitators is recommended, one who has negotiated a cross-cultural transition and represents a credible role model, and the other from the majority culture who provides an authentic explanation and interpretation of pervading cultural and behavioral norms. Overall, program evaluations have shown that the ExceLL intervention produces gains in social self-efficacy, improvements in social interaction skills, and greater preparedness for cross-cultural communication (Knott et al., 2013; Mak & Buckingham, 2007). This is consistent with the feedback we have received from both domestic and international students on the program at our own university.

In other instances, research can be undertaken, findings disseminated, and recommendations made with the objective of advising a public sector. In many cases, there are funds available for this type of applied research. For example, we assembled an interdisciplinary research team with expertise in psychology, linguistics, and communication to apply for funding from Education New Zealand, a Crown agency responsible for international education. We examined the perceptions of and interactions with international students, conducting qualitative and quantitative studies with peers, teachers, and members of the wider community. The final report covered many topics, including how perceptions of international students vary depending on their national origins; factors that contribute to the low level of intercultural friendships between international and domestic students; the gaps between teachers' views of cultural inclusiveness in their classrooms and the perceptions of their students; the challenges of working with international students; and instructors' needs for professional development (Ward et al.,

2005). At Education New Zealand's request, we undertook a "roadshow" taking the findings to the international education sector in various parts of the country, which was well received by those working with international students. Not all of our results, however, were welcomed by high-level management. One of the most important findings of the research for educational institutions was evidence of the curvi-linear relationship between the proportion of international enrollments and attitudes toward and interactions with international students. For domestic students, attitudes became more positive and intercultural interactions more frequent with increasing enrollments when these enrollments were less than 9% of the total. Between 9% and 14%, the attitudes became more negative and the interactions less frequent with increasing enrollments. The trend was similar for teachers where the attitudes toward international students became more negative when enrollments reached 12%–14% (Ward et al., 2009). This is not to say that institutions should limit enrollments to these proportions, but the findings point to the need to prepare staff and students in receiving institutions for increasing numbers. My own conversation with the head of our university's international strategy made it clear that he did not much like our results, and our university's strategic plan at that time aimed for international students to make up 25% of our total enrollments by 2025.

Working with government for program development or policy change essentially involves playing the long game. Do not expect to see immediate results, and it is important to remember that change is not all about the evidence base, but it also involves broader social, political, and economic issues. If you are setting out with a long-term goal in mind, it is important to have at least a basic understanding of government policy, strategies, or visions. Linking your evidence base to government priorities is a crucial step in effecting change—that and repeating your message at every opportunity.

Arising from theory and research on acculturation and intercultural relations, I have highlighted the critical importance of cultural competencies for decades (Ward & Kennedy, 1999; Ward, 2001; Ward & Szabó, 2019; Wilson et al., 2013). These skills are necessary not only for the success of newcomers, such as international students and immigrants, as they engage with a new culture, but also for members of the receiving society who require new sets of cultural competencies for effective intercultural interactions. This is particularly important in New Zealand where one in four residents is overseas-born.

With an evidence base in both basic and applied research, I have repeated the cultural competency message many times and in many ways. I have discussed immigrant experiences at local conferences that bring together government and academic researchers; at summits that mix academics with government and service providers; and at meetings of professional organizations. We have provided evidence that new immigrants' intentions to remain in New Zealand are related to their level of cultural competency (Wilson et al., 2017), an important finding as New Zealand is highly concerned with the retention of skilled immigrants in a globally competitive environment. We have conducted two needs analyses that have highlighted the necessity for cultural competency training, one for immigrant communities and one for public sector employees dealing with immigrant settlement. Importantly, over recent years, our advocacy for cultural competency programs has overlapped with the New Zealand State Services Commission's (2018, p. 1) emerging Diversity and Inclusion vision wherein state services should "reflect, value and understand the communities they serve."

Along these lines, the most striking development within New Zealand government agencies has been the launch of a pilot Intercultural Capability Development Program. The objectives of the program are to support an increasingly diverse workforce within government agencies and to support staff within externally facing customer-focused roles. The development of the online tool, guided by an external advisory group, including academics, consists of a series of intercultural scenarios and behavioral options with feedback to tap intercultural competencies such as cultural empathy, effective communication skills, and cognitive and behavioral flexibility. The online scenarios are accompanied by reflective exercises and face-to-face sessions with coworkers. Although the program evaluation yielded mixed results, *Mana Aki: Building Competence in New Zealand's Public Service* was selected as one of ten highly innovative global integration projects profiled at the 2020 OECD High-Level Policy Forum on Migration and Integration.

Clearly, our research and advocacy did not determine government efforts to enhance cultural competency in public sector employees; however, our efforts, both as researchers and advisors, represented just one stream of influence on this development. As an academic, you should never expect that all you need to do is share your findings. It is never as simple as that. We advocated just as strongly for intercultural training programs for new immigrants on the basis of our research; however, to date there has been no sign of the development of national government-funded cultural competency programs to accompany English language training for newcomers.

In relatively rare instances, there may be opportunities to influence government policies that have major impacts on communities. The Christchurch mosque tragedy, where 51 Muslims at prayer were slaughtered by a white supremacist, devastated our country. Widespread efforts were directed not only to show unity with and support for members of our Muslim community, but also to enact changes to ensure this does not happen again. Government, voluntary organizations, and members of the Muslim community turned to researchers for guidance on a range of topics, from security and gun control to the nature and causes of terrorism, to the definition of hate crimes, and to ways in which to promote social inclusion. The *New Zealand Journal of Psychology* published a rapid-response issue with discussion of diverse topics, including Islamic perspectives on loss and bereavement; national identity and attitudes toward Muslims; screening instruments for assessing psychological distress following disasters; flourishing after tragedy; white nationalism; the experience of being Muslim in New Zealand; and others.

The content of the journal formed the basis of a briefing for the Prime Minister after the terrorist attack. Government departments sprang into action in efforts to collate relevant multidisciplinary research, sometimes resulting in official publications such as the Ministry of Social Development's (2020) *Social Inclusion in New Zealand: A Rapid Evidence Review*. Moreover, a Royal Commission of Inquiry into the terror attack was launched. The report, which was presented to the Governor-General and Parliament in November and December 2021, includes 44 recommendations addressing counter-terrorism efforts; firearms licensing; support for survivors, witnesses, and families; improving social cohesion; and implementation strategies. Since then, the Department of the Prime Minister and Cabinet have invited a multidisciplinary group of interested academics to consult on government's response to the recommendations. Processes such as this offer some of the best opportunities for influence that are available to applied researchers; it is a pity, however, that it was a national tragedy that provided the impetus to open up these lines of communication.

Concluding Comments

Psychologists around the world have often discussed the need for problem-oriented research and making psychology relevant to national priorities. They have also bemoaned the paucity of research designed to solve real-world problems (Kariuki, 1982; Pandey, 2019; Sinha, 1989). I believe this is overly pessimistic. Indeed, Valery Chirkov (2009, p. 89) argued that "modern acculturation psychology has become almost useless for immigrant communities and for the immigrant assisting organizations." I was not convinced then and remain unconvinced now. At the time, Valery's words prompted Cigdem Kağıtçıbaşi and I to prove him wrong. To these ends, we edited a special issue of the *International Journal of Intercultural Relations* titled "Acculturation Theory, Research and Application: Working with and for Communities" (Ward & Kağıtçıbaşi, 2010). The studies were conducted in diverse national and sociopolitical contexts—Spain, New Zealand, Turkey, Australia, Guam, and the United States—and were situated in heterogeneous communities made up of immigrants, international students, refugees, and asylum seekers. The research methods varied with interviews, ethnographic approaches, the use of interventions, and participatory action research. Despite these variations, there was unity in diversity; all studies shared the common objectives of empowering acculturating individuals and communities, enhancing social integration and psychological well-being, and improving interpersonal and intergroup relations. The point is that applied acculturation research is occurring and making a difference.

Of course, there are conditions that can maximize the opportunities to make a difference in the real world. New Zealand, for example, is a small country of 5 million people, where everybody knows everybody, and government departments are just down the road from our university. Moreover, it is an excellent location to conduct research on acculturation and intercultural relations. We have a large proportion of overseas-born residents; the majority of our visibly different immigrants are first generation; and Auckland is now more diverse than New York or London. That said, the possibilities for applied research are almost limitless. Although I have drawn predominantly on social and cross-cultural psychology in this chapter and have highlighted studies on acculturation and intercultural relations, this is not to suggest that applied research must be limited to certain areas. Indeed, at our Centre for Applied Cross-Cultural Research, our indigenous psychologist, Tia Neha, works with Māori (the native peoples of New Zealand) to improve a range of social, educational, health, and well-being outcomes (e.g., Neha et al., 2020). Our cultural psychologist, Rita McNamara, draws on developmental psychology, cognitive anthropology, and behavioral economics in her theory of mind research in the Pacific. She has been a long-standing advocate for positive development in indigenous communities and not only has promoted indigenous approaches to education in the Pacific, but also has explored with the Ministry of iTaukei Affairs in Fiji how her research might support the Kadavu communities (McNamara & Naepi, 2018).

In the end, I encourage you to take up Pandey's (2004, 2019) challenge to pursue and promulgate applied research, whether for the benefit of individuals, organizations, communities, or nations. Despite its trials and tribulations, it can be immensely rewarding, and even small contributions can make large differences. Pettigrew (1998, p. 669) has referred to our neglect of applied research as "missed opportunities." Esses and Dovidio (2011, p. 5) argue that "psychology need not shy away from tackling challenging, broad social issues with our scientific and statistical tools" and that "addressing social issues enriches science." Ultimately, conducting applied research, be it in social, cross-cultural, indigenous, or other areas of psychology, will bring much-needed scientific knowledge to bear on policy formulation and program development in sociopolitical, educational, and economic spheres and across the spectrum of micro-, meso-, and macro-concerns.

References

Berry, J. W. (1997). Immigration, acculturation and adaptation. *Applied Psychology*, *46*, 5–34.

Berry, J. W. (2013). Intercultural relations in plural societies: Research derived from multiculturalism policy. *Canadian Ethnic Studies*, *3*(2), 1122–1135.

Berry, J. W. (Ed.). (2017). *Mutual intercultural relations*. Cambridge University Press.

Berry, J. W., Kalin, R., & Taylor, D. M. (1977). *Multiculturalism and ethnic attitudes in Canada*. Supply & Services.

Berry, J. W., Phinney, J. S., Sam, D. L., & Vedder, P. (Eds.). (2006). *Immigrant youth: Acculturation, identity and adaptation*. Lawrence Erlbaum Associates.

Berry, J. W., Poortinga, Y. H., Breugelmans, S. M., Chasioitis, & Sam, D. L. (2011). *Cross-cultural psychology: Research and applications*. Cambridge University Press.

Berry, J. W., & Sam, D. L. (2016). Theoretical perspectives. In D. L. Sam & J. W. Berry (Eds.), *The Cambridge handbook of acculturation psychology* (pp. 11–29). Cambridge University Press.

Buschini, F., Guimond, S., & Breakwell, G. (2010). Social issues and social psychology: Distinctive pathways to applying social psychology to resolving major social problems. *Revue Internationale de Psychologie Sociale*, *23*(2), 5–15.

Centre for Applied Cross-Cultural Research. (2016). *Social influences on the adaptation to a new cultural environment: A research summary of "Advancing Acculturation Theory and Research" by Colleen Ward & Nicolas Geeraert*. www.wgtn.ac.nz/cacr/research/1-page-research-summaries/Social_influences_on_the_adaptation_to_a_new_cultural_environment.pdf. Retrieved September 30, 2024.

Chirkov, V. (2009). Introduction to the special issue on Critical Acculturation Psychology. *International Journal of Intercultural Relations*, *33*(2), 87–93.

Collie, P., Kindon, S., Liu, J., & Podsiadlowski, A. (2010a). Mindful identity negotiations: The acculturation of young Assyrian women in New Zealand. *International Journal of Intercultural Relations*, *34*(3), 208–220.

Collie, P., Liu, J., Podsiadlowski, A., & Kindon, S. (2010b). You can't clap with one hand: Learning to promote culturally grounded participatory action research. *International Journal of Intercultural Relations*, *34*(2), 141–149.

Corenblum, B., & Stephan, W. G. (2001). White fears and native apprehensions: An integrated threat theory approach to intergroup attitudes. *Canadian Journal of Behavioural Science/Revue canadienne des sciences du comportement*, *33*(4), 251–268.

Dick, B., Stronger, E., & Huxham, C. (2009). Theory in action research. *Action Research*, *7*(1), 5–12.

Diener, E. (2000). Subjective well-being: The science of happiness and a proposal for a national index. *American Psychologist*, *55*, 34–43.

Diener, E., Lucas, R., Schimmack, U., & Helliwell, J. (2009). *Wellbeing for public policy*. Oxford University Press.

Diener, E., & Suh, E. (1997). Measuring quality of life: Economic, social, and subjective indicators. *Social Indicators Research*, *40*, 189–216.

Dovidio, J. F., & Esses, V. M. (2007). Psychological research and public policy: Bridging the gap. *Social Issues and Policy Review*, *1*(1), 5–14.

Esses, V. M., & Dovidio, J. F. (2011). Social psychology, social issues and social policy: What have we learned? *Social Issues and Policy Review*, *5*(1), 1–7.

Fischer, R. (2014, May 6). *Political correctness gone mad: The issue of the 'racist' survey in Auckland*. http://culturemindspace.blogspot.com/2014/05/political-correctness-gone-mad-issue-of.html

Kariuki, P. (1982). The challenge and role of psychology to development in Africa. *Journal of Eastern African Research and Development*, *12*, 151–160.

Kelman, H. C. (1972). The problem-solving workshop in conflict resolution. In R. L. Merritt (Ed.), *Communication in international politics* (pp. 168–204). University of Illinois Press.

Kelman, H. C. (1979). An interactional approach to conflict resolution and its application to Israeli-Palestinian relations. *International Interactions*, *6*, 99–122.

Kelman, H. C. (1995). Contributions of an unofficial conflict resolution effort to the Israeli-Palestinian breakthrough. *Negotiation Journal*, *11*, 19–27.

Kelman, H. C. (1998). Social-psychological contributions to peacemaking and peacebuilding in the Middle East. *Applied Psychology: An International Review*, *47*(1), 5–28.

Kindon, S., Pain, R., & Kesby, M. (Eds.). (2007). *Participatory action research approaches and methods: Connecting people, participation and place*. Routledge.

Knott, V. E., Mak, A. S., & Neil, J. T. (2013). Teaching intercultural competencies in introductory psychology via the application of the excellence in cultural experiential learning and leadership model. *Australian Journal of Psychology*, *65*(1), 46–53.

Kruusval, J., Vetik, R., & Berry, J. W. (2009). The strategies of inter-ethnic adaptation of Estonian Russians. *Studies of Transition States and Societies*, *1*(1), 3–24.

Liu, J. H., McCreanor, T., McIntosh, T., & Teaiwa, T. (2005). *New Zealand identities: Departures and destinations*. Victoria University Press.

Mak, A. S., & Buckingham, K. (2007). Beyond communication courses: Are there benefits in adding skills-based ExcelL sociocultural training? *International Journal of Intercultural Relations*, *31*(3), 277–291.

Masgoret, A.-M., & Ward, C. (2006). Cultural learning approaches to acculturation. In D. L. Sam & J. W. Berry (Eds.), *Cambridge handbook of acculturation psychology* (pp. 58–77). Cambridge University Press.

McNamara, R., & Naepi, S. (2018). Decolonizing community psychology by supporting indigenous knowledge, projects and students: Lessons from Aotearoa and Canada. *American Journal of Community Psychology*, *62*(3–4), 340–349.

Ministry of Social Development. (2020). *Social inclusion in New Zealand: Rapid evidence review*. www.msd.govt.nz/documents/about-msd-and-our-work/publications-resources/research/social-inclusion-in-new-zealand-a-rapid-evidence-review/social-inclusion-in-nz-rapid-evidence-review-report.pdf

Neha, T., Reese, E., Schaughency, E., & Taumoepeau, M. (2020). The role of whānau (New Zealand Māori families) for Māori children's early learning. *Developmental Psychology*, *56*(8), 1518–1531.

New Zealand State Services Commission. (2018). *Diversity and inclusion*. www.publicservice.govt.nz/assets/Legacy/resources/Diversity-and-Inclusion-approach.pdf

Oishi, S., & Diener, E. (2014). Can and should happiness be a policy goal? *Policy Insights from Behavioral and Brain Sciences*, *1*(1), 195–203.

Pandey, J. (2004). Psychology in India enters the 21st century: Movement toward an indigenous discipline. In J. Pandey (Ed.), *Psychology in India revisited: Developments in the discipline, Vol 3: Applied social and organisational psychology* (pp. 342–370). Sage.

Pandey, J. (2019). Psychology and societal development: Indian context. In J. Pandey, R. Kumar, & K. Thapa (Eds.), *Psychological perspectives on diversity and social development* (pp. 163–179). Springer.

Pettigrew, T. F. (1988). Influencing policy with social psychology. *Journal of Social Issues*, *44*(2), 205–219.

Pettigrew, T. F. (1998). Applying social psychology to international social issues. *Journal of Social Issues*, *54*(4), 663–675.

Pettigrew, T. F., & Tropp, L. (2006). A meta-analytic test of intergroup contact theory. *Journal of Personality and Social Psychology*, *90*(5), 751–783.

Riek, B. M., Mania, E. W., & Gaertner, S. L. (2006). Intergroup threat and outgroup attitudes: A meta-analytic review. *Personality and Social Psychology Review*, *10*(4), 336–353.

Riek, B. M., Mania, E. W., Gaertner, S. L., McDonald, S. A., & Lamoreaux, M. J. (2010). Does a common identity reduce intergroup threat? *Group Processes and Intergroup Relations*, *13*(4), 403–423.

Searle, W., & Ward, C. (1990). The prediction of psychological and socio-cultural adjustment during cross-cultural transitions. *International Journal of Intercultural Relations*, *14*, 449–464.

Serpell, R. (2011). Social responsibility as a dimension of intelligence and an educational goal: Insights from programmatic research in an African society. *Child Development Perspectives*, *5*(2), 126–133.

Shaver, J. H., Sibley, C. G., Osborne, D., & Bulbulia, J. (2017). News exposure predicts anti-Muslim prejudice. *PLoS ONE*, *12*(3), e0176406

Sinha, D. (1989). Research in psychology in the developing world: An overview. *Psychology and Developing Societies*, *1*(1), 105–126.

Stephan, W. G., Boniecki, K. A., Ybarra, O., Bettencourt, A., Ervin, K. S., Jackson, L. A., McNatt, P. S., & Renfro, C. L. (2002). The role of threats in the racial attitudes of Blacks and Whites. *Personality and Social Psychology Bulletin*, *28*, 1242–1254.

Stephan, W. G., Diaz-Loving, R., & Duran, A. (2000). Integrated threat theory and intercultural attitudes: Mexico and the United States. *Journal of Cross-Cultural Psychology*, *31*(2), 240–249.

Stephan, W. G., & Stephan, C. W. (2000). An integrated threat theory of prejudice. In S. Oskamp (Ed.), *Reducing prejudice and discrimination* (pp. 23–45). Lawrence Erlbaum Associates.

Stephan, W. G., Ybarra, O., & Bachman, G. (1999). Prejudice towards immigrants. *Journal of Applied Social Psychology*, *29*(11), 2221–2237.

Stevenson, C., Costa, S., Easterbrook, M. J., McNamara, M. N., & Kellezi, B. (2020). Social cure processes help lower intergroup anxiety among neighbourhood residents. *Political Psychology*, *41*(6), 1093–1111.

Stuart, J. (2014). A qualitative analysis of Muslim young adults' adaptation experiences in New Zealand. *Journal of Muslim Mental Health*, *8*(2), 21–46.

Stuart, J. (2019). *How hate came to my hometown*. https://edition.cnn.com/2019/03/15/opinions/christchurch-researcher-muslims-stuart/index.html

Stuart, J., & Ward, C. (2018). The relationships between religiosity, stress and mental health for Muslim immigrant youth. *Mental Health, Religion and Culture*, *21*(3), 246–261.

Stuart, J., & Ward, C. (2019). Exploring everyday experiences of cultural diversity: The construction, validation and application of the normative multiculturalism scale. *European Journal of Social Psychology*, *49*(2), 313–332.

Stuart, J., Ward, C., Jose, P., & Narayanan, P. (2010). Working with and for communities: A collaborative study of harmony and conflict in well-functioning, acculturating families. *International Journal of Intercultural Relations*, *34*, 114–126.

Ward, C. (2001). The ABCs of acculturation. In D. Matsumoto (Ed.), *Handbook of culture and psychology* (pp. 411–446). Oxford University Press.

Ward, C., Bochner, S., & Furnham, A. (2001). *The psychology of culture shock*. Routledge.

Ward, C., Gale, J., Staerklé, C., & Stuart, J. (2018). Multiculturalism in context: A framework for psychological research. *Journal of Social Issues*, *74*(4), 833–855.

Ward, C., & Kağıtçıbaşi, Ç. (2010). Introduction to "Acculturation theory, research and application: Working with and for communities." *International Journal of Intercultural Relations*, *34*(2), 97–100.

Ward, C., & Kennedy, A. (1999). The measurement of sociocultural adaptation. *International Journal of Intercultural Relations*, *23*, 659–677.

Ward, C., Kim, I., Karl, J. A., Epstein, S., & Park, H.-J. (2020). How normative multiculturalism relates to immigrant well-being. *Cultural Diversity and Ethnic Minority Psychology*, *26*(4), 581–591.

Ward, C., Lescelius, J., Jack, A., Naidu, R., & Weinberg, E. (2018). *Meeting the needs and challenges of immigrants and former refugees in the Nelson and Tasman regions*. Report Prepared for the Nelson Tasman Multicultural Council. www.wgtn.ac.nz/__data/assets/pdf_file/0004/1741432/Meeting_the_needs_and_challenges_of_migrants_and_former_refugees_in_the_Nelson_and_Tasman_regions_May2018.pdf

Ward, C., & Lin, E.-Y. (2005). Immigration, acculturation and national identity in New Zealand. In J. Liu, T. McCreanor, T. McIntosh, & T. Teaiwa (Eds.), *New Zealand identities: Departures and destinations* (pp. 155–173). Victoria University Press.

Ward, C., & Masgoret, A.-M. (2006). An integrated model of attitudes toward immigrants. *International Journal of Intercultural Relations*, *30*, 671–682.

Ward, C., & Masgoret, A.-M. (2008). Attitudes toward immigrants, immigration and multiculturalism in New Zealand: A social psychological analysis. *International Migration Review*, *42*(1), 227–248.

Ward, C., Masgoret, A.-M., & Gezentsvey, M. (2009). Investigating attitudes toward international students: Implications for social integration and international education. *Social Issues and Policy Review*, *3*, 79–102.

Ward, C., Masgoret, A.-M., Newton, J., Crabbe, D., Ho, E., & Holmes, P. (2005). *Interactions with international students*. Report prepared for Education New Zealand. www.wgtn.ac.nz/__data/assets/pdf_file/0007/1924882/Interactions_with_international_students.pdf

Ward, C., Masgoret, A.-M., & Vauclair, M. (2011). *Attitudes towards immigrants and immigrant experiences: Predictive models based on regional characteristics*. Department of Labour. www.mbie.govt.nz/dmsdocument/2724-predictive-models-based-on-regional-characteristics-pdf

Ward, C., Ng Tseung-Wong, C., Szabo, A., Qumseya, T., & Bhowon, U. (2018). Hybrid and alternating identity styles as strategies for managing multicultural identities. *Journal of Cross-cultural Psychology*, *49*, 1402–1439.

Ward, C., & Szabó, Á. (2019). Affect, behavior, cognition and development: Adding to the alphabet of acculturation. In D. Matsumoto & H. S. Hwang (Eds.), *Handbook of culture and psychology* (2nd ed., pp. 648–700). Oxford University Press.

Watters, S. M., Ward, C., & Stuart, J. (2020). Does multiculturalism threaten or foster social cohesion? *International Journal of Intercultural Relations*, *75*, 82–94.

Westwood, M. J., Mak, A. S., Barker, M., & Ishiyama, I. (2000). Group procedures and applications for developing sociocultural competencies among immigrants. *International Journal for the Advancement of Counselling*, *22*(4), 317–330.

Wilson, J., Ward, C., Fetvadjiev, V. H., & Bethel, A. (2017). Measuring cultural competencies: The development and validation of a revised measures of sociocultural adaptation. *Journal of Cross-cultural Psychology*, *48*(10), 1475–1506.

Wilson, J., Ward, C., & Fischer, R. (2013). Beyond culture learning theory: What can personality tell us about cultural competence? *Journal of Cross-cultural Psychology*, *44*, 900–927.

Part II

Societal Changes and Social Psychology

4 Addressing Environmental Problems in South Asia and the World

The Need for Multiplism and Policy Relevance

Richard Barry Ruback[1]

Over the period 1988–2009, I was one of the colleagues of Professor Janak Pandey. During this time, we conducted research in villages, cities, large metropolitan areas, and a large religious festival on topics relating to environmental stressors, poverty, and religious beliefs. In several of these studies, Professor Pandey and I examined crowding, addressing a gap in the research, since most studies on the topic had been conducted in North America, where levels of density are less than a fourth of what they are in many of the locations we studied. Four issues characterized our joint work, issues that relate to the future of psychological science in India and the rest of the world.

1) *Psychology should address societal problems.* Throughout his career, Professor Pandey's research has focused on the importance of poverty in affecting the choices of individuals, the workings of communities, and the structure of society. His work on environmental issues reflects his concern with high social and spatial density and with both the direct and indirect effects of economic issues on people's experience of the natural and built environment.
2) *Individual-level variables need to be considered in the larger contexts of culture, especially religion.* At Professor Pandey's suggestion, we conducted studies of the *Magh Mela*, an annual religious festival which has been held for more than 2,000 years at the confluence of the Ganges and Yamuna Rivers. The *Mela* attracts millions of visitors each year, most coming as religious pilgrims, but some because of business opportunities (e.g., store owners, boatmen). Our studies addressed both philosophically significant issues (e.g., what makes a place holy; Ruback et al., 2008) and more empirical questions regarding how religious beliefs and occupational role affect perceptions of the material, social, and symbolic aspects of the environment (Ruback et al., 2009).
3) *Empirical methods should meet the highest standards of reliability, validity, and replicability, but they must also be adapted to the cultural context.* Most of the research methods in social psychology were developed

DOI: 10.4324/9781003461302-7

in the West. Translating these methods to respondents in South Asia, most of whom were illiterate or semi-literate, required sensitivity to their backgrounds and creativity in terms of adapting methods to capture the purpose of the measurement, rather than blindly copying the form. To meet these problems, we used techniques jointly developed by the psychology faculty at the Centre of Advanced Study at the University of Allahabad (Ruback & Pandey, 1991, 1996) and with the extensive cooperation of scholars in three countries regarding translation and back-translation of survey instruments.

4) *Psychological research needs to involve the training of the next generation of social scientists and the education of an informed leadership knowledgeable about the strengths, weaknesses, and usefulness of social science.* Across all of our projects, Professor Pandey brought in other faculty, including junior faculty, and dozens of students—undergraduate and graduate—who helped with the research. More than 20 of these students were PhD students, who have gone on to university and business positions.

Many of Professor Pandey's collaborations were with scholars from abroad. He saw part of his role as sensitizing these foreign researchers, including me, to the unique problems of India and to the more general problems of conducting psychological research with populations that differ in several ways from the educated, English-speaking, wealthy populations that most of these researchers had studied before coming to India. It was with this heightened sensitivity to the necessity of adapting methods to India that changed my approach to research in India and, with other scholars, to my work in South Asia more generally. Most of my research in South Asia with Professor Pandey and others focused on environmental issues, particularly crowding.

Environmental Issues in South Asia

People have lived in South Asia for about 65,000 years, probably arriving by coastal migration (Majumder, 2009), and the region contains some of the oldest continuously occupied cities in the world. Because the area provides all of the necessities for human habitation—abundant water, rich alluvial soil, and a favorable climate for growing crops during both the winter and the monsoon seasons—in recent millennia, the subcontinent has been home to a large number of people. The Indus Valley civilization may be at least 8,000 years old (Sarkar et al., 2016). At the peak of the Indus Valley (Harappan) civilization, about 5 million people, roughly 10% of the world's population, lived in South Asia (http://factsanddetails.com/india/History/sub7_1a/entry-4099.html). At the beginning of the 17th century, estimates for the population in South Asia ranged from 110 to 145 million. By the Census of 1872, there were an estimated 255 million people in British India (Gadgil &

Thapar, 1990). Today, there are more than 1.8 billion people on the subcontinent (United Nations, 2019). I cite this history of humans in South Asia to emphasize the fact that current conditions overlay thousands of years of tradition and culture.

Countries in South Asia have among the most serious social problems in the world. Based on measures of water and sanitation, Bangladesh ranks 128th out of 178 countries, Pakistan ranks 140th, and India ranks 145th (Wendling et al., 2020). In terms of air pollution, of 98 countries, Bangladesh ranks first, Pakistan ranks second, and India ranks fifth (IQ Air, 2020a). Of the world's cities with the worst air pollution, India has six of the top 10, and 21 of the top 30, including Ghaziabad, with the worst air pollution in the world (IQ Air 2020b).

In terms of crowding, more than half of all people in the world live in Asia, and more than one-fifth live in the three most populous countries in South Asia: India, Pakistan, and Bangladesh. In the past 70 years, South Asia had a population growth rate higher than the world average (Macrotrends, 2021). While the world population increased 210% from 1950 to 2021, the population for these three countries increased 295%; while these three countries accounted for 17.8% of the world's population in 1950, they accounted for 22.7% in 2021. This considerable population increase is the result of larger and better-quality food supplies, improved healthcare, lower rates of infant mortality, and longer adult lives.

The projected growth rates for the three countries will mean that they will continue to be crowded. From the 2021 base, by 2050, India's population is expected to grow 18%, Pakistan's population is expected to grow 50%, and Bangladesh's population is expected to grow 16%. By comparison, the world's population is expected to grow 24%. In the year 2050, about 22.2% of the world will live in these three countries, compared to 14.4% who will live in China. In other words, these three countries in South Asia are, and will continue to be, one of the largest concentrations of people in the world.

What is paradoxical is that most of the research on environmental stressors, particularly crowding, has been conducted in North America and Europe, where the problems, not to minimize them, are less serious than those in the developing world. It is important that research be done in the parts of the world where the problems are greatest not only because the absolute level of the environmental stressors is so much higher than in North American and Europe but also because there is a question of whether cultural differences affect how people in different countries evaluate and respond to these stressors.

Related to the overall growth in population in South Asia is the fact that some areas, especially the large cities, are growing much faster than other areas. Just as crowding worldwide is the result of the uneven distribution of the population, so too is the problem of crowding in South Asia the result of concentrations of people in the cities, as people move from rural areas to the big cities (Ruback et al., 2004). By 2050, the three largest urban areas in the world are projected to be Mumbai (42.4 million), Delhi (36.2 million), and Dhaka (35.2 million; Hoornweg & Pope, 2016).

Even though most people in South Asia (about 65%) live in rural areas, most of the problems facing these countries—overcrowding, air pollution, water pollution, and traffic—are in the cities, especially the large cities. Particularly during the past four decades, cities in South Asia have seen large influxes of rural migrants. In South Asia, the urban population grew by 130 million between 2001 and 2011 (Ellis & Roberts, 2016). In India, about 45% of urban growth is the product of rural to urban migration (Todaro, 1989), a trend that has continued since the 1920s (Sharma, 1997). Moreover, especially in less-developed regions like South Asia, this urbanization is often concentrated among a few large cities. When these migrants come to the cities, they are likely to live in high-density slums with inadequate urban services (Rao, 1986). As more and more migrants come to the cities, these slums account for larger and larger proportions of the population. Aside from the crowding resulting from this rural migration, cities in South Asia have been overwhelmed by a considerable increase in the number of motor vehicles and by rapid industrialization, both of which contribute to air pollution and environmental degradation.

It makes sense to think of India, Pakistan, and Bangladesh together because they share borders, climate, and geography. They also share a common history over the past 5,000 years, including being under Mughal rule during the 16th through mid-19th centuries and being part of British India from 1857 to 1947. They differ, however, in the dominant religion and in their political history since independence. Although most of the research we conducted was in India, we also conducted a few studies in Bangladesh and Pakistan. Crowding in these three countries is experienced somewhat differently because of differences in physical geography, culture, gender norms, and location.

Research on Environmental Psychology in India

Most of the research Professor Pandey and I conducted in South Asia concerned the perception and effects of crowding. In particular, we investigated five important issues. First, we were interested in whether people differ in their definition of crowding. In various studies, we tested the possibility of different definitions by comparing husbands and wives within households in Allahabad (Ruback & Pandey, 1991), male and female pedestrians in the capital cities of India and Bangladesh, and different occupational groups at a major religious festival, the *Magh Mela*, held every year at the Sangam, the confluence of the Ganges and Yamuna Rivers. The research was firmly rooted in the literature from social psychology, particularly as our research findings indicated that objective conditions are less important than how people perceive those conditions and whether they believe they can do something to cope with those conditions.

Second, we were interested in whether there are negative cognitive, social, and health-related consequences of crowding. We tested this question by examining mental distress and physical symptoms in multiple situations—villages, a large city (Allahabad), the slums of capital cities (Delhi, Dhaka, Islamabad; Ruback et al., 2002; Ruback & Pandey, 2002), and on city streets in Delhi and Dhaka. We also looked in several studies at the relations between spouses and between parents and children. In some studies, we also looked at indicators of anger and violence between adults, such as quarrels, yelling, and throwing things at each other.

When we started our research, we believed that four general factors would affect reactions to crowding: gender, culture, multiple stressors, and mitigating beliefs, including perceived control. These factors overlap, in that all are related to culture.

Gender

First, we expected that gender would matter. We expected that women would be more upset by crowding because, due to gender role norms, they spend more time than their husbands in crowded home situations. We found that women, compared to men, rated their homes more negatively, experienced more physical symptoms, and thought the supply of resources in their homes was insufficient. Surprisingly, however, women also believed that their homes could house more people and were significantly more likely to want more children (Ruback & Pandey, 1996). In the slums of New Delhi, we found that women rated household stressors more negatively than did men.

One source of differences among individuals arises from cultural expectations for people in different roles. For example, there are likely to be differences between men and women in judgments of stressors if gender roles are different in the two cultures. Such is the case in South Asia, where gender roles are deeply rooted in culture and society (Mandelbaum, 1988), have an important effect on day-to-day life, and appear to be stronger than in many areas of the world (Williams & Best, 1990). Typically, men in South Asia are defined by their occupational roles, as is true in much of the world, but women in South Asia are more often defined only by their kinship ties to men (Mandelbaum, 1988, p. 100). Men and women in South Asia have traditionally lived in different social worlds (Mandelbaum, 1988, p. 4). Inside the home, there is usually a separate area where women spend most of their time performing domestic and child-rearing tasks. Men also have a separate area, often a veranda or area outside the house, where they relax, entertain, and sleep. Women are inside their homes most of the time, leaving occasionally to visit kin and neighbors in the women's areas of these homes. In contrast, men spend much of their free time with friends, coworkers, and kinsmen, often outside or at public food places.

One of the gender differences we did not expect was differences in the number of people who were said to live in the household. Interviewers separately interviewed husbands and wives in 167 households. Although we found that the correlation between the responses of husbands and wives was high, it was not perfect. There were gender differences in who counted as a person (e.g., whether a child under 5 counted). Men tended to count these young children. There were also gender differences in whether relatives who were staying at the home for an extended time were living at the house. In general, women tended to include these individuals, whereas men did not.

Culture

Second, we thought that culture would importantly influence behavior. That is, we expected that South Asians would be less distressed by crowding than are North Americans, whether because they are less likely to define conditions as crowded, because they have different preferences for interpersonal spacing, or because there are differences in psychological impact. However, like Evans et al. (2000), we found no differences in cultural tolerance for crowding. Third, we expected that location would matter. We expected the effects of crowding to be worse in very large cities than in medium-sized cities and worse in medium-sized cities than in rural villages. We questioned cycle rickshaw and autorickshaw drivers in Dhaka about three environmental stressors (noise, air pollution, and crowding) and how they reacted to these stressors (Ruback & Begum, 1995). Compared to autorickshaw drivers, cycle rickshaw drivers reported experiencing more physical symptoms and greater feelings of anomie; autorickshaw drivers earned significantly more money and spent more time outside. Air pollution was judged to be the worst stressor. Compared to a sample of male pedestrians, the rickshaw and autorickshaw drivers rated the noise and air pollution in Dhaka as significantly less aversive.

We also thought that high levels of density, although generally leading to negative effects, might sometimes be desired. Specifically, we expected the crowding at a religious festival would be positively perceived and we found some evidence for that (Ruback et al., 2008).

Overall, we concluded that crowding has negative effects, although the size of these effects depends on the particular sample and particular variable being studied. Contrary to suggestions that South Asians are not affected by crowding, we found that Indians do experience negative effects from crowding, although, when placed in the larger context of other stressors, the effects of crowding are not always large. Also, by asking about different members of the household, specifically about children, we were able to discover that social density per se is not the crucial factor. Rather, who these people are is the more important factor.

Moreover, these negative effects appear even if people say they are not crowded. For instance, in a study of men and women in households in a large city, we found that, compared to their husbands, wives were significantly more likely to say that they wanted more people in their household, but they were also significantly more likely to experience more negative effects of crowding (Ruback & Pandey, 1991). As another example, our investigation of religious bathers at the Sangam found that these individuals reported that it was better for more people to be at the religious festival. However, despite what they said, the more people who were around them, the worse, they said, they felt. This result is consistent with Evans et al.'s (2000) finding that even though, at a given level of density, Mexican Americans and Vietnamese Americans were less likely than African Americans and Anglo Americans to call their households crowded, there was no difference among the groups in the extent to which they experienced negative effects.

Cultural differences in the roles of men and women are likely to exist even when the religion is the same. For example, Pakistan and Bangladesh are both predominantly Islamic countries (Pakistan is 96% Muslim, Bangladesh is 89% Muslim; Central Intelligence Agency, 2020), but their cultures are quite different. Pakistan is a more orthodox Islamic country (it is officially the Islamic Republic of Pakistan, whereas Bangladesh is officially the People's Republic of Bangladesh), and, therefore, one would expect stronger gender differences there than in Bangladesh.

Although Pakistan was under British rule for roughly a century, British institutions of government did not displace older tribal systems in the northwest and feudal chieftaincies in the south (Naipaul, 1998). Particularly since 1973, Pakistan has become a more orthodox Islamic country. In that year, the country adopted a new constitution, which contained numerous Islamic elements, including the observance of Islamic moral standards, the proper organization of religious endowments and mosques, prohibition of the consumption of alcohol, and promotion of the use of the Arabic language (Faruki, 1987). Oil wealth from Saudi Arabia and Libya increased Pakistan's ties to the Middle Eastern Arab countries and to Islamic movements. The 1980s were characterized by continuing efforts of social, legal, and political Islamization (Voll, 1994, p. 341).

Bangladesh, in contrast, generally has a less orthodox view of Islam, in part because the Islam that spread to Bengal after 1201 was not the pristine version of Arabia and in part because Bengal was separated by language and culture from the Arab Islamic tradition (Banu, 1992, p. 182). In modern Bangladesh, about 55% of the population consider themselves to be orthodox Muslims (e.g., they have a total and literal acceptance of the Koran, they strictly observe religious obligations), 5% practice a modern version of Islam, which emphasizes rationalism and individual judgment in interpreting the Koran, and 40% practice a popular or syncretistic version of Islam, which has polytheistic and animistic dimensions (Banu, 1992, p. 66). Although there have been attempts to establish Bangladesh as a fundamentalist Islamic country, most groups see the country as a modern, adaptationist Islamic state (Voll, 1994).

We found gender differences in both Bangladesh and Pakistan, but there were more gender differences, and the gender differences were stronger in

Islamabad than in Dhaka, consistent with the Islamic influence in the two countries. We also compared the responses of men and women in India and Bangladesh. In both India and Bangladesh, female pedestrians rated crowding significantly more negative than males did. Moreover, the fact that the difference between men's and women's ratings of crowding was greater in Bangladesh than in India was consistent with our hypothesis that women would be more upset by crowding in predominantly Muslim Bangladesh than in predominantly Hindu India, because of the greater role restrictions placed on women in Bangladesh, including restrictions on intrusions on their personal space.

Multiple Stressors

Third, we examined the effect of multiple stressors, in order to determine whether the effects of individual stressors are additive or interactive, that is, whether the effect of more than one stressor is simply the sum of the effects of each of the separate stressors, or whether the presence of multiple stressors is much worse than the sum of each stressor considered separately. An alternative possibility is that there is a ceiling effect, such that beyond some point the presence of multiple stressors is no worse than the presence of any one stressor. We examined this question of the effect of multiple stressors using interviews with slum residents in three capital cities and with pedestrian in two of these cities. We also investigated this question using experimental manipulations of crowding in "tempos," multi-passenger autorickshaws, in weather that was pleasant, hot, or very hot. In connection with our investigations of multiple stressors with pedestrians and tempos, we tested an attributional theory of crowding, in that we examined the effect of giving information about one stressor on judgments about another stressor. For example, a study of crowding in the United States titled "Hot and Crowded" examined male college students' attitudes and behaviors in a psychology laboratory in which density and temperature were varied. Our experimental replication in a natural setting (using three-wheeled autorickshaws) was conducted during the summer in India and created extremely high levels of crowding. The title for our paper, "Very Hot and Really Crowded," reflected Professor Pandey's belief that studies in the West often do not fully capture the extreme environmental conditions in India and other developing countries.

Mitigating Beliefs

Fourth, given that there are negative effects of crowding, we examined factors associated with India that might mitigate these effects. Specifically, we were interested in whether a belief in God would reduce the mental distress and physical symptoms associated with crowding. In our interviews with pilgrims and other groups at the *Magh Mela*, we found that belief in God did not reduce mental distress and physical symptoms. We also tested whether the speculation about the culturally unique responses of Indians to stressors, acceptance of these stressors as a reality and becoming helpless, are useful strategies for mitigating the effects of crowding. We found that neither was effective; both strategies were related to greater distress and reporting of more physical symptoms. Related to these potentially mitigating beliefs, we were interested in whether perceived control, a factor shown in the West to be consistently related to lower distress (e.g., Mirowsky & Ross, 1989), was also related to lower distress in South Asia. Across all of our studies, we found that more perceived control was related to better outcomes and less distress; people who cope actively with crowding do better than those who passively accept it. In sum, Indians appear to cope with crowding in the same way that North Americans cope with crowding. We also found that giving individuals information about the effects of stressors did not increase perceived control. Our experimental results suggest, in fact, that this information makes things worse, by pinpointing the source of the distress.

Doing Research Useful for Theory

The world is global, the problems are massive, and the resources for research are limited. Given these pressures, we must conduct research that can be used to advance theory and policy. Such research must be reliable and valid. To meet that goal, we researchers should use a multiplistic approach and should test models that incorporate the indigenous culture.

Multiplism

Multiplism refers to the use of multiple methods to investigate research questions, an approach that has long been advocated by social scientists (Mark & Shotland, 1987), although rarely employed. The rationale behind the approach is that valid answers can be best achieved if answers converge across multiple dimensions. Global problems, like crowding and other environmental issues, require multiplism on multiple dimensions. The goal is to find convergent results across these multiple dimensions because convergence leads to greater confidence. The absence of convergence could mean that a research conclusion is not valid. Alternatively, it could indicate that the world is not flat, that is, that other factors moderate what appear to be main effects. At the very least, the lack of convergence raises questions that call for more research.

The research I have described on crowding and environmental problems in South Asia embodied much of this multiplism. Our concern about the generalizability of results in this research program called for multiple populations in multiple locations using multiple research methods, multiple dependent measures, and multiple types of statistical analyses. We studied the problems using interviews, questionnaires, observations, and experiments. Dependent measures included beliefs, behaviors, subjective attitudes, and objective indicators of environmental stressors, including counts of people, the number of rooms, temperature readings, digital blood pressure monitoring, and electronic decibel measures of noise. Some measures, such as income, are particularly difficult to obtain, especially when respondents do not trust researchers or, in the case of some members of the household, do not know the amount. As a proxy, we counted items in the household (e.g., chairs, beds) that would be related to wealth and income.

The theoretical basis for the research came from multiple disciplinary perspectives: psychology, social psychology, sociology, demography, and urban studies. That is, the questions we investigated required research at multiple levels: individual, small group, large groups, institutions, and cities. The research was conducted at multiple sites: villages, cities (Allahabad, New Delhi, Visakhapatnam, Dhaka, Islamabad), neighborhoods within a metropolis, and multiple countries (India, Pakistan, Bangladesh, Nepal; Pandey et al., 2009) with different cultures and religions. The research involved multiple types of research participants, including rural villagers, migrants, slum dwellers, pedestrians, cycle rickshaw and autorickshaw drivers, riders of public transportation, children (Pandey et al., 2000), and college students (Ruback & Patnaik, 1989). At the *Magh Mela*, we interviewed *kalpavasis* (pilgrims), police, sweepers, boatmen, and police. In two studies, we found that people perceive places differently because of the different material, social, and symbolic aspects of the locations and because individuals have different backgrounds and different reasons for being at the locations (Ruback et al., 2008). We also observed territorial behavior at the *Magh Mela* (Ruback & Kohli, 2005).

Across the research studies, we used multiple types of statistical analyses. Since we conducted our studies, new types of analyses have been developed, such as multilevel modeling, which considers the nested nature of data (e.g., residents within neighborhoods) and which future research should incorporate. Our goal in using this multiplistic strategy was to discover the degree to which findings converge across research methods, types of research participants, and research sites. Our hope was for consistency across these dimensions, so that we would have greater confidence in both the validity and generalizability of the results.

Indigenous Perspectives

The failure to find consistent results could be a methodological problem, or it could be differences in the populations studied. One way to separate those two possibilities is to test whether the differences are cultural. More than 35 years ago, Sinha (1986) characterized the fourth phase of the development of psychology in India as one of questioning Western theories and models and searching for appropriate frameworks that Indian psychologists could use to address the "larger issues and problems facing the country" (p. 63). Coming from the West, it is not surprising that my bias toward behavioral universals is that of most Western psychologists that "what is true locally must be true everywhere" (Smith & Bond, 1994, p. 46), as opposed to the indigenous psychologies approach, which "does not a priori assume the existence of psychological universals" (Pandey, 2004, p. 349). It has been argued that future research in environmental psychology in India needs to incorporate Indian concepts of the person–environment interactional perspective to explain why findings do not generalize across countries. Translating the specific Indian context into testable hypotheses would be of enormous benefit to the development of theory more generally. Pandey (2004) also suggested that indigenous psychology would make research more relevant: "a goal of indigenous psychology is to address primary issues (such as disadvantage and poverty, intergroup relations and identity, rapid social change and management) of national concern, facilitating national development" (p. 350).

Doing Research Useful for Policy

Across countries, research findings are typically dismissed by policy makers who do not like the results. More than 30 years ago, Tripathi (1988) was pessimistic about studies by Indian psychologists that could be useful to policy makers since there was "a dearth of systematic problem-focused studies" (p. 142). Tripathi was particularly concerned about the quality of the research, which tended to be single studies, with small samples and little theory, and which were correlational rather than experimental. As I have suggested, multiplistic research programs would be one way to address some of Tripathi's concerns.

An additional technique would be to explicitly attempt to make the research relevant to policy.

Policy Relevance

Ruback and Innes (1988) suggested that, in terms of practical applications, research can be considered in terms of two dimensions: (a) whether or not the research investigates the effects of policy variables and (b) whether or not the effects of manipulations are measured by useful dependent variables. The first of these dimensions concerns what Ruback and Innes called policy variables, which are those factors that can be changed by policy makers. Arresting drivers of vehicles that violate pollution laws is a policy variable. In contrast to policy variables, non-policy variables are beyond the control of decision-makers. For example, the sex of a person is not a policy variable, because a decision-maker has no control over this factor.

The second dimension of practical research concerns what Ruback and Innes called the utility of the dependent measures. There are numerous variables that could be used to determine whether a manipulation has an effect. However, only some of those variables are of interest to policy makers. For example, the effect of a changed policy for arresting traffic offenders for pollution violations could be measured in terms of whether there are fewer polluting vehicles on the road, whether there is a decrease in air pollution, and whether people have more respect for the government. City officials are likely to care more about fewer polluting vehicles than about greater respect for the city government.

Scope of the Problem

A second aspect of practical research is how the problem under consideration is seen vis-a-vis other problems (Ruback & Pandey, 2010). Thus, for example, overpopulation, although an important problem, cannot be adequately studied without also investigating poverty, illiteracy, the rural/urban base of the population, religion, cultural traditions, environmental degradation, and resource depletion. Because the rewards in academia require researchers to conduct projects of manageable scale, these projects are likely to test relatively small questions and to measure effects on some but not all relevant variables. The limited scope of such research may mean that it is dismissed by policy makers.

Suggested Strategy

To make our research more relevant and useful to policy makers, psychologists might use a two-step research procedure. In the first step, researchers should conduct correlational research to determine if potential policy variables are significantly related to high utility dependent measures. Creativity is called for in this first step, in the sense that potential policy variables should be broadly considered. There should also be focus on what may be mediating variables, as these variables are the likely explanations for why a program does or does not work. Moreover, careful consideration is needed concerning what dependent variables decision-makers care about. If in this first step, potential policy variables are found to be significantly correlated with high utility dependent variables, then the second step of research is required. In this second step, potential policy variables are systematically manipulated to determine if they indeed produce significant changes on the high utility dependent variables. These policy variables are moderators, as they specify the conditions under which a program would or would not work. Knowledge of moderators can help policy makers identify culturally appropriate buffers of crowding effects and evaluate the probability of success of a program, whereas knowledge of mediators can assist in policy decisions.

Conclusion

In this chapter, in honor of Janak Pandey, I have summarized research that he and I and others conducted in environmental psychology, particularly crowding. Studying environmental issues of water shortage, air pollution, and crowding requires study at multiple levels, individual, neighborhood, city, and nation. Understanding the behavior of people facing these problems requires attention to their history and culture and a recognition of the disconnect between the immediate problems of scarce resources, inadequate housing, dirty air, polluted water, noisy neighborhoods, and a "shortage of food, fuel, and fodder" (Jain & Palsane, 204, p. 291) and the more distal global problems facing the world.

Friedman argued that the world of business is becoming flat. But I suggest that the world is not flat in terms of culture and gender norms and perhaps other dimensions. In fact, the world's flatness is an empirical question that social psychologists can continue to address. Our goal as social scientists is to conduct research that is reliable and valid, that considers the local understanding of behavior, and that is useful for policy makers.

Note

1 While presenting this work on environmental psychology, I find it pertinent to briefly outline Professor Pandey's academic journey and disciplinary concerns. He has had enormous influence on Indian psychology and social science. He has investigated important questions and distilled information for students and researchers through his writing and editing, and he has served as a bridge between Western empirical psychology and the indigenous psychologies of developing countries. His career has been an inspiration to younger psychologists. For more than 50 years, Professor Pandey has been involved in social psychological research, beginning with his work in 1964 as an interviewer for a multi-nation project on the impact of industrialization on modernization. A few years later, while a master's student at Patna University, Professor Pandey worked with Professor J. B. P. Sinha on research that showed that in a resource-limited society, increasing Need for Achievement (n-Ach; McClelland, 1961) led to selfishness, the appropriation of assets, and the undermining of collective productivity, causing McClelland to qualify his argument about n-Ach by suggesting that in resource-limited societies, n-Ach training must be combined with cooperative attitudes. Thus, early in his career, Professor Pandey had already provided evidence that the psychological world is not flat. He has published numerous monographs, articles, and reviews, including editing two three-volume editions of *Psychology in India* (1988, 2004), which summarized psychological research in the country.

References

Banu, U. A. B. R. A. (1992). *Islam in Bangladesh*. Brill.

Central Intelligence Agency. (2020). *The world factbook*. www.cia.gov/the-world-factbook/south-asia/

Cone, J. D. (1986). *Environmental problems/behavioral solutions*. Brooks/Cole.

Ellis, P., & Roberts, M. (2016). *Leveraging urbanization in South Asia: Managing spatial transformation for prosperity and livability*. World Bank. https://openknowledge.worldbank.org/handle/10986/22549

Evans, G., Lepore, S. J., & Allen, K. M. (2000). Cross-cultural differences in tolerance for crowding: Fact or fiction. *Journal of Personality and Social Psychology*, *79*, 204–210.
Faruki, K. A. (1987). Pakistan: Islamic government and society. In J. L. Esposito (Ed.), *Islam in Asia: Religion, politics, and society* (pp. 53–78). Oxford University Press.
Gadgil, M., & Thapar, R. (1990). Human ecology in India: Some historical perspectives. *Interdisciplinary Science Reviews*, *15*, 209–223.
Hoornweg, D., & Pope, K. (2016). Population predictions for the world's largest cities in the 21st century. *Environment & Urbanization*, *29*, 195–216.
IQAir. (2020a). *World most polluted countries 2019 (PM2.5)*. www.iqair.com/world-most-polluted-countries
IQAir. (2020b). *World most polluted cities 2019 (PM2.5)*. www.iqair.com/world-most-polluted-cities
Macrotrends. (2021). www.macrotrends.net/countries/WLD/world/population-growth-rate
Majumder, P. P. (2009). The human genetic history of South Asia. *Current Biology*, *20*, R184–R187. www.cell.com/current-biology/pdf/S0960-9822(09)02068-5.pdf
Mandelbaum, D. G. (1988). *Women's seclusion and men's honor: Sex roles in north India, Bangladesh, and Pakistan*. University of Arizona Press.
Mark, M. M., & Shotland, R. L. (1987). Toward more useful social science. In R. L. Shotland & M. M. Mark (Eds.), *Social science and social policy* (pp. 335–370). Sage.
McClelland, D. C. (1961). *The achieving society*. Free Press.
Mirowsky, J., & Ross, C. E. (1989). *Social institutions and social change: Social causes of psychological distress*. Aldine de Gruyter.
Naipaul, V. S. (1998). *Beyond belief: Islamic excursions among the converted peoples*. Random House.
Pandey, J. (2004). Psychology in India enters the twenty-first century: Movement toward an indigenous discipline. In J. Pandey (Ed.), *Psychology in India revisited: Developments in the discipline* (Vol. 3, pp. 342–370). Sage.
Pandey, J., Siddiqui, R. N., Udas, A. K., & Ruback, R. B. (2009). Residents' reactions to environmental stressors in Kathmandu: A comparison of the inner city versus the outskirts. *Psychological Studies*, *54*, 202–212.
Pandey, J., Verma, M., & Ruback, R. B. (2000). Perceived crowding in Indian classrooms: The effects of age, gender and household density. *Psychology and Developing Societies*, *12*, 139–154.
Rao, M. S. A. (1986). *Studies in migration: Internal and international migration in India*. Manohar.
Ruback, R. B., & Begum, H. A. (1995). Environmental stressors in Dhaka: The views of rickshaw drivers. *Bangladesh Psychological Studies*, *5*, 1–14.
Ruback, R. B., Begum, H. A., Tariq, N., Kamal, A., & Pandey, J. (2002). Reactions to environmental stressors: Gender differences in the slums of Dhaka and Islamabad. *Journal of Cross-Cultural Psychology*, *33*, 100–119.
Ruback, R. B., & Innes, C. A. (1988). The relevance and irrelevance of psychological research: The example of prison crowding. *American Psychologist*, *43*, 683–693.
Ruback, R. B., & Kohli, N. (2005). Territoriality at the Magh mela: The effects of organizational factors and intruder characteristics. *Environment and Behavior*, *37*, 178–200.
Ruback, R. B., Kohli, N., & Pandey, J. (2009). Hindus' evaluations of Hindus and Muslims: Religious leaders and pilgrims at the *Magh Mela*. *Journal for the Scientific Study of Religion*, *48*, 375–385.
Ruback, R. B., & Pandey, J. (1991). Crowding, perceived control, and relative power: An analysis of households in India. *Journal of Applied Social Psychology*, *21*, 315–344.

Ruback, R. B., & Pandey, J. (1996). Gender differences in perceptions of household crowding: Stress, affiliation, and role obligations in rural India. *Journal of Applied Social Psychology*, *26*, 417–436.
Ruback, R. B., & Pandey, J. (2002). Mental distress and physical symptoms in the slums of New Delhi: The role of individual, household, and neighborhood factors. *Journal of Applied Social Psychology*, *32*, 2296–2320.
Ruback, R. B., & Pandey, J. (2010). Policy relevant research for development: A conceptual framework and empirical approach. In J. Pandey, T. N. Sinha, & A. K. Sinha (Eds.), *Dialogue for development* (pp. 201–215). Concept Publishers.
Ruback, R. B., Pandey, J., Begum, H. A., Tariq, N., & Kamal, A. (2004). Motivations for and satisfaction with migration: An analysis of migrants to New Delhi, Dhaka, and Islamabad. *Environment and Behavior*, *36*, 814–838.
Ruback, R. B., Pandey, J., & Kohli, N. (2008). Evaluations of a sacred place: Role and religious belief at the *Magh Mela*. *Journal of Environmental Psychology*, *28*, 174–184.
Ruback, R. B., & Patnaik, R. (1989). Crowding, perceived control, and the destruction of property. *Psychological Studies*, *34*, 1–14.
Sarkar, A., Mukherjee, A. D., Bera, M. K., Das, B., Juyal, N., Morthekai, P., Deshpande, R. D., Shinde, V. S., & Rao, L. S. (2016). Oxygen isotope in archaeological bioapatites from India: Implications to climate change and decline of Bronze Age Harappan civilization. *Scientific Reports*, 6–26555. https://doi.org/10.1038/srep26555
Sharma, A. N. (1997). *People on the move: Nature and implications of migration in a backward economy*. Vikas Publishing House.
Sinha, D. (1986). *Psychology in a third world country: The Indian experience*. Sage.
Smith, P. B., & Bond, M. H. (1994). *Social psychology across cultures: Analysis and perspectives*. Allyn and Bacon.
Stiglitz, J. De. (2006). *Making globalization work*. Norton.
Todaro, M. P. (1989). *Economic development in the Third World* (4th ed.). Longman.
Tripathi, R. C. (1988). Applied social psychology. In J. Pandey (Ed.), *Psychology in India: The state-of-the-art* (Vol. 2, pp. 95–157). Sage.
United Nations Department of Economic and Social Affairs. Population Division, Population Estimates and Projections Section. (2019). *World population prospects 2019. File POP/1-1: Total population—both sexes*. https://population.un.org/wpp/
Voll, J. O. (1994). *Islam: Continuity and change in the modern world* (2nd ed.). Oxford University Press.
Wendling, Z. A., Emerson, J. W., de Sherbinin, A., Esty, D. C., et al. (2020). 2020 Environmental performance index. *Yale Center for Environmental Law & Policy*. https://epi.yale.edu/downloads/epi2020report20200911.pdf
Williams, J. E., & Best, D. L. (1990). *Sex and psyche: Gender and self viewed cross-culturally*. Sage.

5 The Deceptive Silence on the Environmental Crisis

Roomana N. Siddiqui

The state of the environment we are witnessing has reached a tipping point and has engulfed the entire planet. It is no longer an issue that attracted attention only of leaders and policy makers in the wake of environmental calamities. As large populations are exposed to the adverse impact of the declining quality of the environment on a regular basis, it has forced people to take cognizance of the problem. The regularity with which one is witnessing the adverse impact of climate change on account of burning of fossil fuel, change in lifestyle, and the developmental agendas of countries to take care of its rising population has made life very scary. We confront the backlash from the environment which is increasingly becoming unpredictable and is causing much suffering and devastation. With every passing day, the situation is getting from bad to worse. Be it the increasing earth temperature, forest fires, incessant and unpredictable rainfall causing flash floods in regions unheard of, rising air pollution, tsunamis, garbage menace, bio-diversity loss, etc., these issues are no longer something that happened in distant places or would happen to future generations. The imprint of the ecological crisis has become so powerful and visible that ignoring or downplaying them will prove fatal for the earth and its inhabitants. It has spread its tentacles all around and people are vulnerable to its consequences. If as a society we do not wake up to its seriousness it might be the next biggest pandemic unleashing havoc and causing a sizeable population to experience fear, rage, grief, and trauma.

A large section of people across the globe have been subjected to some form of hardship on account of the environmental crisis and they have struggled to cope with these unprecedented and deeply frightening environmental calamities and the consequent unsettling emotions. By and large, we acknowledge the severity of the issue but when it comes to doing something about it, we keep quiet. Even in our normal conversations we rarely talk about it or hear others discuss about it. This leads to a "climate spiral of silence," where even those who care about the issue shy away from discussing it because they so infrequently hear other people talking about it (Heald, 2017). The manner in which we discuss issues relating to the environment has a great deal to do with how much and how deeply we think about it. Unless we break this silence, we will not be able to address it with an urgency which is the need of

DOI: 10.4324/9781003461302-8

the hour. This requires identification of the key barriers that act as roadblocks in voicing the eco-fear and anxiety people are enduring on a day-to-day basis.

The Faulty Attitude Accounting for Eco-Silence

The environmental crisis is impacting our life on a day-to-day basis, and people by and large are aware of the severity of the situation and do have a general concern about it, but when it comes to behavioral response to tackle, there appears to be a disconnect. This disconnect between awareness, concern, and behavioral response on environmental issues maybe due to "value-action" or "attitude-behavior" gap (e.g., Blake, 1999; Kollmuss & Agyeman, 2002; Eiser, 1994; Ungar, 1994). Generally at the attitudinal level, we see that people are very pro-environment and would want the problems to be resolved but when it comes to taking action then different set of factors gain salience and outweigh the antecedents factors. Hence, unless those factors that are creating road blocks toward environmentally friendly behavior are addressed, we will not be able to do much on the impending crisis.

The environmental problems feel real for those people who are directly affected by it but a large section of people see them as a temporary phenomenon that may or may not affect them. This tendency to see it as spatially distant as well as temporary do not make people personally threatened. This spatial trap (Osbaldiston & Sheldon, 2002) pushes the issues outside our immediate attention as it is not causing any immediate personal difficulties. In those circumstances where they are daily experiencing distress on account of poor quality of air, water, and lack of hygienic condition even in these situations, they develop a funneling perspective where they pay more attention to other pressing problems and devote less attention to issues that are not accorded greater priority. In such a scenario, people are unlikely to engage in mitigative and adaptive behaviors. Siddiqui and Pandey (2003) demonstrated that when people are faced with intense economic and environmental crisis, then they give precedence to the economic crisis more compared to environmental crisis. It is a matter of priority. In a situation where precedence is given to individual survival, then the collective costs become socially distant, and this according to Jones and Rachlin (2006) accounts for the psychological discounting of the seriousness of the issue and lowers cooperation.

When people put environmental issues on low priority, they do not pay much serious attention to the current scenario. The cues may be there in the surrounding and the social media, but due to lack of interest or attention to these cues, one becomes environmentally blinded. This selectively screening off the relevant environmental cues may be due to ignorance, uncertainty, or skepticism. This screening off proper knowledge makes them incapable of realizing the cause and extent of the crisis. This was noted by Bord et al. (2000) in the context of climate change. In the eventuality of a crisis, such people are caught unawares as they do not know what to do to overcome them as they do not know how to translate them into actions.

This faulty attitude not only absolves people from accepting their responsibility but also accounts for lack of initiative on their part. Many conveniently believe they can do nothing about it at the individual level. People often do not act because they think that they have little behavioral control over the outcome (e.g., Ajzen, 1991; Huebner & Lipsey, 1981) or that their actions will not have much impact (a lack of self-efficacy; Ajzen, 2002). This promotes the status quo and prevents people from coming together and engaging at the collective level. They will defend and justify the status quo and will speak against others trying to "rock the boat" as that will change how things are currently operating. Change in the status quo requires acceptance of their own contribution to the crisis which is not a comfortable state of affairs. They are optimistic that Nature or some Super power will take care of the crisis and nothing will happen to the earth. This optimism bias (Weinstein, 1980) gives us the confidence that in due course of time the environment will rectify itself or the policy makers at the national and international will come up with policies or green technology that will solve the problem. Considerable evidence suggests that people downplay personal risks from environmental hazards (Hatfield & Job, 2001; Weinstein et al., 1988). Thus, it is due to optimistic bias that although global citizens do expect environmental conditions to worsen over the next 25 years but not in places where they live compared to other places (Gifford et al., 2009).

Ironically, though people have this belief that the system will take care of the crisis, yet lack of trust in the system adds to the uncertainty. There is enough evidence to suggest that many people distrust messages that come from scientists or government officials (e.g., Earle, 2004; MacGregor et al., 1994). In times of natural catastrophe, messages given by policy makers may be paid attention to, but after some times, the progress and gains made are diminished or erased by subsequent actions. Thus, a rebounding effect occurs partly because it is based on a lack of trust in those who give the advice or set the policy (Eilam & Suleiman, 2004). Trust is important for changing behavior, and people need to be assured that others will not take advantage of them. The "free rider effect" acts as an inhibitor. People will trust if they perceive that the change is effective, valuable, and equitable (e.g., Brann & Foddy, 1987; Foddy & Dawes, 2008) and the policy-making bodies are genuine and honest. In sum, when trust sours, the probability of adopting positive climate change behavior diminishes.

State of Denial and Apathy

Despite the fact that we have entered a dangerous phase of environmental positioning, we witness a sense of both denial and apathy in tackling the situation. Many people ignore the warnings as either too distant or as wishful thinking by politicians and intellectuals. The logic given by such voices is that it is a natural progression where the old environmental change will lead to a fresh renewed one. The common belief that nature has self-correcting mechanisms and will take care of itself in due course of time often results in apathy. As a result, people are more in the denial mode compared to accepting that the environmental crisis is serious and human being are the main contributor to it. According to the Yale program, only 34% of those surveyed in the United States deny the role of humans in global warming. Yet those who have both the science and public opinion on their side remain astonishingly quiet. Research from Harvard psychology professors suggests that the human brain is simply not equipped to respond to threats so far ahead, but only to more immediate, short-term dangers. Unfortunately, short-termism is also engrained in almost all economic and social institutions within capitalist society, making it even harder to achieve effective change.

Once we deny or reject information relating to the severity of the environmental crisis, we become indifferent toward it. It is well accepted empirically that one must have feelings about an issue then only one can take personally meaningful action regarding it. Apathy literally means "without feeling," and this leads to unconcern. This lack of a compelling feeling fails to sufficiently motivate us to do something about it. Apathy is a feeling but it also refers to an attitude, an attitude of indifference, unresponsiveness, and lack of interest. Such an attitude saps you of so much energy that you feel lethargic, listless, and enervated—almost too "paralyzed" to act—and certainly without the will to do so. Which is why apathetic individuals are easily identified by their very passivity. Their interest in confronting life's challenges is seriously compromised. They just don't care enough. And frankly, they don't care that they don't care. This lends support to the thinking that I am too small to do anything about the environmental crisis, and this results in the "tragedy of the commons" (Hardin,1968).

Despite the visible signs of its impact, we still find a lot of indifference among people. In order to understand this state of denial and indifference, one needs to understand the cognition behind it. The "ostrich effect"—the tendency to selectively reject available inconvenient information, for example by ignoring the environmental impact of one's own behavior—is a way of avoiding guilt and moral imbalance in the first place. This tendency makes it important to inform the public about the climate changes in the right way—to stress the severity of the problem enough to make people understand the problem, but not so much that it makes people reject the information

Discounting the Future

We discount the perils that society is and will be facing on account of the degrading environmental conditions. This is due to the tendency of undervaluing distant or future risks. People believe that environmental conditions were worse in places other than their own (Gifford et al., 2009). According to Gifford (2011), no one wants to believe that their daily activities are responsible for a global disaster that has already turned millions of people into climate refugees and killed scores of others. Herman Daly an ecological economist observed that many of our environmental decisions are made as if the earth "were a business in liquidation" (Gore 1992). It becomes convenient to discount when intergenerational distribution of resources is involved or the future is uncertain and distant (Wade-Benzoni, 1999).

The discounting may occur due to a positive illusion which enables us to see ourselves, our environment, and the future in a more positive light than is objectively the case (Taylor & Brown, 1988). Such positive illusions reduce the quality of decision-making and prevent us from acting in time to address significant problems (Bazerman & Watkins, 2004; Bazerman & Moore, 2008).

Role of Emotions

In the environment behavior link, the focus invariably is on how environmental awareness and attitude influence our response to the environment. The emphasis is more on the cognitive processes with little emphasis on the affective process. Despite the fact that it is well established that emotion plays a significant role in how people have evolved and adapted to the changing environmental conditions during the course of evolution, when it came to research on environmental issues, emotion did not get much precedence. However, recently the role of positive and negative emotions as predictors or mediators of ecological behavior has been recognized (Vining & Ebreo, 2002). Emotions do play a major role in the reactions made to environmental crisis.

Faced with an environmental catastrophe, it is natural to experience the emotions of fear. It is this fear which motivates people to engage in self-protective behavior or enable them to contribute their time and expertise to suggest ways and means to bring about a change. On the other hand, if people do not see it as an issue affecting them and fail to experience an element of fear or anxiety, then they will not take the impending environmental catastrophe seriously, and we might also underplay the fear faced by others as dysfunctional. The "eco-fear" (Chalquist, 2023) is a healthy response to a frightening situation, as it enables a person to recognize that the fear is genuine and realistic, and this acts as an indicator that something must be done and action must be taken.

Direct exposure to environmental calamity does lead to experience of fear, anxiety, and trauma in the person. However, regular occurrence of intense environmental calamities, like flash floods, forest fires, landslides, incessant rainfall, or intense heat waves, also creates panic and stress. Though one may not experience it directly, the coverage on media or social media, along with the visuals of the large-scale destruction and damage caused by it, results in experience of indirect and vicarious emotions of fear. Observing visuals of climate change effects worldwide also leads to anxiety and uncertainty about the unprecedented scale of current and future risks to humans and other species (Kidner, 2007; Maibach et al., 2009; Norgaard, 2009).

Apart from negative emotions, positive emotion, that of empathy, can play a constructive role in managing the crisis. Empathy is considered an approach emotion that motivates the individual to take a proactive approach with the desire to do something about it. Moreover, the success of appeals to guilt or empathy is likely to depend on whether a behavior is viewed as a social issue or a social cause (Bagozzi & Moore, 1994). If a proactive behavior toward the environment is seen as a social cause, for example if anti-plastic drive is accepted by society, then emotional appeals will be more fruitful. However, when a particular environmental behavior is seen as a social issue (using public transport or private vehicle), where people have strong attitude toward either of the two and is controversial, then emotional appeals are likely to have less success. Guilt also becomes a motivator for pro-environmental behavior when people see that the negative affect is not aligning with their internalized subjective norms or personal norms, as outlined within the Theories of Reasoned Action and Planned Behavior (Ajzen & Fishbein, 1980) and the Norm Activation Model (Schwartz, 1977) respectively. So those individuals who have accepted pro-environmental behavior as a value they will be more motivated by guilt. Thus, the feeling of guilt leads the individual to take responsibility for their actions, rather than the other way round (Berndsen & Manstead, 2007). It is also true that guilt is unlikely to achieve the requisite change if there are no effective alternative actions available or the structures and systems are not conducive or facilitative in enabling the individual to act. If there is lack of clarity around the most appropriate behavior to deal with the crisis then it may release the individual from a feeling of guilt. On the other hand, shame is an avoidance motivation where a person would like to deny or hide away from accepting his role in contributing to the crisis.

The Blame Game

The silence or one can say the inaction toward the environmental crisis to a large extent can be linked to the blame game that one witnesses at both the individual and group levels. People and nations have their own assessment of responsibility and blame, and often these assessments are influenced by perceived inequity. This perception often serves as a justification for lack of effective measures that are needed to mitigate the impact. People justify their complacency by putting the blame on others. At the international level, developing countries blame the developed nations for not cooperating while developed nations blame them for contributing to the crisis. Just like the blame game of developing countries on developed nations and vice versa, the same dynamic is visible at the local and individual level. We engage in environmentally maladaptive behavior in terms of the energy we consume and the lifestyle we live. People are not ready to give up those habits and behaviors that are self-serving.

Perceived inequity is often considered as a reason for inaction. "Why should I change if they won't change?" The fear of being victimized by free-riders (Kerr, 1983; Olson, 1965) serves as a barrier for some individuals, who are skeptical that why should they contribute responsibly to the cause of climate change when (they fear) others will not. The fear or suspicion that others expect us to change while they are not changing results in a feeling that others are freeloading on their efforts. In experimental resource dilemmas, when any sort of inequality or inequity (real or perceived) exists, cooperation tends to decline (e.g., Aquino et al., 1992). People lose motivation when they think others aren't pulling their weight—it's known as the sucker effect. Success depends on showing how the effort is shared by other in mitigating the problem. This requires for transparency in the efforts made to tackle the issue.

Role of Media in Side Lining the Environmental Issues

It is said that we cannot form an opinion about any issue unless and until we have the requisite information. It is in this context that the role of media, as an information dissemination agency, becomes critical. The type of issues which media gives coverage has a huge impact in generating opinion and awareness on them. Over the year, large-scale penetration of media within the nook and corner of the country makes it a powerful source of information which influences the reaction and response of the people. The type of issues raised by the media and the nature of information disseminated determines the level of awareness on any issue. This plays a major role in enabling individuals to make appropriate or inappropriate behavior to the issue in question., Unfortunately, one witnesses an eerie silence on the severity of the environmental issues and the coverage given is so scanty that often it gets missed, Morgan (1997) rightly pointed that a significant amount of the public's knowledge of environmental issues is likely to come from the media. Hence, it is not surprising to see that a large portion of the population is not aware about the gravity of the environmental crisis as the media gives very little space to issues related to it. It is not possible to get firsthand experience or knowledge about the vast array of environmental problem like greenhouse effect, ozone depletion, climate change, rising of sea level, and environmental pollution that confronts the earth. One has to depend on agencies for not only information but also the severity of the situation. People do have firm opinion on those issues which they are regularly confronting firsthand but if we restrict ourselves to only those issues then this has a limiting affect.

Over the years, one common trend noticed in the Indian media is that environmental issues get some space mainly during winters when the air pollution of metropolitan cities gets really bad and starts affecting visibility due to dense smog and also during the rainy seasons when the issue of water logging affects the normal routine of people. Otherwise, media pays attention to such issues only at the time of natural calamities which are becoming a regular feature. Looking at the manner in which media covers the environmental issues, it is generally done in a sensationalized manner which is very myopic. Buell (2005) noted that environmental news coverage is typically devoid of scientific explanations and is mainly event oriented. Knowledge of the root causes of environmental crisis is not given much attention. Hiebert (2006) stated that the media has a responsibility to inform, to educate, and to make us aware of the current status along with the future consequences. Media is a powerful medium which can promote and inhibit values and attitudes toward the environment and environmental crisis.

We need more programs with an emphasis on raising public awareness about the environmental problems. Understanding the current status and root cause of the crisis is critically important in spreading awareness among masses. Without awareness it will become difficult to involve and motivate people to engage in environmentally friendly behavior. Often, coverage of environmental issues emphasizes problems and conflicts instead of solutions. According to Gore (2006), the media must provide detailed information in a contextualized, accurate manner so as to equip the public with the knowledge they need to guide their understanding and actions toward the natural environment.

Rightly referred to as mind managers, it is up to the media to present the correct information or create a false sense of reality by presenting the information in such a manner that people find it difficult to understand, and hence, they reject the actual conditions of the situation. The power of media lies not only (and not even primarily) in its power to declare things to be true but also in the power to provide the form in which the declaration appears (Schudson, 1982). Generally, people rely on information given by media as they appear to have a relationship with the real world, and the more outreach the media has over the population, the responsibility becomes manifold to report the correct facts and figures. According to Burgess (1990), the media's ability to change the course of the environmental crisis is immense. It can play a critical role in helping to halt and reverse the future expansion of environmental problems and to maintain existing efforts in the community.

Role of the media should not be restricted to simply transmitting information about any environmental catastrophe but pay attention to the causes of the crisis and how they can be handled at the local as well as global level. It is necessary to increase the public's sensitivity to environmental and development problems. People profit through environment education, by gaining an understanding of how their individual actions affect the environment, acquiring skills that are useful to evaluate various sides of issues, and becoming better equipped to make informed decisions. As the range of issues are quite diverse, it requires an effective articulation. This according to Burgess (1990) will depend on how much we have considered the culturally specific encoded messages which will be decoded and given meaning by their audiences within existing frames of reference.

The Way Ahead

Given the gravity of the situation and the lack of seriousness shown toward the impending environmental catastrophe, one requires to make concerted efforts to mitigate the impact on the planet and its inhabitants. This requires a multipronged strategy and a much proactive approach at all levels ranging from the individual, local, and international levels. This calls for major adjustments, realignment, and collaboration that may require sacrifice and changes in lifestyle. Since it is difficult for people to give up personal gains in favor of collective benefits it is a huge challenge to convince them about the future gains of a sustainable lifestyle and this ultimately will lead to transformation. The critical point is to raise awareness regarding the benefits of a sustainable lifestyle. It is here that the media can play a very active role in spreading awareness about the environmental challenges and its long-term repercussions.

People need to know how the rupture caused to our symbiotic relationship with the natural world is the major cause of the present-day situation. When people were living in harmony with nature and nurturing it, we did not face such a bleak situation. It was the change in approach from living with nature to control over nature that precipitated the crisis manifold. The confrontational approach has to be replaced by new ways of relating with nature. As there cannot be a single strategy that fits all, we need to take into account the cultural beliefs and practices of a particular region so there is more acceptance by the people rather than when it is not relatable. If we pay greater attention to local adaptation and link our efforts with local concerns, then there is more likely that people will engage with environmental issues in a more effective manner. In cases where people have options of interventions that complements and respects the social and cultural environment, there it is helpful in addressing the problems encountered by social barriers. Since cultural norms and institutions are to a large extent responsible for the creation of barriers and restrictions, particularly at the local level, it is important to address these institutions and norms at the local level. A local saliency motivates more effective action and reduces vulnerability.

It is essential to develop sustainable environmental systems for future generations which should focus on protection, restoration, and management of resources. This can be achieved only when people are well informed on the present status of the crisis, its contributing factors and what could be the best way to handle them. If we know more about the environment, we can play a more useful role in solving environmental problems. The failure to recognize the ecological limits of earth will only exacerbate the crisis further. We need to evolve strategies that not only helps in tackling the situation and helping in reduction of the risk of disasters, but they must also be mutually reinforcing. Both reducing the occurrence of disaster and tackling it in the eventuality of its occurrence has to be planned in a way which is complimentary to each other. For example, the thinking that "environmentally friendly" behavior can compensate for unsustainable behavior needs to be changed because if we keep on adding to the problem at one end by our environmentally maladaptive behavior and feel good that we are doing our bit then it might defeat the purpose. In the words of Schumacher (1995) natural resources are capital and cannot be treated as income of the globalized free market economy

In order to address the barriers acting as impediments to sustainable behavior, we need to give up our sense of entitlements both at individual and institutional levels and alter restrictive and maladaptive perceptions, norms, and cultural constraints. Any attempt to address these facets will not be successful if they do not empower and inform individuals who remain comfortable in their adaptive behavior. Despite the fact that people are aware and fearful of the environmental crisis yet it seems the fear or the impending threat is not sufficient to mobilize them for action. The threat will mobilize people toward environmentally friendly behavior only if they are made to realize the personal cost they may incur due to one or the other form of environmental problem be it pollution, natural calamity or climate change. It is only when people realize the personal cost that it may inflict to them and become aware of the dangers lurking in the future that they will make an attempt to change their maladaptive behavior. Along with this people also need to be made aware of the solutions available to them. What's missing is the concrete examples of how to tackle the situation. People will be motivated to adopt a pro-environmental approach if they are informed about strategies that are concrete, doable, and meaningful in removing that threat.

Concluding Comments

Despite the fact that human behavior is at the center of the environmental crisis, the discipline of psychology has not been very effective in contributing toward suggesting impactful interventions to handle the crisis. The approach of psychology has been individualistic where the focus has been on the individual so the suggestions were more on changing individual behavior. But looking at the intensity of the problem genuine attempt on the part of the individual might make some local level difference but might not be able to help tackle the crisis. As an individual, people may be concerned about the environment but they feel helpless in confronting it at the individual level. People often ignore or deny those problems they feel helpless to deal with thus it is important that people feel they have the power to do something about it. As Bandura (1997) pointed out that individuals and groups are not likely to act to solve a problem unless they have a belief—a perceived sense of efficacy—that their individual and collective actions can make a difference. This is applicable to the environmental crisis also. People easily get discouraged and feel that one person's action won't make a significant difference. Thus, in order to persuade people to act in environmentally adaptive manner, we need to communicate in ways that build their sense of self-efficacy and collective efficacy.

It is this change in perspective, that is, from the individual to the collective, that may help break the silence and enable people to come together for a common cause. One way this could be achieved is by mobilizing the collective to respond so as to empower each other. Nobel laureate Ostrom (1990) demonstrated that ordinary people are capable of creating rules and institutions that allow for the sustainable and equitable management of shared resources. She very rightly pointed out that we have ignored what citizens can do and the importance of real involvement of the people involved. When people come together for a cause especially during a crisis, they are able to generate that hope which is very essential to deal with such a situation. If large section of people are motivated and mobilized then they have the ability to imagine many alternative ways of changing the world and establishing a society characterized by more sustainable relations between humans and the rest of nature. This requires an understanding of the significance of the symbiotic relationship between human society and environment, highlighting the symbolic and emotional reasons that the environment is important for humans and not just seen as a source of resources. It is in this domain that psychological research becomes critical to understanding this symbiotic relation between humans and the environment.

References

Ajzen, I. (1991). The theory of planned behaviour. *Organizational Behavior and Human Decision Processes*, *50*, 179–211.

Ajzen, I. (2002). Perceived behavioral control, self-efficacy, locus of control, and the theory of planned behavior. *Journal of Applied Social Psychology*, *32*, 665–683. https://doi.org/10.1111/j.1559-1816.2002.tb00236.x

Ajzen, I., & Fishbein, M. (1980). *Understanding attitudes and predicting social behavior*. Prentice-Hall.

Aquino, K., Steisel, V., & Kay, A. (1992). The effects of resource distribution, voice, and decision framing on the provision of public goods. *Journal of Conflict Resolution*, *36*, 665–687. https://doi.org/10.1177/0022002792036004003

Bagozzi, R., & Moore, D. (1994). Public service advertisements: Emotions and empathy guide pro-social behaviour. *Journal of Marketing*, *58*(1), 56–70.

Bandura, A. (1997). *Self-efficacy: The exercise of control*. W.H. Freeman.

Bazerman, M. H., & Moore, D. (2008). *Judgment in managerial decision making*. Wiley.

Bazerman, M. H., & Watkins, M. D. (2004). *Predictable surprises: The disasters you should have seen coming and how to prevent them*. Harvard Business School Press.

Berndsen, M., & Manstead, A (2007). On the relationship between responsibility and guilt: Antecedent appraisal or elaborated appraisal? *European Journal of Social Psychology*, *37*, 774–792

Blake, J. (1999). Overcoming the 'Value-Action Gap' in environmental policy: Tensions between national policy and local experience. *Local Environment*, *4*, 257–278.

Bord, R., O'Connor, R., & Fisher, A. (2000). In what sense does the public need to understand global climate change? *Public Understanding of Science*, *9*, 205–218.

Brann, P., & Foddy, M. (1987). Trust and the consumption of a deteriorating common resource. *Journal of Conflict Resolution*, *31*, 615–630. https://doi.org/10.1177/0022002787031004004

Buell, L. (2005). *The environmental imagination: The nature writing and the formation of American culture*. Baknap press.

Burgess, J. (1990). The production and consumption of environmental meanings in the mass media: A research agenda for the 1990's. *Transactions of the Institute of Geographers*, *15*(2), 139–161.

Chalquist, C. (2023). *It's not eco-anxiety—It's eco-fear!* www.chalquist.com/post/it-s-not-eco-anxiety-it-s-eco-fear

Earle, T. C. (2004). Thinking aloud about trust: A protocol analysis of trust in risk management. *Risk Analysis*, *24*, 169–183. https://doi.org/10.1111/j.0272–4332.2004.00420.x

Eilam, O., & Suleiman, R. (2004). Cooperative, pure, and selfish trusting: Their distinctive effects on the reaction of trust recipients. *European Journal of Social Psychology*, *34*, 729–738. https://doi.org/10.1002/ejsp.227

Eiser, J. R. (1994). *Attitudes, chaos and the connectionist mind*. Oxford.

Foddy, M., & Dawes, R. M. (2008). Group-based trust in social dilemmas. In A. Biel, D. Eek, T. Ga¨rling, & M. Gustaffson (Eds.), *New issues and paradigms in research in social dilemma* (pp. 57–71). Springer.

Gifford, R. (2011). The dragons of inaction: Psychological barriers that limit climate change mitigation and adaptation. *American Psychologist*, *66*, 290–302.

Gifford, R., Scannell, L., Kormos, C., Smolova, L., Biel, A., Boncu, S., Corral, V., Güntherf, H., Hanyu, K., Hine, D., Kaiser, F. G., Korpela, K., Lima, L. M., Mertig, A. G., Mira, R. G., Moser, G., Passafaro, P., Pinheiro, J. Q., Saini, S., . . . Uzzell, D. (2009). Temporal pessimism and spatial optimism in environmental assessments: An 18-nation study. *Journal of Environmental Psychology*, *29*, 1–12. https://doi.org/10.1016/j.jenvp.2008.06.001

Gore, A. (1992). *Earth in the balance: Ecology and the human spirit*. Penguin.

Gore, A. (2006). *An inconvenient Truth: The planetary emergency of global warming and what can we do about it*. Bloomsbury.

Hardin, G. (1968). The tragedy of the commons. *Science*, *162*(3859), 1243–1248.

Hatfield, J., & Job, R. F. S. (2001). Optimism bias about environmental degradation: The role of the range of impact of precautions. *Journal of Environmental Psychology*, *21*, 17–30. https://doi.org/10.1006/jevp.2000.0190

Heald, S. (2017). Climate silence, moral disengagement, and self-efficacy: How albert bandura's theories inform our climate-change predicament. environment: *Science and Policy for Sustainable Development*, *59*, (6), 4–15.

Hiebert, R. (2006). *Mass media: In Introduction to modern communication*. Madison Printing Press.

Huebner, R. B., & Lipsey, M. W. (1981). The relationship of three measures of locus of control to environmental activism. *Basic and Applied Social Psychology*, *2*, 45–58.

Jones, B., & Rachlin, H. (2006). Social discounting. *Psychological Science*, *17*(4), 283–286. https://doi.org/10.1111/j.1467–9280.2006.01699.x

Kerr, N. L. (1983). Motivation losses in small groups: A social dilemma analysis. *Journal of Personality and Social Psychology*, *45*, 819–828. https://doi.org/10.1037/0022-3514.45.4.819

Kidner, D. (2007). Depression and the natural world: Towards a critical ecology of psychological distress. *International Journal of Critical Psychology*, *19*, 123–146.

Kollmuss, A., & Agyeman, J. (2002). Mind the gap: Why do people act environmentally and what are the barriers to pro-environmental behavior. *Environmental Education Research*, *8*, 239–260.

MacGregor, D., Slovic, P., Mason, R. G., & Detweiler, J. (1994). Perceived risks of radioactive waste transport through Oregon: Results of a statewide survey. *Risk Analysis*, *14*, 5–14. https://doi.org/10.1111/j.1539-6924.1994.tb00022.x

Maibach, E., Roser-Renouf, C., & Leiserowitz, A. (2009). *Global warming's six Americas 2009: An audience segmentation analysis*. www.climatechangecommunication.org/images/files/GlobalWarmingsSixAmericas 2009c.pdf

Morgan, J. (1997). *Geo-graphing: Writing the world in geography classrooms*. Institution of Education.

Norgaard, K. M. (2009). *Cognitive and behavioral challenges in responding to climate change. Policy research working paper; no. WPS 4940*. World Bank. © World

Bank. https://openknowledge.worldbank.org/handle/10986/4134 License: CC BY 3.0 IGO.
Olson, M. L., Jr. (1965). *The logic of collective action: Public goods and the theory of groups*. Harvard University Press.
Osbaldiston, R., & Sheldon, K. M. (2002). Social dilemmas and sustainability: Promoting peoples' motivation to "cooperate with the future". In P. Schmuck & W. P. Schultz (Eds.), *Psychology of sustainable development* (pp. 37–57). Kluwer Academic Publishers. https://doi.org/10.1007/978-1-4615-0995-0_3
Ostrom, E. (1990). *Governing the commons: The evolution of institutions for collective action*. Cambridge University Press.
Schudson, M. (1982). *Discovering the news: A social history of American newspapers*. Basic Books.
Schumacher, E. F. (1995). *A guide for the perplexed*. Random House.
Schwartz, S. (1977). Normative influences on altruism. In L. Berkowitz (Ed.), *Advances in experimental social psychology*. Academic Press.
Siddiqui, R. N., & Pandey, J. (2003). Coping with environmental stressors by urban slum dwellers. *Environment and Behavior*, *35*(5), 589–604.
Taylor, S. E., & Brown, J. D. (1988). Illusion and well-being: A social psychological perspective on mental health. *Psychological Bulletin*, *103*(2), 193–210.
Ungar, S. (1994). Apples and oranges: Probing the attitude-behaviour relationship for the environment. *Canadian Review of Sociology & Anthropology*, *31*, 288–304.
Vining, J., & Ebreo, A. (2002). Emerging theoretical and methodological perspective on conservation behaviour. In R. Bechtel, A. Churchman (Eds.), *Handbook of environmental psychology* (pp. 541–558). Wiley.
Wade-Benzoni, K. A. (1999). Thinking about the future: An intergenerational perspective on the conflict and compatibility between economic and environmental interests. *American Behavioral Scientist*, *42*(8), 1393–1405.
Weinstein, N. D. (1980). Unrealistic optimism about future life events. *Journal of Personality and Social Psychology*, *39*, 806–820.
Weinstein, N. D., Klotz, M. L., & Sandman, P. M. (1988). Optimistic biases in public perceptions of the risks from radon. *American Journal of Public Health*, *78*, 796–800.

6 Social and Individual Concerns in the Life and Work of Mahatma Gandhi

An Informal Essay

Girishwar Misra

Gandhi, born in the late 19th century, was a selfless practitioner of Karma Yoga, who greatly influenced Indian society from the early 1900s to the mid-20th century. He relentlessly pursued liberation for his own land. He advocated for political and social reform. His life exemplified an extraordinary and unparalleled demonstration of human accountability. He held the belief that thoughts possessed significant influence and emphasized the importance of equality and human values (Kool & Agrawal, 2020). Gandhi recognized and valued both the positive attributes and limitations of Indian civilization. He advanced a comprehensive alternative to both communism and capitalism. Gandhi's writings including *'The Story of My Experiments with Truth,' 'Hind Swaraj,' 'Mangal Prabhat,'* and *'Constructive Programme'* provide a comprehensive account of his views, principles, commitments, and observations. He famously stated, 'My life is my message,' thereby exemplifying integrity, bravery, and fearlessness. His ideology was profoundly entrenched in his spiritual ideas and values. He stood for nonviolence, truth, self-discipline, and minimalism, among other principles. He practiced and encouraged many forms of self-control, such as fasting, celibacy, and non-attachment, in order to achieve inner peace and self-actualization. Gandhi also highlighted the importance of physical labor and service to others, seeing them as honorable sacrifices that result in satisfaction and good health. Mahatma Gandhi was an exceptional individual who extensively delved into different facets of personal and societal existence, both on a global scale and within his own country (Kool & Agrawal, 2022). His abstract principles, including truth, faith, nonviolence, and non-stealing, were rooted in his personal encounters. He was inspired by the Bhagavad Gita (BG) and other religious writings, combining lessons from other religions into his own philosophy (Gandhi, 1945c). This chapter explores the experiential journey, philosophical framework, and perspectives on individual and society of Mahatma Gandhi.

A Remarkable Existence: Life and Philosophy of Mahatma Gandhi

Mahatma Gandhi's life was characterized by various challenges and triumphs in the realms of physical, mental, social, and spiritual domains. His

DOI: 10.4324/9781003461302-9

upbringing and life experiences during his formative years influenced his childhood, equipping him with the necessary skills and knowledge to pursue a prosperous career as a lawyer. His English education expanded his intellectual perspectives and nurtured empathy and compassion. Upon his arrival in India, he lacked any instant inclination to achieve independence for India. He initiated his philanthropic endeavors in South Africa, championing the underprivileged and providing assistance to those in need. His first act marked the beginning of a nearly eight-year Satyagraha. Gandhi led a multifaceted existence and became as a prominent figure in the challenging political landscape of South Africa.

After encountering various religions and cultures, he emerged as a leader who propelled civilization forward. By withstanding the allure of temptations, he placed human values at the forefront and remained steadfast in upholding them. Mahatma Gandhi held the belief that thoughts possess the power to transform lives. He promoted global egalitarianism, asserting that God safeguards all of creation and that each individual assumes the role of a guardian. Gandhi advocated for autonomy, concord, and self-governance while accepting the merits and limitations of his culture. His solution to communism and capitalism was a comprehensive system. Gandhi's expansive and analytical perspective was effective in both South Africa and India. Following the footsteps of Gandhi, Nelson Mandela, Martin Luther King Jr., and Suu Kyi advocated for the rights and well-being of their respective communities in south Africa, North America and Myanmar, respectively.

Spiritual Approach to Life

Gandhi's work is groundbreaking. He held a belief in God, possessed a spiritual inclination, and adhered to many perspectives and practices. Gandhi advocated for and adhered to a range of basic principles and undertakings, including the following: *silence, abstinence from food, self-control, veneration for the five elements, devotion to a higher power, celibacy, nonviolence, compassion, minimalism,* and *honesty*. Gandhi advocated for the incorporation of environmental and social constraints and consequences into our living situations. He observed Yudhishthira's melancholy following his victory in the Mahabharata and recognized its pointlessness. Human spirituality reaches its highest point at the pinnacle.

Attaining Gandhi's practical objectives proved to be arduous. He encountered shame, terror, loss, danger, instability, and uncertainty. He thoroughly examined and experimented with all of these principles, and once they proved effective, he devoted his entire life to them. The presence of numerous temptations inside the world made it challenging to uphold one's self-worth. Gandhi's self-control and sincere devotion to God were cultivated through spiritual experiences and mental fortitude.

Gandhi's definition of civilization is the act of fulfilling one's duties, which necessitate adherence to principles. Exercising control of one's thoughts and emotions is an integral aspect of adhering to regulations. It represents the advancement and development of human society. Gandhi advocated for self-restraint and refraining from undue indulgence. He argued that moral and spiritual development allows access to material and cultural resources. It is advisable to not surpass these restrictions as having more desires leads to increased luxury, which hinders personal growth and advancement. Gandhi believed that the pursuit of material wealth or increased desires would not contribute to the betterment of the world.

Mahatma Gandhi practiced yoga on a daily basis. He observed *Yamas* and *Niyamas*. He believed that 'to pursue the truth in the divine form, one must initially adhere to several commitments.' These commitments encompass integrity, non-aggression, abstaining from theft, celibacy, and *aparigraha* (non-possession), among others. Celibacy regulates desires and emotions, nonviolence restricts feelings of anger, animosity, and rage, and *aparigraha* eradicates the act of amassing possessions. He believed that honest individuals enjoy a connection with the divine by refraining from engaging in theft. Gandhi noted that truth and nonviolence are fundamental principles that form the basis of all religions (Gandhi, 1945b).

Gandhi believed that fasting was a great way to cleanse the body, mind, and soul. It entails restricting the senses while liberating the soul to some extent. According to Gandhi, fasting helps us do our jobs more successfully and attain our goals. He initially fasted in 1913 at the Phoenix Ashram in South Africa as a kind of penance for the moral downfall of two ashram inmates. He also fasted for two weeks before his death to promote communal harmony (Parel, 2007). Gandhi fasted 30 times during the course of his life. He also believed that silence is an essential aspect of spiritual practice for individuals seeking truth. He held that humans have a natural tendency to exaggerate, suppress, or overstate the truth, whether deliberately or unknowingly, and that quiet is crucial for overcoming this weakness. According to him adopting a silent attitude permits the soul to achieve clarity and a deeper comprehension of its journey, causing everything that was previously unclear or perplexing to become crystal plain. Mahatma Gandhi emphasized the importance of *Brahmacharya Vrat*, which involves exercising control over the senses—mind, speech, and body. According to Gandhi, it is impossible to attain self-realization without self-restraint. He believed that true Brahmacharya can only be achieved when thoughts are regulated to the extent that no desire develops.

Inspirations From Bhagavad Gita

In his autobiography, titled *The Story of My Experiments of Truth*, Gandhi mentions that he initially encountered the BG by reading Edwin Arnold's English version, which was gifted to him by English theosophists. The concluding lines of Chapter 2 had a significant impact on him. Gandhi thought the BG was an essential text. This belief grew over time, and he considered it the best book on philosophy. This book was helpful to him during times of despair. His devotion to the BG grew with time. He felt compelled to investigate further. He began trying to understand the content of the BG in its original Sanskrit through translations and memorized its lines. Gandhi has stated, 'For me, that book became an adult guide of conduct. The concepts such as *aparigraha* and equanimity, struck a chord with me. How can I cultivate equanimity? Should I burn the house and go on pilgrimage?' The immediate response was that pilgrimage could not be performed without first burning down the house. Gandhi claims that 'English law helped me here. The definition of the word trustee was very clear. Despite the trustee's possession of crores of rupees, he owns none of it. Mumukshu should act like this. I learned this from Geeta. It was evident to me, like a lamp, that in order to become aparigrahi, or equated, a change of heart is required' (Gandhi, 1945c). Gandhi was particularly struck by the concept of *Sthitaprajna* (a person with steady wisdom) and *Bhakta* (devotee) in the 12 chapter of the BG. He had discovered a way to live life. Gandhi began practicing celibacy in 1906. He believed that celibacy begins with physical restriction. However, in genuine celibacy, there should be no filthiness of thought. A full Brahmachari does not have malicious ideas, even in his dreams.

Gandhi claimed that exercising moderation in diet, including fasting, has improved his health and self-control. He observed that in order to get positive results when fasting, one must continually limit oneself and conquer the urge for taste. Individuals who fast stay quiet during the fasting period, but they do not receive spiritual nutrition. Fasting and other forms of self-restraint help people achieve abstinence, but they are not the only components.

In the concluding section of his autobiography, Mahatma Gandhi advocates for a spiritual approach to life, emphasizing the value of truth as a symbol of honor and respect. To have a direct contact with a profound incarnation of truth like Satyanarayan, one must first develop a true and self-realized love for all living beings. Furthermore, someone who wishes to do so must be involved in all aspects of life. He says 'This is precisely why my commitment to the truth has prompted me to participate in politics. It is crucial to highlight that religion and politics are not related; those who are unfamiliar with religion may not grasp this, but I have no reservations or emotions of shame in stating this remark' (Bilgrami, 2002).

Significance of Self-Purification

Union with all living beings is not possible without self-purification. Nonviolence, or dharma, cannot be practiced without self-purification. An unclean soul is unable to perceive God. Thus, purification is required in all parts of one's life path. This purification is possible because of the intimate relationship between the individual and the collective, in which the purity of one equals the purification of many. However, the path to purification is tough. Purity entails freeing oneself from thoughts, speech, and actions motivated by attachment and hatred. Despite regular efforts, he did not achieve this level of constant purity in the initial period. He noted:

> As a result, I am not swayed by others' praise; in fact, it frequently causes me significant distress. I believe that overcoming one's inner turmoil is more difficult than conquering the globe through armed conflict. Even after landing in India, I discovered hidden defects inside myself, which makes me feel ashamed. Nonetheless, I am resolute and committed. I have embraced the search of truth and will continue to do so. However, I am aware that the journey ahead will be arduous. To make progress, I must humble myself and become insignificant. Salvation is only possible when one willingly humbles oneself. Humility is the highest expression of nonviolence. With this in mind, I'll end these remarks by asking for humility and seeking help from the world.

The BG promotes altruistic dedication, and Mahatma Gandhi maintained that actions without renunciation lead to enslavement. Renunciation entails assisting others, and when carried out with genuine selflessness, there is no connection. Hence, actions should be performed for the sake of serving others. Gandhi regarded the Ishavasyopanishad as a significant advancement in knowledge and chose to name his initial mantra 'Gyan Pradeep,' signifying the enlightenment of knowledge.

The entire world is occupied by God, and as a result, no one has authority over anything. When we do not have the right, non-attachment is normal. Taking this principle a step further, Gandhi observed that when a man pays too much attention to the outcome and constantly broods about it, he begins to deviate from the path of action and becomes impatient. Then he becomes angry. In such a situation, he does a variety of inappropriate things. He is unable to complete his tasks because he is preoccupied with his senses. As noted by Gandhi, 'He who gives up his effort falls, and he who gives up the result rises.' However, giving up fruits does not imply that a person should be absolutely neutral toward fruits. He should also be aware of the forthcoming consequences of his activity. Similarly, there should be information regarding the steps necessary to complete that task, as well as the capacity required. Being prepared in this manner allows a person to remain interested in his task even when he does not want the fruits. Gandhi believed that achieving self-realization, which is the pursuit of inner peace and tranquility, was unattainable without the presence of God. The BG provides deep understanding, but it primarily appeals to one's emotions and should be understood on a heartfelt level. The basic idea of the BG is renunciation (Gandhi, 1945c).

Nonviolence and Satyagraha

Gandhi, a pacifist, philosopher, and statesman, held the conviction that nonviolence was the supreme moral principle and advocated for unconditional love toward oneself and all living creatures (Kool & Agrawal, 2020). He steadfastly adhered to nonviolence even in the face of extreme adversity. He interpreted the epic 'Mahabharata' as a narrative illustrating the equivalence of conflict and victory. As everyone knows, the BG is Krishna's teachings to Arjuna on the battlefield. It includes elements such as philosophy, spirituality, and divinity. Gandhi regards Krishna as empirical, pure knowledge, and Arjuna as the appropriate deed. He has freely acknowledged its significance in his life. During his time in prison, he developed a Gujarati version of BG. He saw nishkam yoga as the focus.

The unwavering commitment to the BG transformed this scruffy and frail lawyer into one of the world's greatest leaders (Gandhi, 1945c). On August 16, 1908, 2,000 Indians burned South African credentials in the Transvaal. This protest against the 'Black Act' marked the beginning of 'Satyagraha' (Gandhi, 1928). When Gandhi returned to India, he effectively used it against the British. Gandhi called it 'Atma Shakti' (Soul Power). The discovery of the Gita was the result of Gandhi's dramatic change in life. According to his secretary, Mahadev Desai:

> Every hour of Gandhi's life was spent consciously living the message of the Gita. He was fearless and possessed incredible moral courage, as nonviolence and cowardice do not go together. He saw himself as Arjuna. Mantras and reference texts were discovered. Then, as energy gradually developed, experiments in life began. Controlled the diet and achieved the goal of reducing oneself to a minimum. We began an attempt to fulfill everyone's interests through unselfish service. Aparigraha, or keeping only what is required, adhered to this guideline. Self-strength and independence can only be achieved by letting go of the ego. That's when creativity emerges.

A Satyagrahi must act courageously. Gandhi effortlessly exemplified the renowned qualities of deliberation, eloquence, and unwavering concentration that are associated with the Mahatma, even in the face of several distractions that would have deterred most people. Gandhi believed in the significance of identifying and taking into account the environment and societal limits in our living places, as well as highlighting human spirituality. Gandhi's commitment to nonviolence, as well as his conviction in the power of truth and selflessness, shaped his activities and influenced leaders around the world. Despite various hurdles and personal faults, Gandhi was unwavering in his pursuit of truth and humility. He authored *Hind Swaraj* (Gandhi, 1938), a critique of Western civilization that puts forth an alternative framework for governing India (Bhargava, 2022).

Gandhi's profound affection for India was widely recognized prior to his arrival. His practice of Satyagraha, fasting, humble way of life, and comprehensive socioeconomic approach served as a source of inspiration for the nation. In 1915, he established the inaugural ashram at Kochrab and spearheaded the Satyagraha movement in Motihari, Bihar, in 1916. He addressed social concerns and upheld moral values such as spirituality, honesty, and righteousness. Gandhi, a prominent leader in the Swadeshi and Sarvodaya movements, selected Wardha, a rural town in India, as his destination due to his conviction that empowering India's rural population was crucial for the country's development. He also recognized that attaining independence necessitated not only a shift in governmental authority but also the enhancement of the well-being of all Indians.

Mahatma Gandhi condemned seven societal vices and established an innovative research facility in Sevagram. The Indian National Congress orchestrated numerous gatherings in Wardha, igniting the 'Quit India' movement. In 1946, Gandhi made a visit to Noakhali with the intention of restoring peace during the riots.

Envisioning an Independent India

Mahatma Gandhi brought a human touch to Indian politics and promoted active involvement of citizens in political affairs. He skillfully managed the delicate relationship between India's quest for independence and its social fabric by actively involving the public and giving importance to the well-being of the people. He employed various strategies, for freeing the nation from British rule (Gandhi, 1945d). He referred to his life as 'the experiment with truth' and extensively studied the history of Satyagraha.

Upon his return to South Africa from London in 1909, Gandhi wrote down his sociopolitical thoughts in Gujarati, which were subsequently published as 'Hind Swaraj' (Gandhi, 1938). However, the police in Bombay seized the publication. Following the conclusion of his tenure in South Africa, Gandhi returned to India in 1915, and subsequently, this book was published in English. On this particular instance, the British government decided to refrain from expressing disapproval, so enabling the material to be disseminated to a broader audience. There have been a mix of favorable and unfavorable remarks regarding this book, both within the country and on a global scale. Gandhi, however, stated that his ideals were profoundly ingrained in his spirit. In 1938, Mahatma Gandhi released his book in the English language through the periodical *Aryan Path*, which was based in Sevagram, Wardha. He stated that, despite facing numerous obstacles over the past three decades, he saw no reason to modify the book in light of those experiences. He strongly believed that the prevalent culture in major Western civilizations, especially in Europe and North America, was harmful to humanity. He also discovered that the ancient religious and ethical culture was more captivating. According to his viewpoint, the British withdrawal from India did not succeed in fulfilling Swaraj's aspiration for self-governance. They saw no advantage in embracing their ideals and civilization. Gandhi held that safeguarding India's spiritual essence is the utmost priority (Bhargava, 2022; Gandhi, 1945d). Gandhi articulates his profound skepticism and wariness toward Western education, science, and institutions. He delineated the adverse consequences of railroads, courts, hospitals, and similar establishments. Gandhi ultimately embraced the notion of spiritual self-governance, with the objective of attaining Sarvodaya.

Idea of Swaraja

Swaraja refers to an individual's psychological condition that is based on principles such as Satyagraha, *Atma Bal* (soul force), and Karma (Bhattacharya, 1954). In order to use that power, it is imperative to wholeheartedly adopt Swadeshi. It is incumbent upon us, either morally or legally, to do so. Gandhi's concepts of civilization are particularly relevant in the contemporary period characterized by widespread violence, brutality, and intolerance.

Intellectuals may debate the effectiveness of Gandhi's nonviolence, his opposition to mechanization, and the importance of Satyagraha. Nevertheless, it is widely recognized that *Hind Swaraj* serves as the focal point of Gandhi's life and career (Bhargava, 2022). Moreover, it is imperative to comprehend that the use of non-cooperation, civil disobedience, and Satyagraha played a vital role in shaping the unique nature of India's fight for independence (Gandhi, 1945a). Historical evidence indicates that the nation acknowledged the advantages of self-governance, although it did not possess the requisite dedication to fully adopt that cultural principle and aspiration. Consequently, Gandhi's perspectives were perceived as inconsequential in the contemporary context. The focus on effectiveness in Western scientific methods and technologies is leading to a growing number of inconsistencies being identified. Gandhi held the belief that the pursuit of wealth, rather than the preservation of labor, was the main driving force for the emergence of machines. Consequently, he endeavored to limit the quantity of instruments. He expressed his disapproval of the unwavering desire of wealth. 'Hind Swaraj' acts as a catalyst for human awareness (Bhargava, 2022), directing us toward the road of the future.

Gandhi expressed disapproval of the parliamentary system and contended that Western civilization's emphasis on materialistic pursuits and physical well-being as the primary measure of happiness and worthiness is flawed. This perspective lacks a solid basis in policy or theology and is rooted in the relentless pursuit of bodily gratification. The British employed persuasive tactics and charismatic leadership to accomplish their objectives, but the Indians were motivated by inciting conflicts. Gandhi held the belief that corruption was progressively destroying India's fundamental ideals and creating a growing disconnect from the divine.

Gandhi vehemently resisted the British teachings that India lacked a separate identity. He declared that 'this accusation is completely unwarranted.' According to him, before British colonization in India, the Indian population was cohesive, sharing a common national identity, ideas, and cultural lifestyle. Consequently, the British established a cohesive country in this area.

Gandhi argues that although God has set physical limitations on humans through the construction of the human body, humanity has successfully surpassed these constraints through various methods. Humans possess cognitive faculties that enable them to understand and recognize the existence of a supreme being, commonly referred to as God. Nevertheless, humans have employed it to intentionally dismiss or overlook the existence or significance of God. Gandhi maintained his conviction that in India, individuals of diverse religious faiths can peacefully coexist, and that religious disparities will not undermine the unity of this nation (Gandhi, 1945d). The individuals belonging to the Hindu, Muslim, Parsi, and Christian communities, who have decided to permanently reside in this country, are considered 'Mulki,' which refers to native inhabitants (Gandhi, 1942). These Mulki individuals are fellow citizens who are required to live together harmoniously for the overall welfare of the nation. Various religions provide unique routes to a shared destination. Individuals should possess a comprehensive understanding of their religious beliefs and actively put them into practice. Mahatma Gandhi had the belief that civilization serves as the medium through which individuals fulfill their responsibilities. Meeting these obligations necessitates the preservation of one's cognitive faculties and consciousness. This indicates a highly developed state.

Gandhi promoted the utilization of Satyagraha as a method for attaining Swaraj, which is founded on the principles of truth, celibacy, and fearlessness. Satyagraha is a potent instrument that engenders satisfaction for both the practitioner and the recipient (Gandhi, 1945c). Gandhi had the belief that English education had subjected the nation to a state of domination. Education's presence has resulted in an increase in hubris, anger, and subservience. He holds the belief that genuine education purifies, calms, and fosters fairness in the mind (Gandhi, 1951). The human mind functions based on inherent principles, and individuals possess control over their senses. They possess genuine feelings, abhor immoral activities, and exhibit equal levels of compassion for others as they do for themselves. Mahatma Gandhi advocates for the conservation and incorporation of all languages. The Hindus, Muslims, Parsis, and Christians residing in this nation are fellow citizens who must cohabit harmoniously for their mutual advantage (Gandhi, 1942). Various religions provide unique approaches to attaining a common objective. Individuals should possess a comprehensive view of their religious beliefs and actively put them into practice.

Swaraj in Ideas

While the Congress voted on the 'Complete Swaraja' resolution in Lahore in 1929, it is likely coincidental that Professor Krishna Chandra Bhattacharya, a renowned philosopher, happened to be engaged in a discussion on 'Swaraj in Ideas' under British rule (Bhattacharya, 1954). He emphasized the significance of fostering a change in mindset. He championed India's liberation from the cultural subjugation perpetuated by the British educational system. He asserted that the domain of thoughts and emotions was compelling Indians to embrace a novel, perhaps polarizing mentality. He contended that in the realm of politics, the matter of exercising dominion over others is readily apparent, and it is crucial to counteract it by rendering it perceptible. The impact of different foreign ideas on cognition varies, but it is extensive and has a significant effect, even if it is concealed and influences the subconscious. The contradiction lies in the fact that the prosperous individuals in India during that period possessed a profound longing for and perceived this foreign culture as favorable, due to their apprehension of retrogressing or lagging behind. Bhattacharya noted the absence of inventive methods in British education when it came to studying ancient history, contemporary circumstances, and future goals. This resulted in a lack of awareness or curiosity about India, while our understanding of other countries grew. Consequently, we turned to Western sources for trustworthy information. Lord Macaulay's successful strategic initiatives in the Indian educational domain were accountable for this state of affairs.

After gaining independence, during the post-colonial period, the idea of a unified world, commonly known as 'one globe' and later referred to as globalization, became increasingly popular, akin to a fashionable trend. The amalgamation of cultural plurality and relativism led to cultural subservience rather than autonomy and liberty. The notion of European integration was believed to be globally applicable. We have acknowledged the authenticity of other individuals' viewpoints on Indian society and culture. India's original paradigm was substituted with an alternative paradigm, leading to cultural oblivion and a transformation in individuals' perspectives and cognition. We have gradually become disconnected from our own selves and from our abundant intellectual and cultural legacy to the extent that its significance has disappeared. We neglect and omit it from the entirety of the educational process. We will only endorse a strategy that is beneficial to Western nations, provided that we provide our consent. We were unable to identify the underlying essence of India.

Self-renewal necessitates an ongoing and fluid process of self-exploration. In order to properly assimilate external knowledge, we must actively get, assimilate, and enhance our comprehension of it, rather than passively accepting and replicating it without discerning analysis.

On August 15, 1947, India achieved independence, and Prime Minister Nehru delivered a famous speech symbolizing the liberation of the nation's spirit. He asserted that India is presently engaged in the process of self-exploration. His objective was to eliminate the country's 'poverty, ignorance, and inequality of opportunity.' He asserted that India is both cognizant and autonomous. We take great pride in a number of our past achievements. We have significantly enhanced our influence and achieved remarkable progress in the domains of knowledge, research, and technology. Nevertheless, the current conditions have undergone a transformation, and democracy is currently stable. However, our capacity for creativity and intellectual engagement has been somewhat restricted, and we are uncertain about our link to our indigenous roots. Indian conceptions exhibit a remarkable range of intellectual diversity and a liberal mindset that can be considered on par with, if not surpassing, ideas from other civilizations. The incorporation of multidisciplinary and multisectoral approach was given priority. Shastra, mythology, and experimentation were closely interconnected. We have severed our connection with these sources and placed ourselves in isolation. A significant portion of our society's well-educated individuals are either uninformed of or resistant to acquiring knowledge about indigenous origin.

Gandhi's Cultural Vision

We have not successfully approached tradition and history with a discerning and unbiased perspective. Instead of passively accepting Western ideas without critical thought, we should actively participate in a meaningful exchange between Eastern and Western cultures, respecting their unique characteristics, in order to attain a harmonious integration of different viewpoints. Bhattacharya held the belief that the incorporation of foreign elements has stripped Indian education of its conventional underpinnings. He ardently advocates for the significance of cultivating indigenous knowledge and raising awareness nationwide. While we condemn the caste system, it is crucial to acknowledge that Western-educated Indians have established a novel caste that exhibits greater intolerance than any previous caste and continuously rejects novel concepts. In order to transcend the caste divide and foster a stronger bond between Indians and their cultural heritage, it is imperative to provide a cultural environment that fosters the development and assimilation of Indigenous talent, while also allowing sufficient time for this process to unfold.

The notion of 'Swaraj in Ideas (Thoughts)' was overshadowed by the amalgamation of colonial legacy and globalization. Culture encompasses the actualization of our creative capacity and serves as the basis for their advancement. Cultural achievements are acquired, cultivated, and transmitted via subsequent generations. Evolution and progress occur as information, talents, ideas, and other kinds of art undergo a transformative process. Culture is a dynamic phenomenon that has an impact on every person. Proficiency in language and effective communication are essential for the success of this endeavor. Culture and communication are inherently interconnected. The abundance of thoughts and concepts encompassed by language profoundly influence our perception and understanding of the universe. India's ancient knowledge history encompasses the development of a wide array of knowledge, encompassing both tangible and intangible aspects. *Aano Bhadrah Kratvo Yantu Vishwatah* fosters the embrace and integration of diverse ideas, hence fostering inclusiveness within Indian culture. It has been asserted that truth is singular, however, individuals perceive it from various viewpoints:

Ekam Sat Viprah, Bahudha Vadanti. There is a commonly held belief that there is a robust and interconnected relationship between the individual and the collective, as well as the body and the universe *Yatpinde tad brahmande*. The Shanti Path of the Vedas encompasses a diverse range of elements, such as water, earth, air, fire, and ether. Tranquility and silence are essential for all individuals. It is important for everyone to display courtesy toward one other. '*Vasudhaiva Kutumbakam*' sought to foster empathy by bringing together the entire global community and its residents, highlighting the significance of collective cooperation and the exchange of ideas. Beneath it all was a profound understanding and compassion for people. Philanthropy and communal solidarity hold great significance in Indian society. Our cultural inheritance exerts a beneficial impact on our personal growth, and by establishing a connection with it, we can uncover the path to an independent and autonomous mindset, as exemplified by the teachings of Swaraj.

Gandhi possessed a comprehensive and inclusive social outlook that encompassed all individuals. His perspective on civilization surpassed cultural boundaries, perceiving the 'East' and 'West' as intricately interconnected and continuously merging in his cognitive processes. He maintained that the elimination of modernity would result in equality between the East and West.

Gandhi strongly condemned contemporary Western society and its desire to extend its global influence. He believed that an authentic Western culture and a distinct Eastern culture would emerge, creating an intrinsic link between the two. Although he did not consider himself an expert on non-modern or non-Western nations, his deep skepticism toward modernity led him to provide a harsh critique of it. Gandhi's beliefs underwent a process of development in response to his experiences, rendering his interpretation applicable in certain circumstances. Nevertheless, it is challenging to offer a solitary and compelling interpretation of Gandhi's multifaceted life and actions. Nevertheless, it seems that Gandhi's disapproval of the contemporary Western society was driven by his adoption of the secular scientific approach. He held the belief that only a transcendent spiritual perspective was advantageous and therefore acceptable to humanity. Secularism has placed great importance on science. Irrespective of the various interpretations of Gandhi's refusal to embrace modern science as a result of bias and superstition, it is crucial to acknowledge the limitations of present-day scientific knowledge. His main source of inspiration is the urban-industrial landscape. Modern science is based on secularism, which upholds a clear separation between intellect and information, and emotion and morality. Likewise, the researcher or investigator should maintain an emotional detachment from the subjects involved in the study.

Modern science has integrated various elements of present-day existence, such as a practical approach toward nature, leading to its detachment from religious or moral concerns and a diminishing of emotional significance. Gandhi held the belief that secular movements in nature, society, and history will not achieve success. Acquiring completely unbiased and morally neutral knowledge that is not influenced by the person acquiring it is an unattainable endeavor. Gandhi is deeply preoccupied with technological advancements. Observers have noted that recent technical advancements have led to a strong focus on practicality and control in contemporary research. The advent of modernity provides a platform for the expansion of technology. It is important to remember that physical science is the basis of contemporary secular science. This foundation also supported the study of biological organisms. This perspective views modern civilization as mechanistic. Autonomy should not be granted to technology as it disguises itself as science and encourages societal transformations that undermine the fundamental human and organic characteristics of individuals, communities, and the environment. Regrettably, there is no escape from this intricate technological maze. Technology has the capacity to resolve the issues it creates. Gandhi's criticism is specifically directed on technocracy, not technology itself, which is of utmost importance to emphasize. From this perspective, the 'charkha' surpasses a mill in performance. He advocates for the preservation of the human race and the independence of individuals.

Mahatma Gandhi challenged political authority and resisted the social evolution theories of the 19th century. He dismissed notions of selfhood, utility, materialism, and the dichotomy between 'individual' and 'social' in his nation-building efforts. He held the belief that collective knowledge bestowed individuals with consciousness. The nascent Indian critique, influenced by Gandhi, should seek novel prospects within its historical context. 'Similar to the revered poet, I endorse the notion of unhindered air circulation. I would rather not have shrubbery.'

The concepts put forward by Mahatma Gandhi regarding the interplay between the individual and society hold great significance. He saw that Indian culture, as a whole, was based on traditional ideas and concepts that originated among the general population. This society harbored concerns regarding modern science, which introduced novel methods of subjugation and brutality. Gandhi dismantled the divisions between religion and politics, as well as between objective and method. He firmly believed that individuals without moral ideals could not make any positive contributions to society. In 'Hind Swaraj,' Gandhi highlighted the internal struggle that emerged among Indians in their resistance against British power and the British themselves. This exemplifies our inclination for an independent English government as opposed to a monarch who is exclusively English. You desire the essence or spirit of the tiger, rather than the physical existence of the creature itself. This signifies your aspiration for India to assimilate into British culture, and if accomplished, it will be recognized as authentic England rather than Hindustan. This does not align with the Swaraj vision that I had expected. The allusion pertains to page 12 of the book 'Hind Swaraj' (Gandhi, 1938).

This problem presents itself in several ways. The speech delivered by Mahatma Gandhi in 1916 to commemorate the establishment of Banaras

Hindu University is remarkable. He strongly criticized lectures delivered in languages other than the audience's native tongue, contending that they were excessively challenging for comprehension. Simultaneously, he established the foundation for an educational institution. He strongly held the belief that students should get education in their native language. He expressed that our languages are crucial for our expression. In order to achieve success, it is imperative that our languages are of exceptional quality. Moreover, he lamented the fact that scientific information is not considered the most precious asset of the nation. Despite a span of 73 years since gaining independence, the condition has persisted without any significant alteration. We have not elevated our nation's languages to the degree they merit. Consequently, the two linguistic civilizations existed beside each other without any form of communication or connection.

Gandhi believed that the struggle for independence encompassed a broader objective than the mere establishment of Indian governance. He fundamentally regarded it as a means for ethical metamorphosis. Moreover, he regarded politics as the fundamental basis of ethical principles. Both capitalism and communism originated in Europe, with communism emerging as a result of the transformation of capitalism. Ultimately, in the 20th century, socialist regimes, which were once presented as potential alternatives to capitalism, either collapsed or eventually merged with it. Gandhi demonstrates the limitations of Marxism and puts out an alternate proposition. It is important to mention that he conducted an assessment and discovered the underlying cause of the country's dependence on an unquestioning fixation with foreign cultures, while disregarding the superior characteristics of its own heritage and traditions. The fascination with English and Western civilization experienced substantial acceleration. Gandhi thought that civilization is characterized by conduct that can guide individuals toward fulfilling their obligations. Self-discipline, ethics, and the pursuit of a meaningful life are interconnected. Consequently, his objective was to establish a country founded on the ideals of belief, veracity, and ethics, rather than merely removing the British, who were unable to differentiate between economic and moral principles.

Gandhi's elucidations and evaluations of modernity are dynamic. They prioritize the disassembly of machinery, alterations in lifestyle, optimization, and the condition of rural communities. It is imperative to perceive violence as a tool or weapon in contemporary society. Gandhi's ideology is characterized by his resolute dedication to the well-being and advancement of the nation. He asserted that the utilization of imported materials leads to economic adversity for native weavers and artisans. Humans distinguish themselves from animals by adhering to principles of social equity and morality, rather than being only driven by self-centered impulses. Therefore, it is crucial to prioritize the favorable attributes while reducing or eliminating the unfavorable ones. Gandhi's endorsement of Swadeshi is based on the universal principles of altruism, pacifism, and affection. He harbored a profound animosity for the period of Western hegemony. He advocated for a worldview that was devoid of oppression, urbanization, industrialization, or technological advancements, but instead focused on the principles of faith and science. He remarked that his town is the only provider of his practical need, while the entire globe satisfies his spiritual desires.

Gandhi, being a social scientist, was dedicated to the pursuit of truth. He possessed a vast academic foundation. He derived his ideas from both Indian and Western sources. He presented an innovative option for India, analyzed from the perspective of a social worker. The primary tenets his writing underscores are those of veracity, the quest for veracity, community, individual fortitude, individual integrity, and self-control. He believed that human activities were all-encompassing. Initially, man displays primal tendencies similar to those of animals. However, as he developed his thoughts, he embraced virtuous qualities associated with being human. Ultimately, man contains an inherent longing for divinity. His primary concentration was on cultivating his spiritual and mental abilities. Gandhi's worldview was characterized by his profound reverence for truth as a sacred entity and his conviction in the presence of truth within humanity. He held the belief that every individual possesses an inherent inclination toward benevolence. He highly valued mankind and its inherent virtues and actively promoted the development and enhancement of each person by discussing a change in mindset.

Mahatma Gandhi endorsed various established institutions as a means to articulate his beliefs regarding God, religion, morality, and nonviolence. He specifically emphasized the initial verse of the 'Ishavasyopanishad,' which asserts that the divine essence is present in all manifestations of existence, regardless of whether they are animate or inanimate. 'Find satisfaction in your current possessions and avoid pursuing the success of others.'

He experienced a deeply significant encounter. 'What benefits would you acquire by minimizing your possessions and cultivating less cravings? I am not interested in the indulgences of this world, but rather in the improvement and advancement of my fellow human beings. To experience true joy, one must be willing to make sacrifices.' He emphasized the notion of trusteeship. He led practical and innovative initiatives at the community level, specifically focusing on small-scale and artisanal sectors. They perceived Khadi as an emblem of mankind's victory over technology. He expressed strong disapproval of the reliance on imported commodities rather than domestically produced goods. He strongly held the belief that economics and ethics should be in perfect agreement. He often advocated for individuals in good physical condition to actively seek job and emphasized that sustenance should be obtained via diligent labor. He cautioned against taking free items. Individuals experiencing hunger should be provided with sustenance, but it should be obtained via exertion and diligent effort.

Indian literature demonstrates the profound impact of Mahatma Gandhi on Indian policy, practice, and innovation. Remembering Gandhi's principles and elucidations is crucial for reestablishing our sense of identity (Hardiman, 2003). His perspectives underwent a gradual transformation as he became familiar with Gandhi's ideals, leading to the development of a unique and deep understanding. Gandhi's perspectives gradually evolved to prioritize rationality and the welfare of humanity. As a result, he had a change in his beliefs, which he has now fully embraced. Gandhi delivered speeches on a wide range of subjects, encompassing truth, nonviolence, refraining from theft, fasting, celibacy, character, morality, *Satyagraha* (nonviolent resistance), trusteeship, *Swadeshi* (support for local industries), *Swaraj* (self-governance), health, cleanliness, *Sarvodaya* (welfare of all), *Harijan* (individuals from lower castes), *Antyodaya* (uplifting the poorest), untouchability, religion, equality among all religions, God, and fearlessness. He engaged in the study, debate, and practical application of spirituality, work, ashrams, and civil disobedience (Gandhi, 1945a). He was a trailblazer in the field of applied social science. Each nation will determine its own trajectory of advancement and modernization, guided by its unique array of principles and cultural legacy. Utilizing domestic resources will have a positive impact on the economy. In 1909, Gandhi delivered a cautionary statement regarding the dangers of technology, and the perceived dangers associated with different technologies are still widely acknowledged today.

A novel form of imperialism has emerged, characterized by the imposition of Western values and prerequisites on the global populace. This is the Western capitalist conspiracy, which is gaining strength as technology makes it increasingly difficult for opponents of capitalism to resist its alluring influence. The advent of ATMs, the internet, and mobile devices revolutionized the service industry. Physical exertion is no longer required. The stock market is experiencing a significant upswing, leading to a rise in profits. Socialism provides a greater number of employment prospects for a broader segment of the population, while capitalism generates fewer job chances that primarily benefit a smaller portion of society. Gandhi advocated for 'Production by Masses' rather than 'Mass Production.' Prioritizing labor is crucial due to its ability to foster productive collaboration, ensure compliance with relevant regulations, safeguard worker dignity, acknowledge and respect diverse forms of employment, and combat class prejudice. Colonialism flourished as a result of the capitalist notion of progress.

The gratification derived from our economy, which ranks as the sixth largest globally with a value of $2.59 trillion, is immense. Furthermore, initiatives such as Make in India, Digital India, and Skill India instill a sense of optimism. The field of education is also seeing significant transformations with advancements in e-learning, distance education, and foreign teacher training. We are drawn to each new fashionable color we encounter in the media, and we excitedly anticipate the arrival of the next one. Technological progress and resource utilization have some constraints. Moral elevation can solely be attained by the exercise of self-discipline and the willingness to make sacrifices. On the other hand, moral degeneration can be attributed to Western materialism. Gaining a comprehensive understanding of and enhancing the innate features and characteristics of human beings is of utmost importance. Gandhi asserted that a human who is egocentric and lacks concern for the welfare of others exists in a condition like to that of an animal (Kumar & Kumar, 2022). The ego constructs and sustains deceptive identities, blending intellectual capabilities with assertiveness to enhance dominance and power, so strengthening one's identification with the ego. The development of a shared understanding of identity advances from basic animal behavior to the more refined characteristics of being human, and ultimately to a transcendent essence. Gandhi advocated for the utilization of spiritual force above violence. He defined self-realization as the comprehension of ultimate reality, encompassing the divine. The sole feasible options are nonviolence and love. He identified a connection between plurality and absolutism. Gandhi established Satyagraha in South Africa, and it has been embraced by political activists and leaders globally.

Mahatma Gandhi attempted to build a link between spirituality and science. He saw no distinction between the two and felt that there are two ways to discover the truth. Although many people see these two notions as separate, incompatible, and discordant, Gandhi felt they are mutually reinforcing within the context of human existence. Engaging in spiritual endeavors brings a wonderful sense of contentment and delight. Religion typically relates to communal or external circumstances, but spirituality refers to an internal, subjective, and individual state. Spirituality is the process of getting beyond the ego and sensuality, also known as 'I-ness,' and toward *'Sarva,'* which represents the entire world. This type of tenacity is highly praised in Hindu, Jain, and Buddhist belief systems. This necessitates changing one's concentration away from self-centeredness. When presented with the problem of unconnected minds, the ego plays no part. Gandhi thought that uniqueness exists within the vacuum. This says that an individual should only work after giving up their ego. Taking activity without consideration for the consequence undermines the ego.

In conclusion, Mahatma Gandhi was a selfless practitioner of Karma Yoga who greatly influenced Indian society from the early 1900s to the mid-20th century. He advocated for political and social reform, emphasizing the importance of equality and human values. Gandhi's life exemplified an extraordinary demonstration of human accountability, and his beliefs were deeply rooted in spirituality and nonviolence. He promoted self-discipline, minimalism, and the importance of incorporating environmental and social constraints into our living situations. Gandhi's ideas, as expressed in his writings challenged the dominant Western education and emphasized the need for cultural self-renewal. He believed in the power of truth and selflessness to shape a better world. Gandhi's legacy continues to inspire, and his teachings remain relevant in the contemporary world.

References

Bhargava, R. (Ed.) (2022). *Politics, ethics and the self: Rereading Gandhi's Hind Swaraj*. Routledge.
Bhattacharya, K. C. (1954). Swaraj in ideas. *Visva Bharati Quarterly*, *20*, 103–114.
Bilgrami, A. (2002). Gandhi's integrity: The philosophy behind the politics. *Post Colonial Studies*, *5*, 79–93.
Gandhi, M. K. (1928). *Satyagraha in South Africa*. Navajivan Publishing House.
Gandhi, M. K. (1938). *Hind swaraj or Indian home rule*. Navjivan Publishing House.
Gandhi, M. K. (1942). *To the Hindus and Muslims* (A. T. Hingorani, Ed.). Anand Hingorani.
Gandhi, M. K. (1945a). *Constructive programme: It's meaning and place*. Navjivan Publishing House.
Gandhi, M. K. (1945b). *From Yeravda Mandir: Ashram observances*. Navjivan Publishing House.
Gandhi, M. K. (1945c). *Gita the mother*. Indian Printing Works.
Gandhi, M. K. (1945d). *India of my dreams*. Hind Kitabs Limited.
Gandhi, M. K. (1951). *Basic education*. Navjivan Publishing House.
Hardiman, D. (2003). *Gandhi in his time and ours*. Permanent Black.
Kool, V. K., & Agrawal, R. (Eds.). (2020). *Gandhi and the psychology of non-violence*. Palgrave Macmillan.
Kool, V. K., & Agrawal, R. (Eds.). (2022). *Gandhi's wisdom: Insights from the founding father of modern psychology in the East*. Springer.
Kumar, R., & Kumar, S. (2022). Understanding individuality in Gandhi's moral philosophy. *Gandhi Marg Quarterly*, *44*, 347–358.
Parel, A. J. (2007). *Gandhi's philosophy and the quest for harmony*. Cambridge University Press.

7 Biopsychosocial and Spiritual Aspects of Globalization

Sonia Suchday and Linda Escobar Olszewski

Globalization may be conceptualized as an evolutionary process, which began from the time of early homo sapiens' creation of small communities and societies; over time, these communities and societies were consolidated and divided to maximize the survival of the species (Pirages, 2007). As humans began to inhabit various areas of the world, they adapted to their environs, and developed customs and traditions to harmonize their lifestyles with their surrounding environment. As individuals began to travel, they took their customs with them. The archeological human landscape is rampant with evidence of human adaptation to outside influences (Crowther et al., 2016).

Globalization refers to the intermingling of people, products, and processes (Suchday, 2015; Prilleltensky, 2012). It leads to the introduction of material and non-material influences from all over the globe on local people and communities through intense social contacts (Gupta, 2018). Globalization also results in challenges and opportunity for those in its path (Blanton & Peksen, 2017; Rudra, 2008). This dynamic interaction with societies near and far and the resultant challenges and opportunities create a need for adaptation and integration from individuals and communities (Suchday, 2015). Although globalization has been around for a long time (Pirages, 2007; Crowther et al., 2016), the current era of globalization is marked by the speed at which products, processes, communication, and humans are traveling from one side of the world to the other. This rapid movement of people, products, and processes requires adaptation to new influences at a rapid pace and has dramatically transformed life around the globe.

Globalization in India

India as a culture and society has been global from early times, with earliest signs of economic and social interactions across the globe dating as far back as 320 BC (Edwin & Okpara, 2015; Mazrui, 2001). Migrants and merchants traveling from all over the world arrived introducing new traditions, religions, tools, and techniques (Agwu & Atuma, 2015). The establishment of trade routes such as the Silk Road and religious and philosophical discourse through the ages solidified India's position a global influencer and a country

DOI: 10.4324/9781003461302-10

that had a constant influx of outside influences (Edwin & Okpara, 2015). After 1947, when Indians regained control and power of their country, and as a reaction against outside rule and British control, Indian political and economic policy was one of self-sufficiency. This autonomy lasted until 1991 when the pace of globalization in India once again accelerated through a deliberate policy of opening to global markets and economic opportunities (Pavri, 2018).

Globalization today is associated with fast-paced urbanization due to deliberate (e.g., development of "smart cities") and opportunistic development of urban areas and increased migration from rural to urban areas (Michel, 2020). Rapid rural to urban migration usually occurs in search of newer opportunities, due to adverse conditions, and discrepant benefits of globalization in rural versus urban areas (Michel, 2020). Implications of rapid globalization and urbanization include difficulties in adapting to the urban environment, including both individual difficulties (e.g., poor health habits) and social difficulties (e.g., loneliness, lower socioeconomic status), and the challenges experienced by urban areas in accommodating the many people who migrate seeking a better life (e.g., infrastructure inadequate for the number of people, environmental degradation).

In India, globalization has come with advantages such as burgeoning opportunities, growth of the middle class, as well as challenges such as inequity and potential loss of cultural values and traditions (Rao et al., 2013; Bhatia, 2018). Cultural traditions are frequently slow to change; when change does occur, it may be attributed to structural shifts, associated with availability of products, credit, and opportunities for education and employment, and not due to a deeper cultural transformation (Derne et al., 2014). Implications of this transformation of Indian society by structural changes rather than a cultural transition introduce a dissonance between globalization-related changes and tradition. For example, though the global economy has opened up employment opportunities, women in India have the lowest participation in the labor force globally (Working for Women in India, 2019), and traditional values and ideas, particularly concerning women's status and roles, persist (e.g., Derne et al., 2014).

Intriguingly, recent exploration of data from multiple national surveys (e.g., Pavri, 2018) indicates that India's traditions of tolerance and inclusion have led to increasing tolerance and social inclusion. However, these attitudes are at odds with widely publicized incidents of violence and rape of women and the tepid response of government officials to these incidents. It has been suggested that survey data may not have adequately captured the widespread diversity of Indian people and culture (Pavri, 2018).

Data from our lab indicate the coexistence of both traditional values, particularly around family and social interrelationships, and spirituality continue to permeate all aspects of Indian culture alongside values reflective of neoliberal globalization such as materialism and individual agency (Suchday et al., 2018). The coexistence of both agentic perspectives and traditional, collectivist values is reflective of the dualistic mindset in India (Sinha, 2014). The dualistic mindset refers to the coexistence of seemingly opposed values in individuals' beliefs, thinking, and behavior (Sinha, 2014). Roots of this dualism may lie in an understanding of the Indian theory of mind, which derives from deep spiritual beliefs and value systems inculcated in the Indian psyche. Indian spirituality and its interaction with globalization will be discussed in more depth in the section on spirituality.

Rapid globalization in India was paralleled by psychologists' efforts to invigorate the field and divorce it from its legacy of colonialism based on Western academic traditions and instead to reflect and emphasize an Indian theory of mind-based ancient texts and practices (Dalal & Misra, 2010). This was an active effort by Indian psychologists to expand the field within India to be more culturally sensitive and attuned to its people, beyond the field's western roots. Psychology based on its western roots focused on science and empirical perspectives and on development of universal principles without accounting for cultural influence (Dalal & Misra, 2010). The efforts to have psychology in India reflect its cultural and historical roots led to the creation of Indian psychology, which refers to philosophical, conceptual, and practical contributions of Indian culture to understanding psychology (Cornelissen et al., 2015).

Globalization has led to the creation of opportunity at material, political, social, and personal levels, but it also comes with a cost to individuals and societies (Suchday, 2015). This chapter will explore the interaction of globalization and traditional values within Indian culture, and their manifestations in biopsychosocial and spiritual aspects of functioning.

As we write this chapter, we are facing one of the most significant consequences of globalization—the novel coronavirus (COVID-19). The virus was first documented in Wuhan, China, and has currently reached the status of a global pandemic with all aspects of life and functioning across the globe—biological, economic, psychological, and social—significantly impacted. The section on COVID-19 below will outline these effects.

Biological Considerations Related to Globalization

Globalization has led to a dramatic increase in chronic non-communicable disease (NCD) such as cardiovascular diseases, cancer, chronic respiratory disorders, and diabetes in India accounting for 61% of deaths (Pati et al., 2019). The rise in NCDs may be attributed to an increase in sedentary lifestyles, increased consumption of high-density foods, tobacco and alcohol consumption, and environmental exposure to toxins, and psychosocial transitions that are resulting from globalization (Bhattacharya et al., 2020; Bhargava & Paul, 2018).

Globalization changes the landscape across nations; in low- and middle-income countries (LMICs), the most visible index of globalization is rapid urbanization resulting from global infusion. The rapid urbanization

India is experiencing has outpaced planning for foundational infrastructure. Globalization is accompanied by rapid changes in lifestyle such as reliance on high-density unhealthy foods and less exercise. However, acclimatization to the influx of influence and ideas related to globalization is significantly slower. Hence, rapid urbanization is accompanied by fast-paced adaptation of manifest factors such as consumption of fast foods but slower paced cultural adaptation and integration. Such unfettered and rapid development frequently contributes to a double burden of disease—leading to the simultaneous presence of both communicable disease and NCD (Bhattacharya et al., 2020; Krishnaswamy et al., 2016). Chronic NCDs such as coronary heart disease, diabetes mellitus, cancer, and mental health challenges (e.g., depression, suicide, and substance abuse) are on the rise globally; India is no exception. Medical and public health issues interact with social and psychological realities to influence health in myriad ways. Recent data show that incidence of these debilitating conditions are higher among older parents who have a child, particularly a son, who has migrated either to another state or to another country (Falkingham et al., 2017).

Increases in NCDs and difficulties that ensue are seen across age groups in India as early as childhood through adulthood and the latter part of life (Bhattacharya et al., 2020; Visaria & Dommaraju, 2019). Moreover, the incidence and prevalence of these disorders interact with demographic changes (e.g., rural to urban living, sedentary lifestyle, food environment) related to globalization. For example, cardiovascular disease and diabetes mellitus are the primary causes of morbidity and mortality in India among older adults. In fact, NCDs in general are now estimated to account for over 80% of deaths in LMICs (World Health Organization, 2017).

Lifestyle changes resulting from following economic opportunities to places far from home can result in diminished well-being. Mental health and physical health may suffer due to social isolation, loneliness, depression, and poor health habits. Furthermore, "off-shore" work, or work with multinational companies where the headquarters of the company are in a different time zone, has resulted in a boom of workers working overnight further impacting health. It is known that working the night shift hours negatively impacts health by disrupting hormonal production and the natural circadian rhythm resulting in adverse health effects (James & Sudha, 2016; Söylemez et al., 2019).

Psychological Considerations Related to Globalization

Well-being is broadly defined as individuals' ability to achieve their potential, be productively employed, contribute to their community, and cope with the normal psychosocial stresses presented in their daily living (WHO definition; Schramme, 2023). Despite this sweeping definition of psychological well-being, the concept often differs from culture to culture and may be, influenced by a society's customs and traditions, making a departure from psychology's colonial roots extremely important (White et al., 2016).

With a rapid influx of ideas and influence, psychological adaptation to globalization is essential to the well-being of individuals, families, and societies. As people, products, processes inter-mingle, there is exposure to dissonant information, from cultures and people all over the globe (Chiu et al., 2009). This information is inconsistently absorbed into daily life, resulting in a polarization both internally and societally with conflicting values and beliefs being simultaneously present (Chiu et al., 2011). This incongruent and conflicting information and speed of influence and adjustment may create or result in an active and conscious resistance to globalization (Herrington, 2013). The challenge of this process is that individuals belonging to different demographics (e.g., young, old, women, men, wealthy, poor communities) may absorb and resist the forces of globalization at divergent and inconsistent rates. For example, young people are more likely to absorb and implement novel ideas, beliefs, practices learned through their exposure to globalization, particularly through their exposure to technological advancements, including social media and internet, compared to older generations (Bhatia, 2018).

The psychological implication of the constant presence of local and global influences is most visible in the development of identity (e.g., Arnett, 2002). Identity, in a globalized world, emerges through an interweaving of local and global influences; it is manifested through seamless interactions with ingroups *and* interfacing with national and international communities (Kapoor & Tomar, 2017). The challenge of identity in a globalized world is the struggle to maintain a cultural identity while navigating an international milieu (Kapoor & Tomar, 2017).

The psychology of Indian people in not easily understood. To the outsider, the behavior of an Indian person may appear to be inconsistent and multilayered in diverse situations referred to as the "dualistic Indian mindset" (Panda & Gupta, 2012). Although this dualistic mindset may make it hard for an outsider to understand the Indian people and culture, the dualistic mindset may provide an advantage for Indian people resulting in them being uniquely poised to make the best of globalization. Understanding the interaction of the "dualistic Indian mindset" and the forces of globalization, requires a historical perspective. These historical influences include ongoing and intimate contact with the outside world through invasions, colonization, travel, trade, and education from ancient times (Sinha, 2014). As indicated earlier, globalization has been a force within Indian culture for millennia and the economic incentives of the late 20th century simply acted to accelerate the pace of globalization (e.g., Edwin & Okpara). Adaptation to these rapid external influences are facilitated through traditional Indian perspectives which propose a deep spiritual journey which has many pathways and acceptance of a changing world as real and illusory ("maya"; Sinha, 2014). This dual emphasis on deep internal values and external changing realities translates into behavior that is sensitive to and transforms in response to contextual influences include place, time, and person (Panda & Gupta, 2012;

Sinha, 2014). Indeed, data from our lab support this (e.g., Suchday et al., 2018), demonstrating the recent influence of accelerated globalization in India are manifested in a kind of dualism. Specifically, data confirmed an endorsement of various opposing concepts in the cultural identity of individuals: for example, individuals identified with individualism and collectivism, spirituality and materialism, interdependent and independent identity, and an emphasis on individual agency and ambition and the strong influence of family in all personal preferences suggestive of the dualistic Indian mindset (Suchday et al., 2018).

An important aspect of psychological influences of globalization is also unequal accrual of benefits among rural versus urban areas, and among people who are rich versus those who are poor. Such unequal access to benefits and exposure to the shining promise of globalization through electronic media, often leads to internal feelings of dissatisfaction and frustration. The frustration experienced due resulting from the inability to achieve the promise of globalization (e.g., better jobs and fast upward mobility) may lead to increased depression and increases in high risk behaviors such as alcohol consumption, drugs, smoking, and unsafe sex, particularly among young people (Bhattacharya et al., 2020). Internalization of dissatisfaction is so significant that currently, in India, suicide is the primary cause of death among young people 15–39 years and is on the rise among the elderly and women (Bhargava & Paul, 2018).

Social Considerations Related to Globalization

Like other LMICs, India has a significant divide between how globalization is experienced by rural and urban populations. In urban cities, globalization is rapid while rural villages are left behind. The benefits of globalization may also result in a divide with higher social strata benefitting more than resource-poor individuals and communities, by enriching knowledge and exposure through education, travel, and various other opportunities to integrate global influences into their Indian identity (Bhatia, 2018).

Social changes in India subsequent to globalization are related to structural shifts in society due to increased mobility of youth to opportunity centers (Bhatia, 2018). As young people move away from their families to pursue opportunities, traditional structures such as familial bonds and controls on marital and employment choices loosen leading to changes in family customs and support systems (Bhatia, 2018). Not only are young people and their lives and health impacted by the loosening of these structures (e.g., child care for a young working couple, double burden of work and home on women), but older people are often adversely affected by lack of security in their old age and loneliness as children move away and traditional supports are altered. Additionally, as mentioned earlier, data also suggest that there is greater incidence of chronic disease among parents who have a son living far away from home (e.g., Falkingham et al., 2017).

The loosening of family bonds due to structural changes such as employment in far off geographical locations also has practical implications for the culture. Indian culture was embodied within large undivided families where childcare responsibility fell on the elderly and care of the elderly occurred within the same family system. The family served as a social security, healthcare, childcare, and an insurance system for individuals. The tragedy of globalization for individuals and communities within India arises from the slow rate of infrastructure growth to provide these necessary services that are in demand as a result of the dissolution of the joint family structure.

Spiritual Considerations Related to Globalization

Spirituality has universal dimensions as seen in a three-country study, including India, China, and the United States (e.g., McClintock et al., 2016). These dimensions include love (for each other and the divine), interconnectedness, altruism, spiritual practice (e.g., meditation, prayer, yoga, qigong), and religious and spiritual reflection and commitment (McClintock et al., 2016). Spirituality is embedded in all aspects of life and functioning in India (Suchday et al., 2018) and continues to play a role in coping and health (Santoro et al., 2016).

Spiritualty is interwoven across Indian culture, family, and daily life (Suchday et al., 2018). Although India is a predominantly Hindu country, Indian spirituality contains elements from the Abrahamic faiths, particularly Christianity and Islam. Indian spiritual beliefs may be understood through the lens of values, including Karma (Deeds) and Dharma (beliefs about right and wrong; Tiwari & Pandey, 2013). Karma is readily understood and is embedded within most major religions in the world (Allen et al., 2015). Dharma is a lesser-known concept because it includes concepts of duty and responsibility to self, others, and a higher being as a guiding principle of right actions (Suchday et al., 2018). Data from our lab among young people from Mumbai and Hyderabad indicate that both of these values are ingrained within life beliefs and these values persist even as the country globalizes at a rapid pace (Suchday et al., 2018; Santoro et al., 2016). Furthermore, data from our lab demonstrate that life beliefs also reflect individualist values such as materialism and individual agency, achievement, and ambition (Suchday et al., 2018). People less familiar with the Indian milieu are frequently surprised by captains of industry and "hard-nosed" business leaders in India openly discussing their "Guru," visits to their ashram, and attendance at religious and spiritual services and retreats. Indeed, globalization results in a sophisticated, interweaving of the processes of identity and choice, including the paradox of retaining traditional identity while simultaneously adopting a global perspective (Suchday et al., 2018).

While the 1991 economic reforms assured that India would be influenced by global exchanges. Interestingly, globalization has also resulted in the export of Indian spirituality. Indian spirituality has traveled to all corners of the world; however, it is contextually manifested. Specifically, the adoption of practices such as yoga and meditation have been adopted as exercise and coping techniques, rather than as a way of life as they are in their original context (Suchday et al., 2014).

COVID-19—An example of Biopsychosocial proliferation of Globalization

The COVID-19 pandemic is an embodiment of the best and worst of globalization. The rapid spread of COVID-19 from Wuhan, China, to the rest of the world demonstrates the impact of globalization, including the rapid movement of people and products across borders. The COVID-19 virus represents an infectious disease, which has had an overarching effect on biological, psychological, and social aspects of functioning in the world, and in India (Verma et al., 2020). Cases in India at this time on September 20, 2020, are at 5.31 million and 85,619 deaths (www.google.com/search?q=COVID19+cases+Inida&rlz=1C1GCEA_enUS775US775&oq=COVID19+cases+Inida&aqs=chrome..69i57j0l7.5347j0j15&sourceid=chrome&ie=UTF-8).

Apart from the devastating health and economic impact, the toll in human terms as been enormous. As indicated with urbanization, there has been a migration of labor from rural to urban areas. Due to loss of jobs and shut down of transportation systems during the COVID-19 pandemic, many migrant workers had to make their way back home on foot, losing their lives in some instances (Verma et al., 2020). Anecdotal evidence has also suggested that when these migrant workers did reach their villages, they were frequently required to quarantine and were isolated from their families. Reports of increased incidence of domestic violence but decreases in violent crimes (e.g., Verma et al., 2020) point to the complex impact of the pandemic-related restrictions on movement and social distancing.

Additionally, the lockdown at home has led to a significant increase in psychosocial distress among individuals and within families. There has been an increase in stigma and discrimination toward people who had COVID-19 and self-isolation by individuals due to fear of infecting their family members (Chaturvedi & Sharma, 2020). Interactions within families due to the lockdown and increased distress may get problematic with expression of negative emotions and increased domestic violence (Chaturvedi & Sharma, 2020). The pandemic has generated significant anxiety, depression, social stigma, and generalized distress, potentially suicides, and a dramatic increase in mental health needs within the population (Roy et al., 2020; Thakur & Jain, 2020). Interestingly, the need for social distancing has also led to a resurgence of an ancient Indian tradition of greeting people by joining hands and saying "Namaste" (Chaturvedi & Sharma, 2020).

The next three sections will cover the biopsychosocial and spiritual impact of globalization on young people, older people, and women.

Youth and Considerations Related to Globalization

Globalization has altered the lives of young people at a rapid rate. This speed of influence has resulted in the simultaneous straddling of tradition of their own culture and global cultures. This navigation of old and new results in an alteration in how youths adapt as they work to incorporate new technologies and other forms of globalization into their everyday lives, and traditional cultures. This juxtaposition of old and new results in young people in the rapidly globalizing world facing difficulties across their identity development, There is tension and struggle between long-standing traditions established cultural norms and a neoliberal identity—as defined by a democratic ideal and free market economy (Bhatia & Priya, 2018). This identity challenge is manifested in the search for identity, finding a career, and a life partner in a multicultural world with multiple and sometimes discordant sources of information (Suchday, 2015). Young people, in a rapidly globalizing world, are faced with both the burden of infectious disease, in particular, the pandemic, and NCDs. Young people need to develop healthy lifestyles and manage high risk behaviors associated with globalization. Because there is no roadmap for how to incorporate globalization into everyday life, individuals are left to negotiate and navigate the impacts of globalization on their own. Not surprisingly, individuals' acceptance of global influence varies, individually and even by generations, with younger generations being more apt to embrace globalization, benefitting from the economic and social changes compared to older people (Breaz, 2019).

Though younger generations are exposed to global cultures through technology, they often lack the economic means to truly participate in financial benefits that the global economy has to offer such as consumerism, employment, and education opportunities (United Nations, 2005). There is some indication that the embracing of Western values in LMICs appears to be easier among young people who are more affluent compared to young people with fewer resources who are attempting to attain material success because of their exposure due to travel and technology (Bhatia, 2018). This idea is consistent with cross-cultural application of Bandura's theory of agency, where the young and affluent more easily embrace agentic perspectives compared to older and less affluent individuals (Bandura, 2018).

Young people's relationship with the globalizing world is complex. Younger generations are quicker to identify and embrace both the economic and social benefits of globalization (Breaz, 2019). Youth's ability to be flexible to the changing global landscape plays a role in their ability to adapt and accept the influences from cultures outside and different from their own (Bernardo et al., 2023). With cortexes still in development, youths are incredibly adaptable and are able to quickly learn and gain competence and expertise in new and evolving technologies. Gen Z, or the iGeneration as they are sometimes referred to, are the first generation to have experienced preponderate access and availability of high-speed, wireless internet. Born in a time when communication technologies were readily available and accessible, the youth culture is constantly online, engaged, and entertained (Sharma & Shukla, 2016) earning them the moniker "Digital natives" (Prensky, 2001) making older generations digital immigrants in this new, global landscape. Furthermore, technological advancements are altering how youth learn, socialize, work, and even view themselves; this is particularly true during this time of pandemic.

In India, data indicate that young people continue to uphold their traditional values of interdependence and emphasis on the importance and role of family and community. This is particularly true as they make important life decisions and in their spiritual and religious identities. However, they are also working within the traditional framework and integrating Western values of material success and individual agency into their daily and family lives (Rao et al., 2013; Suchday et al., 2018).

An important influence on Indian youths comes from the creation of multinational industries where young people seek opportunities (Bhatia & Priya, 2018). With the increasing availability of economic prospects through employment, many young people are moving away from home, to following employment possibilities. Living away from their families introduces individuals to a new, independent lifestyle that contrasts the traditional one of interdependence. Young people adapt to work in these multinational industries, either through training to participate in company culture or as a function of needing to function within a corporate culture. Through this process of adaptation, there is a tendency to embrace western values of happiness and achievement, and the development of neoliberal identities, which encompass these values (Bhatia, 2018; Bhatia & Priya, 2018).

Advanced Years and Considerations Related to Globalization

It has been suggested that globalization has had deleterious effects on the geriatric population (Fry, 2005). Globalization is resulting in a reorganization of the family structure in India. Factors which contribute to this re organization include a decline in fertility, increase in longevity, and medical advances which has resulted in the growth of an elderly population (> 60 years; Agarwal et al., 2016). Of note is that in India, ancient texts have provided a guideline of various stages of life, including old age; they depict declining health and facilities and increased dependence on the family as a natural process and part of the normative life experience (Visaria & Dommaraju, 2019). In this scenario, the elderly are held in high regard, and they are valued as providers of spiritual, psychological, and physical support to the family via their engagement in childcare (Visaria & Dommaraju, 2019). Data also indicate that life expectancy is higher among women compared to men leading to significant social and economic challenges (Agarwal et al., 2016), which will be discussed in the section on women below.

India has a rich tradition of "joint" families, which include parents, male siblings and their spouses, and children living together (Samanta et al., 2015;

Rao et al., 2013). Older people in this setting are frequently revered and regarded as the repository of wisdom, traditions, and values. They are responsible for distributing these values and traditions, while simultaneously providing childcare to younger members of the family. Data indicate that living in these multigenerational household accrues many health benefits to older people (Samanta et al., 2015). However, with globalization, and the need to follow economic opportunity, young people are increasingly moving away from the traditional residence, resulting in a reorganization of the family system, and giving rise to income insecurity and isolation among the elderly (Agarwal et al., 2016).

Finally, data on aging in India also comes from research on palliative care among older adults. This data highlight the importance of the roles that spirituality, family, and community play in the lives of the geriatric population in India (Gielen et al., 2017; Inbadas, 2017). The literature indicates that distinct from western countries, in India, spirituality is woven into the family and community; as such, spirituality is also embedded in the economic concerns associated with caring for this group. Specifically, researchers indicate that spirituality is related to beliefs in karma and/or fate, practice of religion (e.g., "puja" or veneration), support from religion, and concerns about family after the individuals' passing (Gielen et al., 2017; Inbadas, 2017). However, it is unclear whether these data (i.e., Gielen et al., 2017), particularly around economic concerns at the end of life, can be generalized across all socioeconomic strata.

Globally, women are overrepresented in the elderly population; this over representation of women among the elderly creates a unique challenge with women. Particularly in India, where women are at a disadvantage in inheriting ancestral property, less likely to be educated; less likely to be economically independent; and more likely to be the victims of discrimination (Agarwal et al., 2016).

Lower-middle-income countries, such as India, do not currently have infrastructure and facilities such as social agencies, security, and healthcare systems that enable older generations to obtain the support necessary without the support of the interdependent and multigenerational family and traditions to support in the management of their everyday lives (Agarwal et al., 2016; Shah & Rajadhyaksha, 2016).

Women and Considerations Related to Globalization

Though globalization has positively influenced the lives of many women in LMICs, women's opportunities remain limited in many aspects of society in LMICs. Women in India have the lowest participation in the labor force globally (Working for Women in India, 2019) and represent only 20% of the workforce. Despite the opening of opportunities with globalization for all, existing social norms, practices, and institutional and structural realities may make it harder for women to benefit from globalization (Fletcher et al., 2017). Discrimination against women in India continues to be rampant and present before birth leading to a poor female to male sex ratio due to female feticide (Banerjee & Biswas, 2016). Reasons for this ratio may be traced to India's patrilineal society where women are considered an economic and social burden who will leave the home requiring an expensive marriage and dowry. Sons and their wives contribute to household expenses, care for the older members, and continue the family lineage. Globalization may have contributed to this scenario through the availability of modern technology leading to easily available sex determination tests and abortion of the female fetus (Banerjee & Biswas, 2016).

In general, India's culture, traditions, and structural and institutional realities make it difficult for women to move past their historical and culture-bound identities (Derne, 2005). Traditionally Indian women enjoyed a high status. However, over time, this position deteriorated limiting their sphere of influence within the home; Historically, women were socialized to sacrifice their own personal needs, or wants, and instead prioritize the needs of their family. They were praised and respected for the sacrifice of their personal aspirations. In fact, in many instances, women's aspirations became the well-being of the family. As young women encounter opportunities in the world around them, they experience an identity crisis as they grapple with these traditional ideals and embracing a new world of opportunities (Yang & Neal, 2006). The continue dealing with external and internalized norms which restrict their role to being caretakers and caregivers (Fletcher et al., 2017).

Gender, social, and economic stratification interact in Indian society with women from higher economic and social status enjoying the benefits of education and engagement in activities outside the home compared to women from a lower socioeconomic background (Dutta, 2016; Twamley & Sidharth, 2019). History provides evidence through the ages of resurgence in the high position of women manifested in the rise of strong women leaders (Dutta, 2016).

In sum, the status of women in India presents a dualistic picture with traditional texts and religion emphasizing female energy as being a key aspect of Indian belief systems and social norms with restrict women' participation in economic and political spheres. With globalization, the norm of an idealized Indian woman incorporates tradition and modernity in that she continues to embody Indian values while being educated (Twamley & Sidharth, 2019).

Conclusion

Globalization has always been an integral part of the Indian psyche through its historical interactions with the world, and perhaps has fed the dualistic mindset, as India has always worked to adapt and incorporate outside influences. Through the ages, Indian traditions have survived through value systems, which enable the absorption of external ideas and products without diluting its traditional beliefs. What differs in current times from the global influences of the past is the rapid speed and the permeation of global influences through media, travel, and the establishment of multinational industries.

Preliminary data from our lab indicate that traditional values continue to exert a strong influence on Indian people and culture. However, these traditions survive and have survived by being flexible and through absorption of outside influences. The effects of globalization are large and far reaching. They have impacted the larger societal, economic, and political systems, the family, as well as the individual through their behaviors and health. The existence of traditions which allow for the absorption of these values have created a novel society which embraces tradition and incorporates modernity through the integration of globalization-related opportunities, values, and beliefs.

References

Agarwal, A., Lubet, A., Mitgang, E., Mohanty, S., & Bloom, D. E. (2016). *Population aging in India: Facts, issues, and options*. IZA Discussion Papers, No. 10162, Institute for the Study of Labor (IZA), Bonn.

Agwu, E., & Atuma, O. (2015). Strategic review of the impact of globalization on the sustainability of communities and business organisations. *International Journal of Business and Management Invention*, *4*(4), 55–62.

Allen, P. M., Edwards, J. A., & McCullough, W. (2015). Does Karma exist?: Buddhism, social cognition, and the evidence for Karma. *The International Journal for the Psychology of Religion*, *25*, 1–17.

Arnett, J. J. (2002). The psychology of globalization. *American Psychologist*, *57*(10), 774–783. https://doi.org/10.1037//0003–066X.57.10.774

Bandura, A. (2018). Toward a psychology of human agency: Pathways and reflections. *Perspectives on Psychological Science*, *13*(2), 130–136. https://doi.org/10.1177/1745691617699280

Banerjee, A., & Biswas, R. (2016). Globalization and violence against women: The missing girls of India. *Journal of Interdisciplinary Economics*, *28*(1), 30–52. https://doi.org/10.1177/0260107915609816

Bernardo, A. B., Albert, J. R. G., Vizmanos, J. F. V., & Muñoz, M. S. (2023). *Toward measuring soft skills for youth development: A scoping study*. PIDS Discussion Paper Series, No. 2023-28.

Bhargava, B., & Paul, V. K. (2018). *Informing NCD control efforts in India on the eve of Ayushman Bharat*. https://doi.org/10.1016/S0140-6736(18)32172-X

Bhatia, S. (2018). *Decolonizing psychology: Globalization, social justice, and Indian youth identities*. Oxford University Press.

Bhatia, S., & Priya, R. K. (2018). Decolonizing culture: Euro-American psychology and the shaping of neoliberal selves in India. *Theory & Psychology*, *28*(5), 645–668. https://doi.org/10.1177/095935431879131

Bhattacharya, S., Juyal, R., Hossain, M. M., & Singh, A. (2020). Non-communicable diseases viewed as "collateral damage" of our decisions: Fixing accountabilities and finding solutions in primary care settings. *Journal of Family Medicine and Primary Care*, 2176–2179. www.jfmpc.com/text.asp?2020/9/5/2176/285092

Blanton, R. G., & Peksen, D. (2017). Dying for globalization? The impact of economic globalization on industrial accidents. *Social Science Quarterly*, *98*(5), 1487–1502. https://doi.org.rlib.pace.edu/10.1111/ssqu.12367

Breaz, A. M. (2019). Attitudes towards globalization and its implications to different categories of age. *Revista de Asistența Sociala*, *18*, 67–78.

Chaturvedi, S. K., & Sharma, M. K. (2020). Psychosocial aspects of Covid-19, the Indian way. *World Social Psychiatry*, 2(2), 129–131.

Chiu, C., Gries, P., Torelli, C. J., & Cheng, S. Y. Y. (2011). Toward a social psychology of globalization. *Journal of Social Issues*, *67*(4), 663–676.

Chiu, C., Mallorie, L., Keh, H. T., & Law, W. (2009). Perceptions of culture in multicultural space: Joint presentation of images from two cultures increases in-group attribution of culture-typical characteristics. *Journal of Cross-Cultural Psychology*, *40*(2), 282–300.

Cornelissen, M., Misra, G., & Varma, S. (Eds.). (2015). *Introduction to foundations and applications of Indian psychology*. Pearson Education.

Crowther, A., Lucas, L., Helm, R., Horton, M., Shipton, C., Wright, H. T., Walshaw, S., Pawlowicz, M., Radimilahy, C., Douka, K., Picornell-Gelabert, L., Fuller, D. Q., & Boivin, N. L. (2016). Ancient crops provide first archaeological signature of the westward Austronesian expansion. *PNAS*, *113*(24), 6635–6640. https://doi.org/10.1073/pnas.1522714113

Dalal, A. K., & Misra, G. (2010). The core and context of Indian psychology. *Psychology and Developing Societies*, *22*(1), 121–155.

Derne, S. (2005). The (limited) effects of cultural globalization in India: Implications for culture theory. *Poetics*, *33*, 33–47.

Derne, S., Sharma, M., & Sethi, N. (2014). Structural changes rather than the influence of media: People's encounter with economic liberalization in India. In Mathur, N. (Ed.). *Consumer culture, modernity, and identity* (pp. 145–167). Google Books.

Dutta, S. (2016). The changing patterns and lived experiences of women pursuing higher education post-marriage in India. *Journal of International Women's Studies*, *17*(1), 169–185. http://vc.bridgew.edu/jiws/vol17/iss1/12

Edwin, A., & Okpara, A. (2015). Strategic review of the impact of globalization on the sustainability of communities and business organisations. *International Journal of Business and Management Invention*, *4*(4), 55–62.

Falkingham, J., Qin, M., Vlachantoni, A., & Evandrou, M. (2017). Children's migration and lifestyle-related chronic disease among older parents 'left behind' in India. *SSM—Population Health*, *3*, 352–357. https://doi.org/10.1016/j.ssmph.2017.03.008

Fletcher, E. K., Pande, R., & Troyer, C. M. (2017). *Women and work in India: Descriptive evidence and a Review of potential policies*. Center for International Development Faculty Working Paper No. 339. Harvard University.

Fry, C. L. (2005). Globalization and the experiences of aging. *Gerontology & Geriatrics Education*, *26*(1), 9–22. https://doi.org/10.1300/J021v26n01_02

Gielen, J., Bhatnagar, S., & Chaturvedi, S. K. (2017). Prevalence and nature of spiritual distress among palliative care patients in India. *Journal of Religion and Health*, *56*, 530–544. https://doi.org/10.1007/s10943-016-0252-5

Gupta, A. (2018). How neoliberal globalization is shaping early childhood education policies in India, China, Singapore, Sri Lanka and the Maldives. *Policy Futures in Education*, *16*(1), 11–28. https://doi.org/10.1177/1478210317715796

Herrington, L. (2013). Globalization and religion in historical perspective: A paradoxical relationship. *Religions*, *4*, 145–165. https://doi.org/10.3390/rel4010145

Inbadas, H. (2017). The philosophical and cultural situatedness of spirituality at the end of life in India. *Indian Journal of Palliative Care*, *23*(3), 338–340. https://doi.org/10.4103/IJPC.IJPC_61_17

James, F. A., & Sudha, S. (2016). Adverse effects of night & rotational shift on Circadian Rhythms. *Advances in Natural and Applied Sciences*, (9 SE), 248. http://search.ebscohost.com.rlib.pace.edu/login.aspx?direct=true&db=edsgao&AN=edsgcl.466051306&site=eds-live&scope=site

Kapoor, B., & Tomar, A. (2017). Psycho-social implications of globalization: An opportunity-based perspective. *Indian Journal of Positive Psychology*, *8*(2).

Krishnaswamy, K., Vaidya, R., Rajgopal, G., & Vasudevan, S (2016). Diet and nutrition in the prevention of non-communicable diseases. *Proceedings in the Indian National Science Academy*, *5*, 1477–1494. https://doi.org/10.16943/ptinsa/2016/48881

Mazrui, A. (2001). *Pan Africanism the era of globalization*. W.E.B Dubois Memorial Lecture.
McClintock, C. H., Lau, E., & Miller, L. (2016). Phenotypic dimensions of spirituality: Implications for mental health in China, India, and the United States. *Frontiers in Psychology*, 7, 1600. https://doi.org/10.3389/fpsyg.2016.01600
Michel, J. P. (2020). Urbanization and ageing health outcomes. *Journal of Nutrition Health and Aging*. *24*(5), 463–465.
Panda, A., & Gupta, R. K. (2012). Deconstructing context-sensitive nature of Indians' behaviour: A preliminary attempt to develop a taxonomy for three work contexts'. *International Journal of Indian Culture and Business Management*, *5*(6). https://doi.org/10.1504/IJICBM.2012.049342
Pati, S., Sinha, R., & Mahapatra, P. (2019). Non-communicable disease risk reduction teaching in India: A curricular landscape. *Frontiers Public Health*, 7, 133. https://doi.org/10.3389/fpubh.2019.00133
Pavri, T. (2018). Is India becoming more liberal? Globalization, economic liberalization, and social values. *Journal of Global Initiatives*, *13*(1), 115–127.
Pirages, D. C. (2007). Nature, disease, and globalization: An evolutionary perspective, *International Studies Review*, *9*(4), 616–628. https://doi.org/10.1111/j.1468-2486.2007.00726.x
Prensky, M. (2001). *Digital natives, digital immigrants*. Retrieved September 9, 2020, from www.marcprensky.com/writing/Prensky%20-%20Digital%20Natives,%20Digital%20Immigrants%20-%20Part1.pdf
Prilleltensky, I. (2012). The what, why, who, and how of globalization: What is psychology to do? *Journal of Social Issues*, *68*(3), 612–629.
Rao, M. A., Berry, R., Gonsalves, A., Hastak, Y, Shah, M., & Roeser, R. W. (2013). Globalization and the identity remix among urban adolescents in India. *Journal of Research on Adolescence*, *23*(1), 9–24.
Roy, D., Tripathy, S., Kar, S. K., Sharma, N., Verma, S. K., & Kaushal, V. (2020). Study of knowledge, attitude, anxiety & perceived mental healthcare need in Indian population during COVID-19 pandemic. *Asian Journal of Psychiatry*, *51*, 102083. https://doi.org/10.1016/j.ajp.2020.102083
Rudra, N. (2008). *Globalization and the race to the bottom in developing countries: Who really gets hurt?* Cambridge University Press.
Samanta, T., Chen, F., & Vanneman, R. (2015). Living arrangements and health of older adults in India. *The Journals of Gerontology: Series B*, *70*(6), 937–947. https://doi.org/10.1093/geronb/gbu164
Santoro, A. F., Suchday, S., Benkhoukha, A., Ramanayake, N., & Kapur, S. (2016). Adverse childhood experiences and religiosity/spirituality in emerging adolescents in India. *Psychology of Religion and Spirituality*, *8*(3), 185–194. https://doi.org/10.1037/rel0000038
Schramme, T. (2023). Health as complete well-being: The WHO definition and beyond. *Public Health Ethics*, *16*(3), 210–218. https://doi.org/10.1093/phe/phad017
Shah, G., & Rajadhyaksha, U. (2016). Global cities, work and family collectivism and work-family conflict in India. *South Asian Journal of Global Business Research*, *5*(3), 341–361.
Sharma, A., & Shukla, A. K. (2016). Impact of social messengers especially WhatsApp on youth-a sociological study. *International Journal of Advance Research and Innovative Ideas in Education*, *2*(5), 367–375.
Sinha, J. B. P. (2014). *Psycho-social analysis of the Indian mindset*. Springer.
Söylemez, S., Sivri, A. B., Şimşek, E., Polat, E., & Çakır, B. (2019). Melatonin, leptin, and ghrelin levels in nurses working night shifts. *Journal of Surgery and Medicine*, (*1*), 22. https://doi-org.rlib.pace.edu/10.28982/josam.443902

Suchday, S. (2015). Anger and globalization among youth in India. *New Directions in Child and Adolescent Development*, 77–84.
Suchday, S., Ramanayake, N. P., Benkhoukha, A., Santoro, A. F., Marquez, C., & Nakao, G. (2014). Ayurveda: An alternative in the United States. *Multicultural Approaches to Health and Wellness in America*, *1*, 151–170.
Suchday, S., Santoro, A. F., Ramanayake, N., Lewin, H., & Almeida, M. (2018). Religion, spirituality, globalization reflected in life beliefs among urban Asian Indian youth. *Psychology of Religion and Spirituality*, *10*(2), 146–156. http://dx.doi.org/10.1037/rel0000161
Thakur, A., & Jain, A. (2020). COVID 2019-suicides: A global psychological pandemic. *Brain Behavior & Immunology*, *88*, 952–953. https://doi.org/10.1016/j.bbi.2020.04.062
Tiwari, S. C., & Pandey, N. M. (2013). The Indian concepts of lifestyle and mental health in old age. *Indian Journal of Psychiatry*, *55*(Suppl 2), S288–S292.
Twamley, K., & Sidharth, J. (2019). Negotiating respectability: Comparing the experiences of poor and middle-class young urban women in India. *Modern Asian Studies*, *53*(5), 1646–1674. https://doi.org/10.1017/S0026749X17000816
United Nations. (2005). *Globalization WPAY for youth*. Retrieved August 31, 2020, from www.un.org/development/desa/youth/globalization-wpay.html
Verma, S., Saharan, A., Polcumpally, A. T., & Biswas, M. (2020). Tentacles of COVID-19 in India: Impact on Indian economy, society, polity and geopolitics. *Journal of Humanities and Social Sciences Studies*, *2*(3), 54–61.
Visaria, A., & Dommaraju, P. (2019). Productive aging in India. *Social Science & Medicine*, *229*, 14–21. https://doi.org/10.1016/j.socscimed.2018.07.029
White, R. G., Imperiale, M. G., & Perera, E. (2016). The capabilities approach: Fostering contexts for enhancing mental health and wellbeing across the globe. *Globalization and Health*, *12*(16). https://link-galecom.rlib.pace.edu/apps/doc/A451554401/AONE?u=nysl_me_pace&sid=AONE&xid=970b0b03
Working for Women in India. (2019, March 8). Retrieved August 30, 2020, from www.worldbank.org/en/news/feature/2019/03/08/working-for-women-in-india
World Health Organization. (2017). *Global action plan for the prevention and control of noncommunicable diseases 2013–2020*. Retrieved August 30, 2020, from http://apps.who.int/iris/bitstream/10665/94384/1/9789241506236_eng.pdf
Yang, R., & Neal, A. G. (2006). The impact of globalization on family relations in China. *International Journal of Sociology of the Family*, 113–126.

Part III

Identity and Intergroup Relations

8 Gender and Age Stereotypes From a Cross-Cultural Perspective

Deborah L. Best, Corinne R. Scannell, and Ariel G. Gianukakis

Our first research collaboration with Professor Pandey was in an investigation of psychological traits associated with women and men, gender-trait stereotypes. For example, women are often described as more affectionate and gentler than men, and men are described as more aggressive and adventurous than women. To investigate these gender-trait stereotypes, the 300-item Adjective Check List (Gough & Heilbrun, 1980), a large, diverse group of adjectives descriptive of human personality, was used, and participants were asked to identify the adjectives generally associated with men or with women in their cultures. In the early studies of gender stereotypes in the United Stated, England, and Ireland (Williams et al., 1977) and in France, Germany, and Norway (Williams et al., 1979), there was a high degree of similarity in the traits ascribed to women and men by young adults in these Western countries. In addition to looking at adults' views, a picture-story measure was employed in these countries to assess 5- and 8-year-old children's awareness of the adult-defined stereotypes (Best et al., 1977; Williams et al., 1981). For both the adult and child studies, there was some variation among countries, but there was a high degree of agreement among adults and among children in the traits associated with women and men.

These findings led to the question of whether there would be such similarity found in countries with greater cultural diversity, such as India with its Hindu traditions and Pakistan with its traditional Muslim culture. Professors Pandey and Haque (Williams et al., 1982) used the same adult and child methodologies that had been previously used in the Western countries by Williams, Best, and colleagues. They found many similarities in the gender stereotypes (Williams et al., 1982) that were consistent with those found in the Western countries, with many of the same items associated with women (e.g., affectionate, dependent, gentle, complaining) and men (e.g., adventurous, aggressive, independent, realistic). However, there were some interesting differences when looking at the affective meaning of the stereotype descriptions. The relatively favorable female stereotype in India and the relatively favorable male stereotype in Pakistan differed from the findings in Western countries where the male-associated items were higher in strength and activity but did not differ in favorability from the female-associated items. The

DOI: 10.4324/9781003461302-12

children's data indicated that gender stereotypes developed much earlier in Pakistan than in India and the Western countries, perhaps related to the high degree of differentiation of gender roles in Pakistani society. However, there was an overall high degree of pan-cultural similarity in the characteristics associated with women and men in all countries studied.

Professor Pandey's contribution to the gender stereotype research of Williams and Best led to the expansion of studies to 30 countries (Best & Williams, 1997; Williams & Best, 1982/1990). Looking across both these adult and child studies, Berry and colleagues (1992) suggested that "the degree of consensus is so large that it may be appropriate to suggest that the researchers have found a psychological universal when it comes to gender stereotypes" (p. 60). Currently a large-scale 42-country replication of this early research is underway to see how gender stereotypes have changed over the past 40 years (Kosakowska-Berezecka et al., 2020, 2022, 2024).

Aware of the differential effects that culture may have for women and men, Professor Pandey's later research examined gender differences when looking at social and environmental stressors, such as poverty and crowding. In India with its high density and interdependent collective culture, Ruback and Pandey found that in urban areas (Ruback & Pandey, 1991) and villages (Ruback & Pandey, 1996) when compared with men, women were more negatively affected by crowding (e.g., loss of privacy), spent more time in crowded households, and had less control and social support to buffer the stress. In spite of such stress and crowding, women wanted more children, consistent with their traditional views of their roles as wife-mother.

Pandey and Ruback (Ruback et al., 2002) extended their examination of gender differences in reaction to environmental stressors, examining crowding and the number of families sharing a water source, to two Muslim countries that differed in orthodoxy and the conventional nature of gender roles. They found more gender differences in more traditional Islamic Pakistan than in less traditional Bangladesh. Pakistani women reported higher levels of mental distress, less satisfaction with their children, less satisfaction with their houses, and less satisfaction with the supply of resources in their houses. This research underscores the importance of contextual cultural factors for understanding social psychological theory and methodology in the examination of life concerns.

Current Views of Gender Stereotypes and Their Impact on Behavior

Gender Stereotypes and Self-Concept

When looking at how children and young adults perceive gender stereotypes, a number of similarities continue to be found across cultures, as was shown in the earlier studies described previously. Recent research has demonstrated that children begin to perceive genders and gender differences at a very young age, and this impacts their development and interactions with others. For example, as early as age five, negative stereotypes about one's own gender can influence a child's performance (Ambady et al., 2001). Such stereotypes become deeply rooted into self-identity and may have powerful effects on how children perceive their own abilities. In many cultures, even when young female students perform better than their male counterparts, they tend to downplay or underestimate their achievements, rating themselves as equal to boys, but not higher (Stetsenko et al., 2000). This is just one way that these gender differences are seen in schools today. Such negative perceptions could influence how children continue to perceive themselves and others as they grow into adulthood.

Gender Stereotypes and Leadership

Recent research has also examined how gender stereotypes impact adult behaviors, looking at their influence on perceptions of women and men in leadership roles (Sczesny et al., 2004). For example, both Indian and Western men perceive executive leadership positions as being "male" positions. However, Indian women did not fall in line with these beliefs, viewing these positions as more balanced between genders. This could be due to the actual opportunities and presence of women in leadership positions in different countries (Sczesny et al., 2004). Nevertheless, women across cultures have shown an increased desire to possess previously considered "masculine" and task-oriented leadership qualities, perhaps signifying a shift toward a more gender-balanced leadership workforce.

Women in the Workplace in India

Examination of women in the workplace in India illustrates some of the changes that have taken place in gender stereotypes and roles since the early studies conducted by Pandey, Williams, and Best. Research shows that women now are more likely to pursue managerial educational studies and opportunities in 2005 than they were in the 1980s (Budhwar et al., 2005). Additionally, gender roles in India have slowly shifted so that now it is more acceptable for Indian women to work in STEM (i.e., science, technology, engineering, mathematics) and political fields (Wesarat & Mathew, 2017). Women's increased presence in the workplace underscores the positive contributions women make in the workplace. Women demonstrate greater empathy in work relationships, greater multitasking skills, greater composure in crisis situations, and greater social skills related to networking, power sharing, and receiving input (Budhwar et al., 2005).

As much as women enrich the professional atmosphere, they still face challenges of unequal pay and career advancement difficulties in the workplace. Tripathy (2018) suggests that women earn salaries that are 20% less than those of men who perform the same job (Tripathy, 2018). A 2009–2010 study revealed that some of the wage gap between men and women in India is due to unexplained or discriminatory reasons, such as the belief that men are more reliable because they are not expected to split work and domestic responsibilities (Deshpande et al., 2018). This discriminatory portion of the wage gap has increased, even though women increasingly present valuable work characteristics, such as experience and reliability (Deshpande et al., 2018). Apart from women performing jobs equal to those of men, women also receive lower pay because their family obligations often necessitate that they work part-time. This can also limit their opportunity for promotion (Böhmer & Schinnenburg, 2018).

Tripathy (2018) has identified career advancement as a challenge for women working in India and attributes it largely to a glass ceiling effect. The glass ceiling prevents women from earning respected management positions, which accordingly prevents women from earning higher wages (Wesarat & Mathew, 2017). Others' perceptions of women's work also hinder their ability to attain managerial careers. For example, men dislike granting managerial positions to women, but they do not mind having women work with them in lower positions (Budhwar et al., 2005). Men's professional preferences contribute to the maintenance of subordinate positions for women. Additionally, women's decisions are met with more scrutiny than men's decisions, which prevents them from moving up quickly in their careers (Tripathy, 2018). Lastly, women's beliefs about the glass ceiling negatively impact their professional success through decreased job satisfaction and decreased psychological well-being (Wesarat & Mathew, 2017). To combat these outcomes, organizations can work to alter the presence of a glass ceiling and women's glass ceiling beliefs. Increasing women's psychological well-being in the workplace is likely to lead to greater productivity for women and the organization at large (Wesarat & Mathew, 2017).

Although women in India currently occupy more professional roles than in the past, traditional Indian religious values still influence gender expectations, such that motherhood and child-rearing are viewed as the most important jobs for an Indian woman (Böhmer & Schinnenburg, 2018). Consequently, motherhood is seen as mandatory, while career development is secondary, making it difficult for working women to balance their professional life with traditional housewife duties (Budhwar et al., 2005). Because women's careers receive divided attention, they are sometimes evaluated as less efficient workers (Wesarat & Mathew, 2017).

Ironically, characteristics that women employ in motherhood and family situations are beneficial in the work environment. When women were told that particular jobs required a caring, relationship-oriented, humble individual, they were more likely to pursue entrepreneurial ventures (Gupta et al., 2013) This highlights the importance of marketing jobs to women's strengths and those that align with traditional motherhood skills. Other workplace changes that could increase women's presence in the workforce would be to provide flexible work options that would help women balance their motherhood and professional roles. This balance has been shown to decrease work–life conflict and increase job satisfaction (Merlin & Agarwal, 2019).

It is also important to recognize the influence that mothers can have in socializing their daughters to pursue careers. Mothers tend to provide support and motivation for daughters to acquire a career in the future. While fathers give direct instruction for professional life, mothers provide daughters with the emotion regulation tools to pursue those careers (Shenoy-Packer, 2014). Family support of working women can override negative societal opinions of working women and encourage female family members to pursue careers (Howell, 2016). Men view their careers as their contribution to the family, and women view child-rearing as their contribution. However, there is no monetary compensation for child-rearing. In order to broaden gender equality in the workplace, it would be beneficial to redefine men's contribution to the family, adding fatherhood along with redefining the mother's contribution by adding her professional role (Fernandez et al., 2016).

Gender Stereotypes and STEM

Another area where gender stereotypes have impacted adult behavior can be seen in the gender balance found and promoted in educational and work areas. Such balance is particularly important in areas that are emphasized around the globe in today's world where the centrality of technology and science are expanding. Research suggests that stereotypes about the cultural roles and abilities related to STEM (science, technology, engineering, and mathematics) deter women from pursuing STEM-related careers (Shapiro & Williams, 2012) Cultural stereotypes pertain to work, values, and the sorts of people involved in STEM. For example, the STEM field is typically portrayed as being socially isolated and run by "naturally intelligent" men (Cheryan et al., 2015). These notions do not align with the typical female stereotype which emphasizes women's role as social and community-oriented helpers (Luong & Knobloch-Westerwick, 2017). Stereotypes that assume women's lesser ability to attain success in an STEM field has discouraged women's entry into the field. Although not all women identify with traditional stereotypes, the misalignment of STEM and female stereotypes often prevents women from entering the STEM field (Makarova et al., 2019). Looking at gender stereotypes and STEM in the United States, Cheryan, Master, and Meltzoff (2015) focused on the ways in which threatening academic environments affect women's STEM participation and self-concept. Their model asserts that female gender stereotypes can lead to women's uncertainty about entering an STEM field. Then, if they enter a STEM academic environment, stereotype threat can lead to females experiencing lower perceived control, lower persistence and engagement in the STEM field, which ultimately leads to lower self-esteem (Casad et al., 2019). In order to encourage women to enter STEM fields, establishing female role models has been effective in decreasing uncertainty regarding STEM (Lockwood, 2006). Female role models attest to women's ability to succeed in an STEM field (Lockwood, 2006).

Modern gender stereotypes extend globally from the United States to India affecting self-concept, leadership, women's role in the workplace, and women's progress in STEM. While women face challenges such as unequal pay, advancement difficulties, lack of academic representation, interventions such as increased female role models, support from mothers, flexible professional options, and marketing jobs to women can be effective in helping women overcome the present challenges. Not only do gender stereotypes impact the professional and personal modern world, but age stereotypes are prominent as well.

Age Stereotypes: Views of Older Adults in India and the United States

Following their studies of gender stereotypes, Williams, Best, and Pandey turned their attention to examining views of older adults, a particularly interesting issue given the cultural differences that appeared to exist in views of aging. When thinking about stereotypes, research generally has compared participants descriptions of their own group with descriptions of an outgroup which is different from that of the participants. This ingroup–outgroup comparison is clearly seen when looking at gender, racial, or ethnic group comparisons. Participants in such studies will never be members of the "other" group they are asked to describe. However, asking young adults about their stereotypes and attitudes toward the elderly is quite different. Unlike outgroup descriptions, when young adults are asked to describe older adults, they are being asked to describe a group that they will someday be a part of. They must look forward and see themselves in the future. This notion of looking at whom they may become certainly influences their attitudes and stereotypes about aging, as well as how they define age categories, estimates of life expectancies, and life satisfaction when they are older. Growing older is a process experienced by everyone. Williams, Best, and Pandey first looked at age stereotypes in India and the United States (Williams et al., 1987) and later expanded their study to include 19 countries (Best & Williams, 1996).

The ways that older adults are viewed by younger adults in different cultures is influenced by cultural values and beliefs about aging as well as by family structure, contact between age groups, and economic development (Best & Puzio, 2019; Gardiner, 2019). In many individualistic cultures, nuclear families are common, contact with older adults may not occur on a daily basis, and older adults are financially stable and may live independently. This contrasts with what is seen in many developing, collectivistic cultures where extended families may live together in the same household, and older adults contribute, often on a daily basis, to childcare and the shared family economy and decisions.

Comparing younger adults' perceptions of older adults in India and the United States in the late 1980s, Williams et al. (1987) provided a look at two different cultures, the more traditional, developing society of India, and the more modern, developed society of the United States. At that time, the typical family living arrangement in India was the joint family in which grandparents, parents, and children resided in a single household, giving children extensive daily experience with older people of their grandparents' generation. On the other hand, in the United States, the nuclear family was the norm, and the typical child did not live in the same household with grandparents. Close family relationships were found in both family living arrangements, but the typical young adult in India had more personal daily experience with older adults than young adults in the United States.

Looking at the stereotype adjectives associated with old adults and young adults in India and the United States, Williams, Best, and Pandey (Williams et al., 1987) found that there was a substantial degree of agreement between the countries, with some small, but interesting differences. In both countries, young adults were viewed as stronger and more active than old adults. Interestingly, old adults were considered less favorable than young adults in India, but the reverse pattern was found in the United States. Indian participants reported living with grandparents and other older relatives longer ($M = 10.22$ years) than did U.S. participants ($M = .78$ years). However, Indian participants' longer living experiences with older adults were not related to their views of older adults. Relative to American participants, Indian participants viewed older adults as more critical and demanding while American participants viewed older adults as more nurturing and reality-oriented. The researchers attributed these differences to the transitions in Indian society that was moving from a traditional joint family, agricultural society to a more industrialized economy. Yet older adults continued to play central roles in the control of family resources and decision-making which may have been seen unfavorably by the younger generation.

This initial study examining stereotypes of the elderly and the aging process was expanded to include young adults in 19 countries representing six continents (Best & Williams, 1996). Participants in these countries were asked to identify the ages associated with being old and middle aged, and to identify life expectancies for themselves and the average person in their country. They were also asked to identify the decade of their lives that would be the most satisfying, how they felt about growing older, and to answer questions about expected life satisfaction when they were old. The results indicated that the ages used to define age categories were somewhat higher in more developed countries and those with larger Christian populations. Overall, men perceived aging to occur earlier but they expected to live longer than women, contrary to the actual life expectancies and mortality in their countries. Both men and women indicated that the twenties and thirties would be the most satisfying, productive period of their lives. Responses to life satisfaction questions were mixed, with some positive attitudes (e.g., would not be bored or sad) but also some negative views (e.g., not happy or satisfied with life). Women were more positive about growing older in countries that were more urbanized, that were no longer dependent upon agriculture, and where education was emphasized, all indicators of economic-social development. As life expectancy has increased around the world with advances in healthcare and economic circumstances, understanding the aging process and the elderly has become increasingly important.

Current Views of Older Adults and of Aging

Age stereotypes continue to exist in families, in the workplace, and in society as a whole across different countries and cultures. This is an increasingly important issue for understanding how these stereotypes impact quality of life and discrimination against older people. It is also beneficial to understand how different groups of people view the idea of aging and what they expect for that time of life in different cultures. Many of the discoveries made by Pandey, Williams, and Best have laid the foundation for new investigations of these stereotypes as countries and cultures continue to develop.

Changes in Age Stereotypes

In looking at Indian and American beliefs regarding intergenerational communication, recent research has shown that both Indian and American young adults provide increasingly more respect and benevolence to adults as they age (Giles et al., 2007). This is a notable difference in perspective from the research conducted by Williams and colleagues in 1987 that determined that old adults were considered to be less favorable in India than in the United States. This would seem to show that there has been a change in the respect that Indian young adults possess for the older population. The previous research also found that Indian young adults often viewed their elderly as "critical and demanding." However, more recently research has shown that Indian young adults view their elderly as more benevolent and possessing more vitality than young adults do in the United States. It is possible that this change in views has come with the development of India which has become a more industrialized economy since the 1980s.

An interesting development in understanding how youth of a country view their older counterparts is the presence of grandparents. Recent studies have shown that young adults show increasing respect to adults as they age (Giles et al., 2007). Although respect for grandparents is a common value in many cultures, this does not directly relate to viewing them positively. This may explain the results found in 1987 that although intergenerational living was more common in India, Indian young adults still found older people to be less favorable (Williams et al., 1987).

Indeed, a long-held cultural norm has been changing in India over the last few decades as an increase in homes for the elderly are appearing across the country (Choolayil & Putran, 2020). As nuclear family structures become more common in India, the respect and acceptance of aging adults are not as widely seen. However, a recent discovery suggests that young Indian adults who live with grandparents, or have frequent quality exposure to grandparents, show significantly lower ageism (Choolayil & Putran, 2020). Although culture may instill values of respect, negative views may still be present. Nevertheless, having intergenerational communication and interactions does increase positive attitudes toward elderly people and aging in India.

When comparing the intergenerational relationships seen in India to those of the United States, interesting connections can be drawn. One study with university students in the United States found that their perceived closeness with their closest grandparent did not impact positive attitudes toward older adults (Freeman, 2002). However, there was a strong relationship between students' favorable attitudes toward their closest grandparent and their favorable attitudes toward older adults in general. Interestingly, the amount of time and the types of activities they shared with grandparents was not as predictive of students' positive attitudes toward older adults as was their perceptions of grandparents' current and future influence on their lives.

Another study in the United States (Stricker & Hillman, 1996) found that young adults gave mildly positive evaluations of all older adults. However, they viewed older adults as less instrumental, autonomous, and pleasant than typical grandparents who were viewed less positively than their own grandparents. Interestingly, they reported greater liking and closeness with grandmothers than grandfathers which is consistent with other U.S. studies (Eisenberg, 1988). These studies suggest that age stereotypes may follow a gradient of familiarity such that stereotypes about the elderly, particularly negative ones, may not apply to older adults with whom one has a close relationship.

Views of the Aging Process

To understand how people view aging adults, it is important to acknowledge how they view the process of aging in general. In 1996, Best and Williams examined attitudes toward aging from people across 19 different countries. Expanding on this work, Reich and colleagues aimed to identify how different cultures perceive "successful aging" (Reich et al., 2020). They found that across cultures, the ideas of social engagement and positive attitudes were important aspects for being successful in old age. Other important themes included independence, physical health, and good cognitive function (Reich et al., 2020). A notable cultural difference was that adults from the Middle East, Asia, and Oceania placed more emphasis on the importance of giving back to their families in old age. This idea of the importance of human connection and interaction is a theme that appears consistently in regard to positivity about old age.

A study that investigated 26 different cultures looking at college students' perceptions of aging found that culture was an important indicator of their views. Many of the perceptions that were consistent across cultures were aligned with biological age-related declines, such as decreased physical and cognitive ability (Löckenhoff et al., 2009). An interesting note is that increased socioeconomic development predicted more negative views of aging, possibly contrasting with the results previously noted that women in more urbanized countries had more positive views of aging (Best & Williams, 1996). However, the current study also found that the influence of socioeconomic development on perceptions of aging was not as relevant as factors such as educational enrollment and population aging (Löckenhoff et al., 2009). There was general cross-cultural consensus about aging trajectories (e.g., increases in wisdom, decreases in physical abilities). Shifts toward more progressive values that accompany economic development may erode traditional beliefs that older adults deserve respect and authority simply due to their age.

One theme found when examining the changes in attitudes toward older adults across cultures is that socioeconomic development may lead to more rational tolerance (Löckenhoff et al., 2009). Modernization Theory suggests that as societies develop, people may become more socially progressive and tolerant while shifting toward more secular rational viewpoints (Inglehart & Baker, 2000). This presents an interesting paradox when looking at India and other traditionally collectivist cultures. While shifting toward a secular rational viewpoint may promote more tolerance, it also signifies a movement away from religious and traditional family values seen in collectivistic communities. Moreover, when considering views of older adults, it is unclear whether future increases in modernization and development will continue to influence the way that people view aging in different cultures.

Conclusions

Gender and age stereotypes have been relevant in the past and continue to be important as the world becomes increasingly industrialized. It is useful to assess current cross-cultural gender and age stereotypes with the foundation established by earlier research. Past research on gender stereotypes displayed support for similarity in the pan-cultural assessment of male and female traits. These universal views were evident despite differences in the affective meaning of male- and female-associated traits and differing developmental timelines for gender stereotypes in India and Pakistan. This underlined the idea that some gender stereotypes persist across cultures, while others appear to be culture specific. Past research by Ruback and Pandey (1991, 1996) also highlighted the importance of considering environment stressors such as poverty and crowding in sociocultural research.

Current research on gender stereotypes tends to focus on self-concept, leadership, women in the workplace, and women's participation in STEM fields. Research on self-concept is consistent with past research that the development of gender stereotypes begins at a young age and extends throughout the lifespan. In adulthood, Indian women are more likely to pursue professional roles than in the past, but they are still expected to take care of domestic duties, as are women in other countries. This dual responsibility may be partially responsible for an Indian wage gap and less advancement opportunities for women. Although gender stereotypes bring challenges for women in India, family support can help them overcome societal expectations.

In the United States, current research focuses on women's participation in STEM. Gender stereotypes prevent women from entering the STEM fields in the first place, and they prevent women from continuing in those STEM fields. Research has shown that providing women with female role models in STEM settings can increase female STEM participation and decrease female withdrawal from these fields in the future.

Past research on older adults and aging by Williams, Best, and Pandey examined young adults' views of older adults in India and the United States. Although Indian young adults were more likely to live with their grandparents than Americans were, Americans rated older adults more favorably than Indians did. Indians' lower favorability ratings of older adults were attributed to socioeconomic shifts in India from more traditional values to more industrialized influences. Other past research suggested that differences in gender and industrialization status affect individuals' views of aging. Current research on age stereotypes focuses on a shift toward greater respect for older adults with age in both India and the United States. It also underlines the impact of intergenerational living, relationships with grandparents, successful aging, and socioeconomic factors.

In order for researchers to assess current gender and age stereotypes, it is crucial to understand the foundation that was laid by researchers in the 1970s and 1980s. While certain gender and age stereotypes have been maintained throughout time, socioeconomic change and intentional interventions can help to reduce restrictive perceptions of gender and age across cultures.

References

Ambady, N., Shih, M., Kim, A., & Pittinsky, T. L. (2001). Stereotype susceptibility in children: Effects of identity activation on quantitative performance. *Psychological Science*, *12*(5), 385–390. https://doi.org/10.1111/1467-9280.00371

Berry, J. W., Poortinga, Y. H., Segall, M. H., & Dasen, P. R. (1992). *Cross-cultural psychology: Research and applications*. Cambridge University Press.

Best, D. L., & Puzio, A. R. (2019). Gender and culture. In D. Matsumoto & H. C. Hwang (Eds.), *Oxford handbook of culture and psychology* (pp. 235–291). Oxford University Press.

Best, D. L., & Williams, J. E. (1996). Anticipations of aging: A cross-cultural examination of young adults' views of growing old. In J. Pandey, D. Sinha, & D. P. S. Bhawuk (Eds.), *Asian contributions to cross-cultural psychology* (pp. 274–288). Sage.

Best, D. L., & Williams, J. E. (1997). Sex, gender, and culture. In J. W. Berry, Y. H. Poortinga, J. Pandey, P. R. Dasen, T. S. Saraswathi, M. H. Segall, & C. Kagitcibasi (Series Eds.) & J. W. Berry, M. H. Segall, & C. Kagitcibasi (Vol. Eds.), *Handbook of cross-cultural psychology: Vol. 3: Social behavior and applications* (2nd ed., pp. 163–212). Allyn & Bacon.

Best, D. L., Williams, J. E., Cloud, J. M., Davis, S. W., Robertson, L. W., Edwards, J. R., Giles, H., & Fowles, J. (1977). Development of sex-trait stereotypes among young children in the United States, England, and Ireland. *Child Development*, *48*, 1375–1384.

Böhmer, N., & Schinnenburg, H. (2018). Preventing the leaky pipeline: Teaching future female leaders to manage their careers and promote gender equality in organizations. *Journal of International Women's Studies*, *19*(5), 63–81.

Budhwar, P. S., Saini, D. S., & Bhatnagar, J. (2005). Women in management in the new economic environment: The case of India. *Asia Pacific Business Review*, *11*(2), 179–193. https://doi.org.go.libproxy.wakehealth.edu/10.1080/1360238042000291199

Casad, B. J., Petzel, Z. W., & Ingalls, E. A. (2019). A model of threatening academic environments predicts women STEM majors' self-esteem and engagement in STEM. *Sex Roles*, *80*(7–8), 469–488. http://dx.doi.org.go.libproxy.wakehealth.edu/10.1007/s11199-018-0942-4

Cheryan, S., Master, A., & Meltzoff, A. N. (2015). Cultural stereotypes as gatekeepers: Increasing girls' interest in computer science and engineering by diversifying stereotypes. *Frontiers in Psychology*, *6*. https://doi.org/10.3389/fpsyg.2015.00049

Choolayil, A., & Putran, L. (2020). Ageism among undergraduate students: Do grandparents make a difference? *Indian Journal of Gerontology*, *34*(3), 333–342.

Deshpande, A., Goel, D., & Khanna, S. (2018). Bad Karma or discrimination? Male–female wage gaps among salaried workers in India. *World Development*, *102*, 331–344. https://doi.org/10.1016/j.worlddev.2017.07.012

Eisenberg, A. R. (1988). Grandchildren's perspectives on relationships with grandparents: The influence of gender across generations. *Sex Roles*, *19*, 205–217.

Fernandez, B., Gopal, M., & Ruthven, O. (2016). *Land, labour and livelihoods: Indian women's perspectives*. Springer ProQuest Ebook Central. http://ebookcentral.proquest.com/lib/wfu/detail.action?docID=4751440

Freeman, P. L. (2002). *College age students' attitudes towards the older adult; Grandparents fit with older adult stereotypes and the closeness of the grandparent/grandchild relationship* (Publication No. 3067113) [Doctoral dissertation, University of Oklahoma Graduate College]. Proquest Information and Learning Company.

Gardiner, H. W. (2019). Culture, context, and development. In D. Matsumoto & H. C. Hwang (Eds.), *Oxford handbook of culture and psychology* (2nd ed., pp. 235–291). Oxford University Press.

Giles, H., Dailey, R. M., Sarkar, J. M., & Makoni, S. (2007). Intergenerational communication beliefs across the lifespan: Comparative data from India. *Communication Reports*, *20*(2), 75–89. https://doi.org/10.1080/08934210701643701

Gough, H. G., & Heilbrun, A. B. (1980). *The adjective check list manual*. Consulting Psychologists Press.

Gupta, V., Turban, D., & Pareek, A. (2013). Differences between men and women in opportunity evaluation as a function of gender stereotypes and stereotype activation. *Entrepreneurship Theory and Practice*, *37*(4), 771–788. https://doi.org/10.1111/j.1540-6520.2012.00512.x

Howell, J. (2016). India's working women and career discourses: Society, socialization and agency. *Journal of International Women's Studies*, *17*(1), 222–224.

Inglehart, R., & Baker, W. E. (2000). Modernization, cultural change, and the persistence of traditional values. *American Sociological Review*, *65*(1), 19–51. https://doi.org/10.2307/2657288

Kosakowska-Berezecka, N., Besta, T., Zadkowska, M., Zawisza, M., Safdar, S., Vandello, J. A., Bosson, J., Włodarczyk, A., Best, D. L., & Anjum, G. (2020). *Towards Gender Harmony project*. www.towardsgenderharmonyproject; www.researchgate.net/project/Toward-Gender-Harmony-Understanding-the-Relationship-between-Masculinity-Threat-and-Gender-Equality-Across-Cultures

Kosakowska-Berezecka, N., Bosson, J. K., Jurek, P., Besta, T., Best, D. L., Zukauskiene, R., & Zadkowska, M. (2022). Gender self-views across 62 countries: A test of competing models. *Social Psychological and Personality Science*, *14*(7), 808–824.

Kosakowska-Berezecka, N., Sawicki, A., Celikkol, G., Bosson, J. K., Van Laar, C., Van Rossum, A., Best, D. L., Jurek, P., Besta, T., Olech, M., & Glick, P. (2024). Does culture moderate gender stereotypes? Individualism predicts communal (but not agentic) prescriptions for men across 62 nations. *Social Psychological and Personality Science*, *0*(0). https://doi.org.wake.idm.oclc.org/10.1177/19485506231221913

Löckenhoff, C. E., De Fruyt, F., Terracciano, A., McCrae, R. R., De Bolle, M., Costa, P. T., Aguilar-Vafaie, M. E., Ahn, C.-K., Ahn, H.-N., Alcalay, L., Allik, J., Avdeyeva, T. V., Barbaranelli, C., Benet-Martínez, V., Blatný, M., Bratko, D., Cain, T. R., Crawford, J. T., Lima, M. P., . . . Yik, M. (2009). Perceptions of aging across 26 cultures and their culture-level associates. *Psychology and Aging*, *24*(4), 941–954. https://doi.org/10.1037/a0016901

Lockwood, P. (2006). "Someone like me can be successful": Do college students need same-gender role models? *Psychology of Women Quarterly*, *30*(1), 36–46. https://doi.org/10.1111/j.1471-6402.2006.00260.x

Luong, K., & Knobloch-Westerwick, S. (2017). Can the media help women be better at math? Stereotype threat, selective exposure, media effects, and women's math performance. *Human Communication Research*, *43*(2), 193–213. https://doi.org/10.1111/hcre.12101

Makarova, E., Aeschlimann, B., & Herzog, W. (2019). The gender gap in STEM fields: The impact of the gender stereotype of math and science on secondary students' career aspirations. *Frontiers in Education*, *4*(60), 1–11. https://doi.org/10.3389/feduc.2019.00060

Merlin, M. S., & Agarwal, B. (2019). Support perceptions, flexible work options and career outcomes. *Gender in Management*, *34*(4), 254–286. http://dx.doi.org.go.libproxy.wakehealth.edu/10.1108/GM-12-2018-0157

Reich, A. J., Claunch, K. D., Verdeja, M. A., Dungan, M. T., Anderson, S., Clayton, C. K., & Thacker, E. L. (2020). What does "successful aging" mean to you?—Systematic review and cross-cultural comparison of lay perspectives of older adults in 13 countries, 2010–2020. *Journal of Cross-Cultural Gerontology*, *35*(4), 455–478. https://doi.org/10.1007/s10823-020-09416-6

Ruback, R. B., Begum, H. A., Tariq, N., Kamal, A., & Pandey, J. (2002). Reactions to environmental stressors: Gender differences in the slums of Dhaka and Islamabad. *Journal of Cross-Cultural Psychology*, *33*(1), 100–119.

Ruback, R. B., & Pandey, J. (1991). Crowding, perceived control, and relative power: An analysis of households in India. *Journal of Applied Social Psychology*, *21*, 315–344.

Ruback, R. B., & Pandey, J. (1996). Gender differences in perceptions of household crowding: Stress, affiliation, and role obligations in rural India. *Journal of Applied Social Psychology*, *26*(5), 417–436.

Sczesny, S., Bosak, J., Neff, D., & Schyns, B. (2004). Gender stereotypes and the attribution of leadership traits: A cross-cultural comparison. *Sex Roles*, *51*. https://doi.org/10.1007/s11199-004-0715-0

Shapiro, J. R., & Williams, A. M. (2012). The role of stereotype threats in undermining girls' and women's performance and interest in STEM fields. *Sex Roles*, *66*(3–4), 175–183. http://dx.doi.org.go.libproxy.wakehealth.edu/10.1007/s11199-011-0051-0

Shenoy-Packer, S. (2014). *India's working women and career discourses: Society, socialization, and agency*. Lexington Books. ProQuest Ebook Central, http://ebookcentral.proquest.com/lib/wfu/detail.action?docID=1767180

Stetsenko, A., Little, T. D., Gordeeva, T., Grasshof, M., & Oettingen, G. (2000). Gender effects in children's beliefs about school performance: A cross-cultural study. *Child Development*, *71*(2), 517–527.

Stricker, G., & Hillman, J. L. (1996). Attitudes toward older adults: The perceived value of grandparent as a social role. *Journal of Adult Development*, *3*(2), 71–79. https://doi.org/10.1007/bf02278773

Tripathy, M. (2018). Breaking the code of gender barrier to leverage the position of women in Indian workplaces. *Space and Culture, India*, *6*(3), 180–193. https://doi.org/10.20896/saci.v6i3.328

Wesarat, P., & Mathew, J. (2017). Theoretical framework of glass ceiling: A case of India's women academic leaders. *Paradigm*, *21*(1), 21–30. https://doi.org/10.1177/0971890717700533

Williams, J. E., & Best, D. L. (1990). *Measuring sex stereotypes: A multination study* (1990 Rev. ed.). Sage. (Original work published 1982)

Williams, J. E., Best, D. L., Haque, A., Pandey, J., & Verma, R. K. (1982). Sex-trait stereotypes in India and Pakistan. *Journal of Psychology*, *111*, 167–181

Williams, J. E., Best, D. L., Tilquin, C., Keller, H., Voss, H. G., Bjerke, T., & Baarda, B. (1981). Traits associated with men and women: Attributions by young children in France, Germany, Norway, The Netherlands, and India. *Journal of Cross-Cultural Psychology*, *12*, 327–346.

Williams, J. E., Daws, J. T., Best, D. L., Tilquin, C., Wesley, F., & Bjerke, T. (1979). Sex-trait stereotypes in France, Germany, and Norway. *Journal of Cross-Cultural Psychology*, *10*, 133–156.

Williams, J. E., Giles, H., Edwards, J. R., Best, D. L., & Daws, J. T. (1977). Sex-trait stereotypes in England, Ireland, and the United States. *British Journal of Social and Clinical Psychology*, *16*, 303–309.

Williams, J. E., Pandey, J., Best, D. L., Morton, K. R., & Pande, N. (1987). Young adults' views of old adults in India and the United States. In C. Kagitcibasi (Ed.), *Growth and progress in cross-cultural psychology* (pp. 227–234). Swets & Zeitlinger.

9 Being a Kalpwasi

Pilgrimage and Identity on the Banks of the Ganga[1]

Nick Hopkins, Steve D. Reicher, and Narayanan Srinivasan

The focus for this chapter is an exploration of the social psychology of pilgrimage. For many researchers located in Europe or North America, this would likely appear an esoteric interest. A quick glance through the index pages of our discipline's textbooks would imply there is little of interest to be found in such a topic. Indeed, you would be hard-pressed to find any entries at all. However, this absence says little about the social significance of pilgrimage. For example, it has been estimated that of all domestic travel in India, over one-third is for the purpose of performing pilgrimage (Singh, 2011). Nor does this absence say anything about the relevance of psychology for understanding pilgrimage. The fact that so many people take enormous pleasure from subjecting themselves to the demanding routines associated with pilgrimage suggests there is much here for psychologists to address. Surely the experience of pilgrimage is crying out for our discipline's attention?

Rather sadly, it seems hard to avoid the conclusion that the absence of entries addressing the psychology of pilgrimage in our standard textbooks speaks volumes about the limits of our discipline's claim to be a truly international discipline. Understandably, these disciplinary limits have been most keenly felt by those located outside North America and Europe. Certainly, many in India have expressed concern about the limited relevance of much psychological theory and research for the phenomena before them (Pandey & Singh, 2005). In turn, there has been much written about the potential of indigenous alternatives (Sinha, 1997, 1998). In what follows we hope to contribute to such ongoing debates. Specifically, we wish to consider the utility of a particular social psychological approach to identity for those working in India. Although this approach has its roots in European Social Psychology, we believe it has a relevance for researchers working in India and elsewhere, and we seek to illustrate our case through discussing an Indo-British project which sought to address the experience of an Indian Hindu pilgrimage. Inevitably, such activities are highly distinctive cultural events, yet we believe that the conception of identity employed in our research allowed us to both respect the cultural particularities of the event and develop analytic insights into collective processes that could allow generalizations from this particular event to others across the globe.

DOI: 10.4324/9781003461302-13

Psychology and Culture

Psychology has long struggled to take culture seriously. Take, for example, Misra and Gergen's (1993) observation that psychology's vision of a universally applicable analysis of behavior based upon experimentation has led to "a culturally de-contextualised science of behaviour" (p. 227). Indeed, they maintain that given this methodological commitment, culture (if considered at all) is routinely conceptualized as a source of error that should be controlled for so that more universal claims about behavior can be identified. Moreover, they argue that to the degree that psychology has sought to address the culture-bound nature of claims about behavior, the research agenda remains skewed to privilege a particular cultural perspective such that much cross-cultural work takes the form of "an ancillary enterprise—checking the validity and local limitations of otherwise universal assumptions" (p. 229). Compounding these problems, they observe that even when cultural distinctiveness is investigated, cultural differences are reduced to a limited number of dimensions of comparison, which are conceptualized and defined from the vantage point of the (Western) mainstream.

Such concerns are not only voiced in India. Increasingly there is a realization that psychology's habit of wanting to make generalized claims about behavior on the basis of research conducted with psychology undergraduates recruited in North America and Europe is deeply problematic because they are so unrepresentative. Indeed, this point is emphasized in Henrich et al.'s (2010) characterization of such samples as being fundamentally WEIRD (Western, Educated, Industrialized, Rich, and Democratic) and thus atypical. Moreover, responding to calls for psychology to take culture seriously, Virgina Kwan (cited in Snibbe, 2003) ironically observes that the discipline as it stands does address culture—however, it is the very specific culture of North America. As she puts it: "mainstream psychology is really cultural psychology, dealing with a very particular cultural context."

All the above suggests that anyone interested in the social psychology of pilgrimage in India would be well-advised to start afresh. However, we believe that there are aspects of contemporary European social psychological theorizing that can shed light on topics and phenomena that are absent from the standard textbooks, but which have enormous personal and social significance in India. Specifically, we believe that the social identity tradition as developed in European social psychology (Tajfel, 1978, 1982; Tajfel & Turner, 1979; Turner, 1982; Turner et al., 1987) may be used in contextually relevant and culturally sensitive ways (Hopkins & Reicher, 2005, 2011, 2013). Indeed, there is a sense in which Tajfel himself shared some of the concerns articulated by Misra and Gergen (1993) described above. He too was seriously troubled by what he saw as the tendency for experimental researchers to treat "the experimental episode as if it were a 'social vacuum', in which the norms and values that normally guided human social behaviour no longer applied" (Condor, 2003, p. 156–157). Indeed, and as we will see, as a framework for exploring group behavior, the social identity perspective emphasizes the need to attend to group members' own understandings of their identities and their associated collective beliefs, values, and norms.

Investigating the Magh Mela

The history to our pilgrimage project is long. It originated in an Advanced Refresher Course (2005) held under the auspices of the Centre of Behavioural and Cognitive Sciences (CBCS) at the University of Allahabad and led by Prof. Janak Pandey. The course brought together a team of UK and Indian researchers, and the difficulties we experienced in discussing theory and research practice in the abstract prompted the idea of a joint exploratory research project. The decision to focus on pilgrimage was in part opportunistic: Allahabad is the site of the annual Magh Mela which attracts hundreds of thousands to a culturally distinctive month-long gathering on the banks of the Ganga. However, it was also inspired by the desire to investigate the utility of social psychological theory in understanding aspects of this culturally distinctive collective assembly.

This exploratory project was conducted over two years (2006–2007) and involved almost 30 researchers (many of whom were PhD scholars) who proceeded to publish a set of outputs under a team name (the *Prayag Magh Mela Research Group* or PMMRG) in a special issue of *Psychological Studies* (PMMRG, 2007a, 2007b, 2007c). As a learning experience, it was challenging (in the best sense of the word) and exciting. It was also a particularly sociable and enjoyable enterprise. Indeed, in the introduction to the PMMRG papers, Cassidy et al. (2007) observed:

> We also hope that these papers convey something of the pleasures of our own experience of another collective—the Prayag Magh Mela Research Group. Although a fraction of the size of the Prayag crowds, we too have had occasion to enjoy the experience of collectivity made possible through this Indo-British research collaboration.

Needless to say, much of the success of this phase of our research collaboration is directly attributable to the remarkable leadership provided by Prof. Janak Pandey. Prof. Pandey had much knowledge and research experience of the event (Elderling & Pandey, 2007; Ruback et al., 2008), and it was he who steered the PMMRG through many of the conceptual and logistical challenges that we faced (all of which needed to be managed within the incredibly tight time constraints associated with the fact that the Magh Mela is an annual month-long event). It was also Prof. Pandey's leadership that allowed the team to cohere and function, and it is testament to the success of this exploratory work and capacity-building exercise that a new and more sustained project was possible (2009–2012). Again, the project was based in the CBCS at the University of Allahabad. It involved a team of four

Postdoctoral researchers in India and one in Scotland. As Prof. Pandey had taken on the challenging role of Vice Chancellor at the newly inaugurated Central University of Bihar, the Allahabad-based team now worked alongside Prof. Narayanan Srinivasan.

Below we outline some of the themes explored in our 2009–2012 research project. In doing so, we draw upon findings obtained using a variety of research methods (interviews, surveys, and experiments). Throughout, our core argument is that the concept of social identity does have a relevance for psychologists addressing a range of phenomena in India and that this relevance is possible precisely because it is a model of process that requires attention to the culturally specific content associated with group identities.

Social Identity

Initially, the concept of social identity was elaborated in order to conceptualize the processes involved in intergroup relations and their transformation (Tajfel, 1978, 1982; Tajfel & Turner, 1979). However, the concept has since been developed to offer an account of what makes group behavior possible (self-categorization theory: Turner, 1982; Turner et al., 1987). This proposes that the self can be defined at different levels of abstraction. In some contexts, we may define ourselves in terms of our individual uniqueness (e.g., "I" vs. "you"). At other times, we may define ourselves in terms of specific group memberships (e.g., "us" vs. "them"). These social identities can vary in terms of their inclusiveness from those that are narrowly defined and include a small number of known others to those that include many millions of others who remain personally unknown to us (e.g., as when we define ourselves in terms of a national identity).

The importance of these collective identities cannot be overemphasized. There is no sense in which they are to be regarded as superficial or as detracting from one's individual identity. They can be deeply felt and potent motivators of behavior. Moreover, they are fundamentally social and cultural products. What it means to be an academic, British, Indian, Muslim, Hindu, or whatever, is the product of wider social processes such that when we act in terms of a social identity we act as socially constituted beings. Indeed, the logic to this social psychological perspective is that the behavioral consequences of identifying in terms of a social group depend on social and cultural factors. As Turner puts it, "process theories such as social identity and self-categorization require the incorporation of specific content into their analyses before they can make predictions either in the laboratory or the field and are designed to require such an incorporation" (Turner, 1999, p. 34). More specifically the theory states that the behavior of those identifying in terms of a particular group membership is shaped by, and conforms to, their cognitive representation (or stereotype) of the beliefs and values associated with that membership.

The merits of such an approach are many. It places individuals' subjective self-categorization at the center of our analysis, which implies we must attend closely to any identity's cultural particularities. We are also invited to investigate the social and cultural practices that make particular identifications and identity definitions cognitively available. Indeed, as Brubaker et al. (2004) observe, the domain of the "mental" and the "psychological" is not identical with the domain of the individual, and the promise of a cognitive approach to identity (such as self-categorization theory) is that it "may help connect our analyses of what goes on in people's heads with our analysis of what goes on in public" (p. 46). The social identity approach also emphasizes that the group memberships employed in self-definition are multiple and that at different times people may act in terms of different social identities. This helps explain both the variation in an individual's behavior in terms of variation in the psychological salience of particular identities and also the homogeneity to group members' behavior. So too, we are drawn to consider the degree to which individuals invest in any particular social category (and on this we can expect between-individual variability). Attending to this level of identification with a particular group membership is important because it is only when individuals see themselves as group members that the cognitive and behavioral corollaries of group membership follow.

The Multiple Implications of Identification

Over the years, the implications of such group-based social identifications for behavior have developed. Originally, the emphasis was on the ways in which a shift in self-definition from an individual to a group-level identity impacted the basis for our behavior (such that we no longer think and act in terms of our individual and idiosyncratic beliefs and values, but in terms of group-based beliefs and values). More recently, there has been increased awareness of the importance of such identities for one's social relations with others—even unknown others (Reicher, 2017). As people come to define themselves in terms of a social identity and see others as sharing that identity, they come to see and treat each other as "fellows" rather than as "other" (Neville & Reicher, 2011). This results in increased helping (Levine et al., 2005) and in the anticipation of social support should one need it (Haslam et al., 2012).

So too there has been growing awareness of how social identity processes shape one's affective experiences. When acting in terms of a particular social identity, one's emotional experience is no longer based on idiosyncratic factors but social identity-related considerations. This means that whether something is to be evaluated positively or negatively depends on its relationship with the values and beliefs associated with the currently salient identity. More specifically, identity-congruent and identity-affirming experiences contribute to positive affect. Furthermore, there is growing awareness of how the sense of social support associated with a shared identification with others contributes to group members' sense that they can cope with the demands placed upon them. Indeed, identification with social groups has been characterized as a basis for improved psychological health and well-being (Jetten et al., 2012).

Applying the Social Identity Approach to Mass Gatherings

The fact that people are in proximity does not mean that they self-categorize as a group. The crowds to be found in Indian railway stations are unlikely to have a sense of collective identity. However, when people assemble at mass gatherings such as the Magh Mela there is potential for the emergence of a shared social identity on the basis of their common faith and purpose. At the same time, just because people are at the same pilgrimage event guarantees nothing. Pilgrimage events are routinely sites of factional dispute as the followers of different traditions struggle to assert their own vision of the event over others (Coleman, 2002; Eade & Sallnow, 1991; Sallnow, 1981). It is also important to note that such events attract all manner of people, and those attending the event may differentiate between various categories of attendees. For example, at the Magh Mela, there are people who visit for a day or two (normally the more auspicious days of the lunar calendar), beggars, market traders, an army of workers who service the Mela's infrastructure (removing rubbish, cleaning latrines, etc.), and others who commit to live at the site for the entire month. One cannot assume that such a diverse range of actors would necessarily identify with each other—their motivations for attending are diverse and can be experienced as incompatible. Yet there remains the potential for some form of shared identity among some attendees, and in our own work, we found that those committing to live on the site for the full month as Kalpwasis (Buzinde et al., 2014; Elderling & Pandey, 2007) could indeed develop a shared identity on the basis of their common pursuit of particular religious practices and spiritual goals (Hopkins et al., 2016b, 2019; Khan et al., 2015; Reicher et al., 2021).

Shared Identity and Social Support

This potential for a shared identity was readily apparent in the interviews conducted with Kalpwasis attending the Mela. First, we found evidence that Kalpwasis did not identify with all others present on the Mela site. Take, for example, one interviewee's characterization of those they met in the market area of the Mela site[2]:

> They come to eat *golgappa* [a street snack]. They would not look at a religious place for two minutes, would eat golgappa, snacks, eat roasted gram [a type of chickpea]. This is why I believe that they come for tourism, mostly they come to picnic. This is why I don't like the road crowd.
>
> (P7M38, Hopkins et al., 2019)

In turn, they routinely contrasted Kalpwasi from these others in terms of their values and behavior. For example, one drew a contrast between the young men who come to watch the crowds of bathers or to work as boatmen ferrying pilgrims to the confluence of the Ganga and the Yamuna, and Kalpwasis:

> Young guys come. They run and move around. Some boatman are also like this who run and move around. The youngsters do this. They do not realize that some old man might fall over because of their [behaviour]. But the Kalpwasis who are there, they do not do this.
>
> (P20F60, Reicher et al., 2021)

Building on such a contrast, other interviewees routinely spoke of Kalpwasis as having something of a shared identity. One question routinely asked by the interviewers invited respondents to compare and contrast their experience of the Mela with their experience of other crowded locations such as the railway station. Typically, a clear contrast was drawn. For example, one explained:

> In the railway station every person has a different purpose, going to different places, going to another country, going to separate stations. But here there is only one purpose, one *dharma* is to be performed, that is why the crowd here and outside are different [] There everyone has separate purposes but here the purpose becomes only one!
>
> (P30M40, Hopkins et al., 2019)

In similar vein, another observed that whereas those at the railway could be characterized as a collection of individuals pursuing their own idiosyncratic goals, the common purpose among Kalpwasis resulted in mutually supportive behavior:

> At the railway station people are not helping each other, [they] fulfil their own aim. When the train arrives, immediately, if they have a reservation, people will board. Suppose it is the General class [a basic level of rail travel], someone is taking their own luggage and facing problems, they [other passengers] will not care. And here [in the Mela], people take much care of this thing!
>
> (P11M72, Hopkins et al., 2019)

This sense of commonality and mutual support was a common feature running throughout our Kalpwasi interviews, and it was common to find references to Kalpwasis' relations with each other as "family-like":

> Relations become good here. Connections with brothers would not be as good as they are here! There might be some problems, but here no matter whoever he is, people help as if like family!
>
> (P3M74, Hopkins et al., 2019)

It was also clear that this support (both actual and anticipated) was welcomed. The daily routine followed by Kalpwasis is demanding (Buzinde et al., 2014; Elderling & Pandey, 2007). They live in canvas tents with little by way of comfort, eat one simple meal a day, and rise early for what can be a long trek for their pre-dawn bathing in the Ganga. Moreover, this routine is pursued at a time of the year (January–February) when the temperature can be cold and the prospect of the pre-dawn Ganga dip is particularly challenging (Pandey et al., 2014). One Kalpwasi spoke of the challenges involved in undertaking this pilgrimage and of the importance of others' identity-related behavior in motivating her own.

Interviewee: The people of the early days, like the kings and saints and all, they would go to mountains like the Himalaya and do penance. Where do we get such stamina? One sparrow will chirp and we will run from fear. Where do we get that courage? If no one bathes in *Gangaji* [the Ganga, venerated as a god] at midnight and we are asked to go for a dip, will we have the strength to go? First, we see [others] and only then do we go

Interviewer: Ok, so you won't go?

Interviewee: See, I won't tell a lie, only when we see the public do we go. If you do not have the courage, how will we go?

(P20F60, Reicher et al., 2021)

Taken together, these brief extracts from our interviews illustrate the point that Kalpwasis attending the Magh Mela undergo something of a social psychological transformation. Rather than thinking of themselves and others in terms of their unique individuality, there is evidence that they tend to think of themselves and other Kalpwasis in terms of a shared social identity and that this has multiple implications. First, there is a shared understanding of the values and norms that should guide their behavior. Second, there is a sense of relational connectedness and family-like intimacy with other Kalpwasis. Third, this sense of connection between Kalpwasis is manifested in behavior that is respectful and helpful. Indeed, as the last quote above hints, there is a sense in which others' action in accordance with their Kalpwasi identity motivates their own. That is, their sense of common purpose gave each the confidence to fulfill the identity-related injunctions associated with being a Kalpwasi.

Enacting Identity

The significance of a shared identity for our participants' ability to fulfill these injunctions was often illustrated when participants reflected on the contrast between their everyday lives and their lives in the Mela. Reflecting on their daily village routines, interviewees routinely reported how they often struggled to orient to spiritual concerns because their interactions with others drew them into more mundane material issues. For example, farmers reported how village interactions resulted in them being drawn into local disputes about land access whilst others referred to interactions in which they were required to address domestic issues. However, in the Mela they described being in a social environment in which their shared identity as Kalpwasis resulted in an alignment of their interests with those around them. Accordingly, they were less likely to be surrounded by identity-incongruent behavior and demands, and more likely to be exposed to identity-congruent behavior and demands. This is well illustrated in one interviewee's response to a question asking about their Mela experience and what aspect of it brought the most pleasure:

> Now, here the best is doing prayers. Here at least, we get time, with full devotion we have to perform prayers. We get time, we devote ourselves entirely to praying, we don't have to go anywhere, nobody is going to come, nobody is going to come and ask you to go with him, give responsibility of some work. So, we sit with full peace of mind and perform prayers.
>
> (P5M55, Reicher et al., 2021)

The wider point here is that the successful completion of one's obligations as a Kalpwasi is not simply an individual accomplishment. Rather, the behavior of one's fellows is relevant to one's ability to realize and enact the values and ideals of this identity. Put simply, one is surrounded by others who recognize one's motivations and concerns which allows one the social space to pursue one's religious rituals and pursue one's spiritual concerns.

Another example concerns the issue of gossip. If one is to free oneself of jealousy and experience a sense of harmony in which the spiritual worth of all is recognized, gossip is to be avoided. Yet avoiding gossip is not so easy, for if one hears others' engaging in it one is inevitably drawn into that which one wishes to avoid (everyday evaluation and judgment). In other words, the pursuit of spiritual concerns depends on the behavior of others and the alignment of interests associated with a shared Kalpwasi identity makes this so much easier. Small wonder then that our interviewees referred to the pleasures of being in the company of others with a shared commitment to speaking spiritual truths:

> And the most important here is the satsang. No one gossips about others. No one wants or looks for awful things in others. Whether it's a Brahmin or whatever caste, all become like one family. This is what is called satsang. Kalpwas means just this—that you do not criticize [gossip about] each other.
>
> (P37F62, Reicher et al., 2021)

Thus far, this outline of our interview data suggests that Kalpwasis could indeed conceptualize themselves in terms of a distinctive social group membership and that this sense of shared social identity resulted in a sense of mutual social support that was both actual (participants could give examples of how they had been helped by their fellow Kalpwasi) and anticipated (participants reported how they had a sense that support would be forthcoming if help were needed). Such support is important in giving Kalpwasis the confidence to undertake what is a physically and psychologically challenging challenge and provides a social context in which an individual's efforts to pursue their spiritual and religious concerns are scaffolded by the actions of others. Our wider point then is that the pursuit of spiritual concerns is not simply a personal choice. It requires the cooperation of those in the immediate vicinity, and a shared identity transforms a collection of individuals with disparate and potentially conflicting concerns and interests into a group with norms that mean that the actions of each support others in their pursuit of identity-related values and practices.

Investigating the Impact of Participation

Inevitably, these claims about the role of a shared identity in facilitating the enactment of participants' spiritual and religious commitments must be regarded as suggestive. However, our confidence in such claims is augmented by quantitative data obtained through a survey with Kalpwasis. Moreover, as these survey data were longitudinal—gathered before (T1), during (T2), and after (T3) their participation—we were able to explore whether the experience of a shared identity during the event had any wider social significance for participants once they had returned home.

This questionnaire survey involved participants completing measures concerning their identification as a Hindu, their performance of religious practices, and their self-assessed health. These data were gathered before and after the Mela. Parallel data were gathered from a Control sample of villagers who did not attend the Magh Mela (Khan et al., 2015; Tewari et al., 2012). In order to explore the social psychological processes relevant to participation in the Mela, our Kalpwasi sample also completed measures during the Mela itself (T2). These concerned their identification with other Kalpwasis; the degree to which they felt their relations with other Kalpwasis were close and supportive; the degree to which they felt able to enact their religious and spiritual values; and their affective experience of the event.

Unsurprisingly, participants' identification as a Hindu was very high (many were at ceiling on this measure) which constrained our opportunity to measure longitudinal changes in identification as a function of participation. However, among those whose pre-Mela level of identification as a Hindu was not at ceiling, we found a pre- to post-event (T1-T3) increase in Hindu identification that was absent among the Controls (Khan et al., 2016). Moreover, Kalpwasis (but not Controls) reported performing more religious practices after the Mela than before. These data therefore provide evidence that participation in the Magh Mela was cognitively and behaviorally consequential.

With regards to the processes involved in producing these psychologically and socially important changes we considered the role played by a sense of shared identity experienced during the Mela (T2). Focusing solely on the Kalpwasis sample, we found variation in the degree to which participants experienced a shared identity. In turn, this variation was consequential: The more participants experienced a shared identity with other Kalpwasis, the more they reported being able to fulfill their religious and spiritual concerns. Furthermore, these process variables helped explain the pre- to post-event increase in their identification as a Hindu and the increase in the frequency of their religious practice. More specifically, perceptions of a shared Kalpwasi identity had a (modest) indirect effect on the post-participation outcomes *via* the sense that they were able to fulfill their religious and spiritual concerns.

Analyses also revealed an impact of participation on Kalpwasis' self-assessed health (Tewari et al., 2012). Our measures of health included items from the core module of the Centres for Disease Control and Prevention Health Related Quality of Life Measure (CDC HRQOL-14: "Over the last week, how would you describe your . . .": "physical health"; "state of mind"; "energy levels?"), and items from a scale developed for use in South Asia (Ruback et al., 1997) capturing the somatization of stress observed in non-Western settings (e.g., "Over the last week, to what extent have you . . .": "suffered from body-aches and pains"; "suffered from breathlessness"; "suffered from headaches?"). We found that whereas one month prior to the event (T1), there was no difference on these health-related measures, there was such a difference one month after the event (T3) (Tewari et al., 2012). Specifically, there was a positive increase in pilgrims' self-reported health and an improvement in symptomology that was absent among the Controls. We also found the more pilgrims perceived a shared identity, the more they experienced positive and supportive social relations with others and the more positive these latter, the greater the pre-event (T1) to post-event (T3) improvements in health and well-being (Khan et al., 2015). Furthermore, mediation analysis showed that the perception of a shared identity had an indirect effect on well-being as measured by the CDC HRQOL-14 *via* the improvements in social relations. Taken together, these data show that participation in the event improved well-being and that this was partly attributable to pilgrims' perceptions of shared identity and the associated transformation of inter-pilgrim relations.

As these quantitative data complement the insights obtained through our qualitative (interview) data, we can have some confidence that a shared identity can emerge among Kalpwasis and that, when it does, it is consequential—both for one's social relations during the Mela (i.e., the development of supportive social relations and one's abilities to enact one's religious and spiritual identity) and for one's post-event life. Again, this underscores the social significance of pilgrimage (overlooked in a discipline that so often exhibits a parochial focus on North America and Europe). So too it underscores the relevance of the social identity approach for understanding important features of such a pilgrimage.

Identity-Based Appraisals

As described in the introduction, the logic to the social identity approach to group behavior is to prioritize the investigation of participants' cultural beliefs and perspective. This is clearly apparent in the analysis of identity-based behavior (group members' behavior is in conformity with their stereotype of the beliefs and values associated with that membership). It is also apparent in the analysis of how people interpret their physical and social environment.

Take something as simple as the experience of one's auditory environment. Noise can be conceptualized as "unwanted sound" (Westman & Walters, 1981) or as "sound out of place" (Bailey, 1996: 50) which implies that our auditory experiences are not simply a reflection of a stimulus's intrinsic properties but vary according to whether the sound is wanted and judged identity-appropriate. This means that rather than assuming a certain auditory environment is stressful we need to understand how people perceive the relationship between that auditory input and the norms and beliefs associated with their social identity.

Data relevant to such observations are available from our interviews conducted at the Magh Mela. The event features hundreds of sound systems broadcasting songs, speeches, and announcements throughout the day (at a level approximating a busy city street: 85–90 dB). The role of cultural beliefs in shaping the experience of this auditory environment was apparent in various ways. For example, we found that some Kalpwasis interpreted this environment through reference to their beliefs about the spiritual significance of the site. Thus, one of our early interviewees described the auditory environment as the "sound of the Saraswati"—the river of knowledge which joins the Yamuna and the Ganga and which further contributes to making the Allahabad Mela such a sacred site (interviewee cited in Prayag Magh Mela Research Group, 2007c). In other words, their identity-related cultural beliefs and values shaped the meaning given to stimuli such that what could otherwise be judged as "noise" was transformed into meaningful (and wanted) "sound." Others differentiated between the sounds comprising the auditory environment such that those judged congruent with their religious and spiritual purpose were rated more positively than those that were judged incongruent. For example, participants often differentiated between sounds that might be enjoyed in the village such as popular (commercial) songs and more spiritually acceptable songs appropriate for the Mela. Thus, when asked about the auditory environment, one interviewee (and her friend) explained:

Interviewee: There is no disturbance for us
Interviewer: No trouble?
Interviewee: No
Interviewer: Like there is this noise all the time, there is this crowd, people are coming
Interviewee: No. No disturbance

Friend: It feels so nice
Interviewer: It feels so nice?
Interviewee: It is pure joy
Friend: You get *darshan*. There are discourses from morning to evening. This is pure joy. This is what we have come for, no?
Interviewee: Religious songs play around the clock
Interviewer: Ok. If they didn't play religious songs and just play any other songs, then you wouldn't like it?
Interviewee: No, no, then my heart would not be in it
Interviewer: Then you wouldn't?
Interviewee: No.

(P22F51, Shankar et al., 2013)

In addition to investigating how participants interpreted their auditory environment as a function of their identity-related cultural beliefs, we conducted a series of experiments in which we explicitly labeled this auditory environment. The number of competing sound systems at the Mela is such that there are many sites where the messages of each are lost and merge into an indistinct cacophony. Capitalizing on this, the researchers produced a sound clip that was sufficiently ambiguous that it could be labeled as coming either from the Mela or from a busy city street. In one study, we played the clip to Kalpwasi participants with the instruction that they should decide for how long they wished to listen to it. When it was labeled as coming from the Mela (rather than the city), participants found the clip more interesting and chose to listen to it longer when it was labeled as coming from the Mela (Shankar et al., 2013). This suggests that when labeled as Mela-related, the clip was experienced as a socially meaningful sound rather than an intrusive annoyance.

In another set of studies, Srinivasan et al. (2013, 2015) investigated how the social meaning of a sound shaped its processing. In these experiments the same clip as above was played for a set duration which our Kalpwasi participants were asked to reproduce in a subsequent task. Participants produced longer estimates when the clip was labeled as coming from the Mela than the city which implies the clip attracted more attention (resulting in richer encoding) when designated as Mela-related. This interpretation is supported by two manipulations introduced into these studies. First, in addition to manipulating the labeling of the sound clip (city-related vs. Mela-related), Srinivasan et al. (2013) manipulated when participants were given the information concerning its origin (either pre-stimulus or post-stimulus) to allow investigation of whether the effect was bound up with encoding or retrieval processes. The results implied the effect was associated with encoding which supports an interpretation of the effect in terms of the Mela-related labeling resulting in a richer and more elaborated memory trace. Second, Srinivasan et al. (2015) manipulated participants' attentional load by asking half the sample to perform a concurrent task. The results showed that reproduced durations were longer when the clip was attributed to the Mela but only when participants completed a single task. This implies the increased duration estimates when the sound was labeled as Mela-related depends on attentional resources being available. Again, these experimental data highlight the importance of taking identity-related cultural belief seriously: Whether an apparently simple auditory stimulus is evaluated positively or negatively, and how it is processed, depends on the cultural meanings attached to it.

Related observations may also be made about our participants' affective experience of the Mela's social environment. Data addressing Kalpwasis' affective experience during the Mela were gathered in the large-scale questionnaire study described earlier, and analysis showed that the positivity of this experience was predicted by our identity-related measures (Hopkins et al., 2016a). First, participants' positive experience of the event was predicted by the degree to which they felt able to express and enact their religious and spiritual values and the degree to which they experienced positive and supportive social relations with other Kalpwasis. Second, both these effects had a basis in participants' experience of a shared Kalpwasi identity. These findings return us to our earlier observations that a shared identity results in both more intimate social relations which are a source of pleasure (Neville & Reicher, 2011) and in an alignment of interests such that group members are better able to coordinate their behavior such that they can more easily enact their shared culturally defined values and norms (Reicher et al., 2021).

All this helps explain something of the pleasure of participation. Among all the diverse contributory factors that are relevant to such pleasure are the social identity processes that make the enactment of culturally defined values and priorities a possibility. It is these processes that transform an aggregate of individuals into a psychological group characterized by a shared understanding of their environment and how they could and should behave in order to realize their culturally defined values and beliefs.

Discussion

Throughout this chapter, we have reported a program of research which sought to take seriously our participants' lived experience of a specific, culturally distinctive event. Throughout, we have focused on the degree to which our participants experienced a shared social identity as Kalpwasis. Here, we made no assumptions about whether such an identity did emerge and with what consequence: These were empirical questions and we found evidence that to the degree a shared identity did emerge, it impacted their social relations and their ability to coordinate the enactment of important culturally specific values and beliefs.

Inevitably, our analysis of these pilgrims' experiences is partial and more could and should be said about how they make sense of undertaking this demanding pilgrimage. Most obviously, our analysis could be complemented by others which explore how participants make sense of their experience through reference to the concepts and categories associated with Hindu belief and practice. That is, our etic analysis of this event could be complemented by an emic perspective. However, we believe that the social identity perspective offers an analytic framework that allows us to capture significant features of our participants' experience of the Mela's social environment (e.g., the potential for a shared social identity) and how it has long-term impacts once our participants returned home. Moreover, we believe that this analytic utility is possible because the social identity approach places so much emphasis on people's *own* understandings of their social identities, their social relations, and their beliefs and values. In turn, we hope this work can contribute to Indian psychology's debates about how best to bring culture center stage.

Our understanding of the social psychology of pilgrimage has come a long way since our early conversations following the Advanced Refresher Course held in Allahabad in 2005. We believe our analysis is not only relevant to those interested in this culturally distinctive Indian event but also holds all manner of lessons for those interested in the pleasures and significance of collective assembly (Ehrenreich, 2006) across the globe. Although it is too early to say whether pilgrimage will start to appear in our discipline's standard textbooks, two things can be said with certainty. The first is that work conducted in India has enormous potential to internationalize Social Psychology. The second is that none of the work described here would have been possible without Prof. Janak Pandey's academic leadership, commitment to Indian psychology, and the internationalization of Psychology. His enthusiasm, generosity, and imagination enabled our Indo-British research team to come into existence. His contribution is indeed one to be celebrated collectively.

Notes

1 The authors wish to acknowledge the financial support of the ESRC ("Collective participation and social identification: A study of the individual, interpersonal, and collective dimensions of attendance at the Magh Mela" RES-062-23-1449). They also wish to thank Sammyh Khan, Mark Levine, Gozde Ozakinci, Kavita Pandey, Shail Shankar, Tushar Singh, Clifford Stevenson, and Shruti Tewari for their input into this project.

2 Where we quote from our interviewees, we identify them with a participant code number and information on their sex and age. For example, P1M82 refers to Participant no. 1, who was male and 82 years old.

References

Bailey, P. (1996). Breaking the sound barrier: A historian listens to noise. *Body & Society*, *3*, 49–66. http://dx.doi.org/10.1177/1357034X96002002003

Brubaker, R., Loveman, M., & Stamatov, P. (2004). Ethnicity as cognition. *Theory & Society*, *33*, 31–64. https://doi.org/10.1023/B:RYSO.0000021405.18890.63

Buzinde, C. N., Kalavar, J. M., Kohli, N., & Manuel-Navarrete, D. (2014). Emic understandings of Kumbh Mela pilgrimage experiences. *Annals of Tourism Research*, *49*, 1–18. https://doi.org/10.1016/j.annals.2014.08.001

Cassidy, C., Hopkins, N., Levine, M., Pandey, J., Reicher, S., & Singh, P. (2007). Social identity and collective behaviour: Some lessons from Indian research at the Magh Mela at Prayag. *Psychological Studies*, *52*, 286–292.

Coleman, S. (2002). Do you believe in pilgrimage? Communitas, contestation and beyond. *Anthropological Theory*, *2*(3), 355–368.

Condor, S. (2003). "The least doubtful promise for the future"? The short history of Tajfel's "sociopsychological" approach to laboratory experimentation. In J. Laszlo & W. Wagner (Eds.), *Theories and controversies in societal psychology* (pp. 153–179). New Mandate.

Eade, J., & Sallnow, M. (Eds.). (1991). *Contesting the sacred: The anthropology of Christian pilgrimage*. Routledge.

Ehrenreich, B. (2006). *Dancing in the streets*. Metropolitan.

Elderling, L., & Pandey, J. (2007). Experiencing the Mahakhumb Mela—The biggest Hindu fair in the world. *Psychological Studies*, *52*, 273–285.

Haslam, S. A., Reicher, S. D., & Levine, M. (2012). When other people are heaven, when other people are hell: How social identity determines the nature and impact of social support. In J. Jetten, C. Haslam, & S. A. Haslam (Eds.), *The social cure* (pp. 157–174). Psychology Press.

Henrich, J., Heine, S. J., & Norenzayan, A. (2010). The weirdest people in the world? *Behavioral and Brain Sciences*, *33*, 61–83. http://doi.org/10.1017/S0140525X0999152X

Hopkins, N., & Reicher, S. (2005). Culture, social identity and the organisation of collective action: Developing a culturally sensitive social psychology. *Psychological Studies*, *50*, 217–225.

Hopkins, N., & Reicher, S. (2011). Identity, culture and contestation: Social identity as cross-cultural theory. *Psychological Studies*, *56*, 36–43.

Hopkins, N., & Reicher, S. (2013). Social identity and group behaviour: A social psychological contribution to the social sciences. In G. Misra (ed.) *Psychology and psychoanalysis* (pp. 795–826). Centre for Studies in Civilization.

Hopkins, N., Reicher, S. D., Khan, S. S., Tewari, S., Srinivasan, N., & Stevenson, C. (2016a). Explaining effervescence: Investigating the relationship between shared social identity and positive experience in crowds. *Cognition and Emotion*, *30*, 20–32. https://doi.org/10.1080/02699 931.2015.1015969

Hopkins, N., Reicher, S. D., Stevenson, C., Pandey, K., Shankar, S., & Tewari, S. (2019). Social relations in crowds: Recognition, validation and solidarity. *European Journal of Social Psychology*, *49*, 1283–1297. https://doi.org/10.1002/ejsp.2586

Hopkins, N., Stevenson, C., Shankar, S., Pandey, K., Khan, S., & Tewari, S. (2016b). Being together at the Magh Mela: The social psychology of crowds and collectivity. In Gale, T. Maddrell, A., & Terry, A. (Eds.), *Sacred mobilities* (pp. 19–39). Farnham.

Jetten, J., Haslam, C., & Haslam, S. A. (Eds.). (2012). *The social cure: Identity, health, and well-being*. Psychology Press.

Khan, S., Hopkins, N., Reicher, S., Tewari, S., Srinivasan, N., & Stevenson, C. (2015). Shared identity predicts enhanced health at mass gatherings. *Group Processes and Intergroup Relations*, *18*, 504–522. https://doi.org/10.1177/1368430214556703

Khan, S. S., Hopkins, N., Reicher, S., Tewari, S., Srinivasan, N., & Stevenson, C. (2016). How collective participation impacts social identity: A longitudinal study from India. *Political Psychology*, *37*, 309–325. https://doi.org/10.1111/pops.12260

Levine, M., Prosser, A., Evans, D., & Reicher, S. (2005). Identity and emergency intervention: How social group membership and inclusiveness of group boundaries shapes helping behavior. *Personality and Social Psychology Bulletin*, *31*(4), 443–453. https://doi.org/10.1177/0146167204271651

Misra, G., & Gergen, K. (1993). On the place of culture in psychological science. *International Journal of Psychology*, *28*, 225–243. https://doi.org/10.1080/00207599308247186

Neville, F., & Reicher, S. D. (2011). The experience of collective participation: Shared identity, relatedness and emotionality. *Contemporary Social Science*, *6*, 377–396, https://doi.org/10.1080/21582041.2012.627277

Pandey, J., & Singh, P. (2005). Social psychology in India: Social roots and development *International Journal of Psychology*, *40*, 239–253. https://doi.org/10.1080/00207590444000186

Pandey, K., Stevenson, C., Shankar, S., Hopkins, N., & Reicher, S. (2014). Cold comfort at the Magh Mela: Social identity processes and physical hardship. *British Journal of Social Psychology*, *53*, 675–90. https://doi.org/10.1111/bjso.12054

Prayag Magh Mela Research Group. (2007a). Living the Magh Mela at Prayag: Collective identity, collective experience and the impact of participation in a mass event. *Psychological Studies*, *52*, 293–301.

Prayag Magh Mela Research Group. (2007b). Revisiting research practice in India. *Psychological Studies*, *52*, 302–310.

Prayag Magh Mela Research Group. (2007c). Experiencing the Magh Mela at Prayag: Crowds, categories and social relations. *Psychological Studies*, *52*, 311–319.

Reicher, S. D. (2017). "La beauté est dans la rue": Four reasons (or perhaps five) to study crowds. *Group Processes & Intergroup Relations*, *20*, 593–605. https://doi.org/10.1177/1368430217712835

Reicher, S. D., Hopkins, N., Stevenson, C., Pandey, K., Shankar, S., & Tewari, S. (2021). Identity enactment as collective accomplishment: Religious identity enactment at home and at a festival. *British Journal of Social Psychology*, *60*(2), 678–699. https://doi.org/10.1111/bjso.12415

Ruback, R. B., Pandey, J., & Begum, H. A. (1997). Urban stressors in South Asia: Impact on male and female pedestrians in Delhi and Dhaka. *Journal of Cross-Cultural Psychology*, *28*, 23–3. https://doi.org/10.1177/0022022197281002

Ruback, R. B., Pandey, J., & Kohli, N. (2008). Evaluations of a sacred place: Role and religious belief at the Magh Mela. *Journal of Environmental Psychology*, *28*, 174–184. https://doi.org/10.1016/j.jenvp.2007.10.007

Sallnow, M. J. (1981). *Communitas* reconsidered: The sociology of Andean pilgrimage. *Man*, *16*, 163–182.

Shankar, S., Stevenson, C., Pandey, K. Tewari, S. Hopkins, N., & Reicher, S. D. (2013). A calming cacophony: Social identity can shape the experience of loud noise. *Journal of Environmental Psychology*, *36*, 87–95. https://doi.org/10.1016/j.jenvp.2013.07.004

Singh, R. P. B. (2011). Pilgrimage and religious tourism in India: Countering contestation and seduction. In R. P. B. Singh (Ed.) *Holy places and pilgrimages: Essays on India* (pp. 307–334). Shubhi Publications.

Sinha, D. (1997). Indigenizing psychology. In J. W. Berry, Y. H. Poortinga, & J. Pandey (Eds.), *Handbook of cross-cultural psychology* (Vol. 1, pp. 129–169). Allyn and Bacon.

Sinha, D. (1998). Changing perspectives in social psychology in India: A journey towards indigenisation. *Asian Journal of Social Psychology*, *1*, 17–31. https://doi.org/10.1111/1467-839X.00003

Snibbe, A. C. (2003). *Cultural psychology: Studying more than the 'exotic other'*. American Association for Psychological Science. www.psychologicalscience.org/observer/cultural-psychology-studying-more-than-the-exotic-other

Srinivasan, N., Hopkins, N. P., Reicher, S. D., Khan, S. S., Singh, T., & Levine, M. (2013). Social meaning of ambiguous sounds influences retrospective duration judgments. *Psychological Science*, *24*, 1060–1062. https://doi.org/10.1177/0956797612465293

Srinivasan, N., Tewari, S., Makwana, M., & Hopkins, N. (2015). Attention mediates the effect of context-relevant social meaning on prospective duration judgments. *Timing & Time Perception*, *3*, 189–200. https://doi.org/10.1163/22134468-00002032

Tajfel, H. (Ed.). (1978). *Differentiation between social groups: Studies in the social psychology of intergroup relations*. Academic Press.
Tajfel, H. (Ed.). (1982). *Social identity and intergroup relations*. Cambridge University Press and Paris: Maison des Sciences de L'Homme.
Tajfel, H., & Turner, J. C. (1979). An integrative theory of intergroup conflict. In W. G. Austin, & S. Worchel (Eds.), *The social psychology of intergroup relations* (pp. 33–47). Brooks Cole.
Tewari, S., Khan, S., Hopkins, N., Srinivasan, N., & Reicher, S. D. (2012). Participation in mass gatherings can benefit well-being: Longitudinal and control data from a North Indian Hindu pilgrimage event. *PLoS ONE*, *7*(10), e47291. https://doi.org/10.1371/journal.pone.0047291
Turner, J. C. (1982). Towards a cognitive redefinition of the social group. In H. Tajfel (Ed.), *Social identity and intergroup relations* (pp. 15–40). Cambridge University Press.
Turner, J. C. (1999). Some current issues in research on social identity and self-categorisation theories. In N. Ellemers, R. Spears, & B. Doosje (Eds.), *Social identity: Context, commitment, content* (pp. 6–34). Blackwell.
Turner, J. C., Hogg, M. A., Oakes, P. J., Reicher, S., & Wetherell, M. (1987). *Rediscovering the social group: A self-categorisation theory*. Blackwell.
Westman, J. C., & Walters, J. R. (1981). Source noise and stress: A comprehensive approach. *Environmental Health Perspectives*, *41*, 291–309.

10 Women, Work, and Health

Perspectives From India

Urmi Nanda Biswas

Examining women's lives in India through a gender lens, this chapter addresses the multifaceted challenges they face. Gender equality intersects with all 17 Sustainable Development Goals (SDGs). United Nations SDG 5 is dedicated to gender equality and empowerment, fostering equitable and inclusive development opportunities. The chapter showcases research studies that illuminate the status of women in India concerning equitable growth, development, and workforce participation, informed by three significant research projects undertaken by the author and her colleagues.

The World Economic Forum's Gender Gap Report 2023 ranks India 127th out of 146 countries in gender parity, marking an eight-place improvement from the previous year. India has achieved gender parity in educational enrollment, closing 64.3% of the overall gender gap. Yet economic participation and opportunity parity stand at only 36.7%. India's ranking on the Gender Gap Index lags behind many Southeast Asian neighbors (Global Gender Gap Report, 2023). Despite a rise in wage and income parity, women's representation in senior and technical roles has seen a slight decline since 2022. The Health and Survival Index notes a 1.9 percentage point improvement in the sex ratio at birth, signaling progress after years of stagnation. Nonetheless, skewed sex ratios contribute to low scores on the Health and Survival sub-index. Health indicators reveal concerning statistics: 53.5% of women of reproductive age (15–49) suffer from anemia, and 33% experience intimate partner violence, surpassing the regional average (WHO, Health Information System, 2023).

Launched in 2015, the United Nations' SDGs urge action to eradicate poverty, protect the planet, and secure peace and prosperity by 2030. SDG 5, advocating for gender equality and the empowerment of women and girls, is pivotal for sustainable and inclusive development. It seeks to eliminate discrimination against women and girls, empowering them to contribute to economic growth and a sustainable future. Against this backdrop, the chapter outlines the challenges confronting Indian women, with a particular emphasis on issues stemming from their social and work contexts, which influence their growth and development from a sustenance perspective.

DOI: 10.4324/9781003461302-14

Changing Demographics for Women in India

Das Sharma (2023) quotes the World Economic Forum's (2022) Global Gender Gap Report to highlight the fact that in India, the educational attainment by men and women is nearly equal, but the divide widens when it comes to economic participation. World Economic Forum's (WEF's) Global Gender Gap Report considers the parity between women and men in educational attainment. Indian women scored 0.961, but when it came to parity in economic participation and opportunity, it sharply fell to 0.350 (WEF, 2022). Since the 1990s, the Indian economy has grown more than 10-fold, but female education and its labor force participation outcomes are complex and not directly correlated with economic growth. Desai and Joshi (2019) report that amidst India's economic growth, a "job deficit" is to be blamed for a decline in female labor force participation (FLFP). Many women from this population who have completed their college education and aspire to white-collar jobs are disappointed. White-collar jobs have declined and not increased in proportion to the working-age population, which increased from 11% to 21% by 2019. These women tend to compete in a small pool of formal sector jobs. Desai and Joshi (2019) state that suitable jobs are absent rather than a withdrawal of educated women from the labor force. The occupational and sectoral segregation by gender has confined women to search for work in particular sectors, which prevails in line with sectoral norms. Prominent Indian corporate houses, such as Accenture with a 300,000-strong workforce, assert that they are determined to achieve their goal of 50% women's representation in their workforce by 2025, by providing flexible work options, supporting women to resume work after maternity leave or off ramping, redesigning parental leaves, providing comprehensive medical insurance coverage, and enabling caregivers through structured training (Das Sharma, 2023). In support of this, Das Sharma (2023) notes that younger women are emerging as more aspirational than their predecessors, contributing to a changed workforce profile of the Millennials and GenZ. Most of the women from this generation are digitally savvy and have emerged through the habit-altering pandemic, which has opened new ways of working, including migrating to other countries for better opportunities and working in the gig economy, which has become very popular, particularly among educated women in the post-pandemic world. Furthermore, government reports show a rise in the proportion of unmarried Indian youths (15–29 years) from 17.2% in 2011 to 23% in 2019. In the case of female Indian youths, the proportion increased from 13.5% in 2011 to 19.9% in 2019 (The Economic Times, 2022)

Primary Roles of Women in Modern India

India is often characterized as a modern nation, boasting the world's ninth-largest industrial economy, rapid urbanization, improved educational access and literacy rates, increased life expectancy, basic healthcare availability, and a democratic political system. Despite these advancements, certain social and economic sectors remain resistant to change due to long-standing ideologies and practices.

The vastness and diversity of India mean that social change is uneven, with urban areas and certain states adopting new societal norms more swiftly than rural counterparts. This blend of traditional and contemporary elements is a testament to India's resilience and stability, yet it also perpetuates deep-rooted gender inequalities.

Surveys indicate that male dominance is prevalent and accepted in both domestic and public realms across various demographics, despite legal reforms against discrimination initiated in the 1950s (Evans et al., 2022; Haq, 2013; the patriarchal and collectivist nature of society continues to influence women's lives, limiting their work opportunities, economic independence, and social liberties; Joshi et al., 2020).

Contemporary research consistently highlights the primary roles of women as wives and mothers, often relegated to subordinate positions in domestic settings. Education is increasingly seen as a means to improve marital prospects rather than career advancement (Barhate et al., 2021, p. 411; Li, 2022, p. 9). Consequently, while educational attainment has led to later marriages, it has not translated into lasting benefits for women, particularly after entering motherhood.

Marriage customs like patrilocal exogamy and joint family systems grant significant control to the husband's family over a woman's employment, healthcare, and personal freedoms. Although education significantly impacts marriage timing, caste and religion also play crucial roles in life choices.

With more couples living in nuclear families, the traditional family obligations persist, albeit from a distance. Studies reveal that even when husbands support their wives' careers, societal pressures often hinder public endorsement. Gender norms also place considerable pressure on men, where a working wife may be perceived as a failure to provide (e.g., the Government of India, 1974; High Level Committee on the Status on Women, 2015; Khanna, 2022). But Dhar (2018) notes that the political will to make the necessary transformation in gender relations and inequalities has so far been absent. Despite some progress, there is still no comprehensive anti-discrimination law that is able to address all the various intersectional factors that lead to women's inequality. Nagpal and Viswanath (2023) report findings from interviews done with 6,600 women from 16 cities of India, highlighting the importance of views of family members which constrain women's ability to work outside the home, and push women to work from home or engage in small businesses to be able to allocate more time to household responsibilities.

In some instances, women contribute to family businesses without formal recognition (Das Sharma, 2023). As men's incomes increase, the necessity for women to work diminishes, reinforcing the cycle of dependency.

Girl Child in India

In India, the natural sex ratio at birth is around 105 girls per 100 boys. However, historically, there has been a skewed ratio favoring boys due to factors like sex-selective abortions. There has been some improvement in recent years. According to the latest National Family Health Survey (NFHS-5, 2019–21), the sex ratio at birth is around 108 boys per 100 girls. The sex ratio at birth is slightly better in rural areas (1,037 females per 1,000 males) compared to urban areas (985 females per 1,000 males) based on NFHS-5 data.

Apart from this, there has been significant progress in terms of acknowledging the legal rights of girls, laws prohibiting female infanticide and child marriage. More girls are attending school than ever before.

Girls in Indian society are often neglected, subjected to maltreatment, and abused. A survey of 1,060 adolescent girls from government schools in Delhi found that seven in every ten girls had experienced some form of maltreatment, including physical, emotional, and sexual abuse (Daral et al., 2016). Furthermore, generalized discrimination is prevalent regardless of the birth order or gender of the siblings; however, evidence regarding selective discrimination is inconclusive (Rajan & Morgan, 2018). Moreover, sons are more likely to receive good-quality education, whereas daughters are either withdrawn from schools or enrolled in free public schools (Sekher & Hatti, 2010). The school dropout rate among girls, especially in rural areas, is higher than boys (Gouda & Sekher, 2014).

In India, women who give birth to a male child are held in high esteem as they contribute to the continuation of the lineage, and consequently, women are pressured to get married and provide a male child to the family. For working women, even though they have modern families, women have to balance families and careers constantly. They are required to put their families first, which ironically brings the stigma at the workplace that Indian women don't take work seriously. Additionally, women often suffer domestic abuse, violence, sexual harassment, maltreatment, and neglect, even during pregnancy. Research carried out on the impact of domestic violence reports that households with a high prevalence of domestic violence also concur with reproductive health problems in women and asthma in children (Biswas & Essau, 2012).

The following section highlights some of the findings from the author's work, demonstrating the causes of low sex ratio at birth in Indian society

Save the Girl Child Campaign: Perspective of Stakeholders

The author carried out an impact assessment research to understand the impact of a public campaign, "Save the Girl Child" on the attitude and behavior of people which was funded by the Indian Council of Social Science Research (ICSSR). The study focused on the attitude and perception of stakeholders responsible for the sex ratio at birth in two states of India, Gujarat and Odisha, during 2012–2016. The research employed a multi-method design and was carried out in three stages. We interviewed gynecologists, paramedical staff, pregnant mothers, their husbands, mother-laws, and immediate kin in the first stage. Gynecologists interviewed in both states thought that almost 50% of pregnant mothers and their families knew the Pre-Conception & Pre-Natal Diagnostic Techniques (PCPNDT) act. However, families from a lower socioeconomic background with less education generally ask questions about the sex of the child, and mostly if it is a second or third pregnancy. Despite the success of Janani Suraksha Yojana and various policies for maternal and child health, in rural areas, pregnant women come for pre-natal consultation quite late, almost at 5/6 months of pregnancy compared to their counterparts in the urban population. Doctors from Gujarat and Odisha suggest that sex determination and sex-selective abortion are seen as a demand–supply phenomenon. Doctors from both states agreed that the "Save the Girl Child" campaign had a positive impact (Biswas, 2016).

The interviews with paramedical staff from anti-natal clinics suggested that the child's health is of primary concern to the families. The paramedics from Gujarat believed that the campaign against sex-selective abortion had contributed to improving the sex ratio. In contrast, their counterparts were from Odisha, where the public campaign was not in practice.

Almost 40–45% of expecting mothers from Odisha reported that they see their future better if they have a male rather than a girl child. Almost similar percentage of mothers (45%) from the urban sample in Gujarat admitted that their families would offer worship and do rituals to have a male child. About 33–50% of pregnant mothers confided that they are concerned about the girl child's security, education, and life as against that of a male child. Between 15% and 20% of expectant mothers thought that giving birth to a male child would elevate their status in the household. About 20% of the expectant mothers said that if the first child is a son, they will not go for a second pregnancy. About 5–7% of the expectant mothers admitted that they would continue to give birth till they gave birth to a male child (Biswas, 2016).

The study also carried a questionnaire survey that assessed the level of awareness about the PCPNDT Act, 1994. Attitude and perception toward male and female children, preferences for the sex of the child, attitude toward education, the liberation of the girl child tried exploring the cause of choice of a male child. The sample comprised 860 parents within an age group of 25–40 across Gujarat and Odisha. The first three highly ranked perceived causes of sex-selective abortion were; (a) the potential of male offspring providing financial security than the female offspring, (b) the son as a natural heir to family wealth—the wealth stays with the "family," and (c) girl as "parayadhan" or a liability collectively. Whereas in Odisha, (a) lack of medical facilities, (b) fear of pressure of dowry in future, and (c) fear of shame to the family which the girl child can bring were considered as the first three causes for sex-selective abortion. Gujarat is a business community; a son is perceived as a guardian and heir to the family businesses. The research reported younger couples reported more positive attitude toward having girl child compared to elder couples. The study interviewed 17 project managers from Gujarat and Odisha, to understand the perspectives of non-government organizations (NGOs) employees engaged with issues related to female feticide or low sex ratio at birth. They reported a significant difference among couples from urban and rural toward sex selection, the attitude being more positive in the urban than rural due to better financial conditions, education, and advanced technological services. Most NGO members from Gujarat and Odisha thought that gender discrimination at the societal level had been the root cause for sex-selective abortion (Biswas, 2016).

A similar study on "Effectiveness of India's National Programme Save the Girl Child: experience of Beti Bachao Beti Padao program from Haryana State" by Gupta et al. (2018) reported that there was a significant increase in sex ratio at birth in the state due to program. These findings suggest that policies and legislation at the system level (government) impact attitude and behavior change at the community level. The findings strongly recommend psycho-educational programs, community participation, and public and private partnerships to fight female feticide and sex-selective abortion.

Adolescent and Young Women in India: Health Issues

A poor start in life can lead to poor health, nutrition, and inadequate learning, resulting in future health implications that are not evident in the present. Particularly, there is a dearth of research on adolescent reproductive health and well-being, emphasizing the need to create knowledge and awareness focusing on India and Southeast Asia (see Biswas, 2021). The lack of knowledge and awareness about health issues related to menstruation, reproductive health, sexually transmitted infections (STIs) accompanied by lifestyle-related factors results in many serious health disorders starting from polycystic ovary syndrome (PCOS), problem pregnancy, reproductive tract infection (RTI), unsafe abortion leading to maternal mortality, cervical cancer and stigma around discussion on menstruation and sex causing serious health risks among women in Southeast Asia (Biswas, 2021).

In rural India, families invest more in the nutrition of male children than females, leading to stunting and thinness among adolescent girls, further leading to reproductive health issues in the future (Alam et al., 2010; Barcellos et al., 2014). Adolescent girls and young women in India are facing two serious health problems that are yet to be researched enough, documented, and prevented. PCOS and Cervical Cancer have been the two most dreadful health issues for today's young women. When PCOS has high morbidity issues accompanied by reproductive health implications, Cervical Cancer is the top most of death among women suffering from cancer in India.

Unhealthy eating and lifestyle habits can be a risk to women and can cause various chronic diseases in women, such as PCOS, and hormonal imbalances.

The last decade has seen a phenomenal increase in the rate of PCOS/Polycystic Ovarian Disease (PCOD) across the globe. In India, it varies from 3.5% to 22.5%. Diagnosis of PCOS/PCOD in adolescence is a challenge because of overlapping symptoms of PCOS with normal pubertal changes in adolescents. PCOS is the most commonly reported endocrine issue in women of reproductive age. PCOD is mostly caused by a combination of hormonal imbalance and genetic tendencies. The prevalence of women suffering from PCOS was researched to be less in comparison in the rural populations to those living in urban areas. It may be because of the rural population's lack of awareness and minimized exposure to junk foods, pollution, and other disruptors. The research also mentioned that even though not diagnosed, 20% of the rural population were symptomatic (Vidya Bharathi et al., 2017). Moreover, it is asserted that up to 70% of women with PCOS remain undiagnosed (Hajivandi et al., 2020).

The most prevalent disease in women and the major cause of death in developing nations, cervical cancer affects one in every eight women. Several research conducted to study the awareness about cervical cancer and its risk among adolescents and young girls from schools and colleges report very little awareness. In addition, parents in both urban, rural, and slum areas of various states of India have reported their hesitancy against cervical cancer screening, and vaccination (Chandana et al., 2020; Mittal & Pokale, 2021; Kataria et al., 2022). In the Budget 2024, the finance minister of India has announced a major budget allocation for screening and vaccination for cervical cancer in India under gender budgeting.

Adolescence is a critical phase in life; the information they receive during adolescence shapes up their behavior patterns and define their future trajectory of health. The transition during adolescence is characterized by significant physical, psychological, and psychosocial changes that involve both risks and opportunities related to health and well-being. The habits and behavior patterns that are formed during adolescence can influence the life prospects of young people, thereby affecting long-term health and social implications that require explicit attention (Sawyer et al., 2012; Liang et al., 2019).

This ground reality highlights the importance of adolescent health and well-being as important milestones in achieving SDGs (WHO, Child and Adolescent Health: fact sheet on SDGs: health targets, 2021). The inclusion of adolescent reproductive and sexual health in the WHO's SDGs acknowledges the fact that there is a need for discussions around reproductive health and well-being from an early age. Although the topic's importance has been recognized since the 1960s, awareness about the topic remains low in the mainstream. Thus, information is not transferred generationally for women. The sociocultural and demographic restrictions on women's education remain the same in large parts of the world. Globally, adolescent girls possess variable and often little information regarding reproductive health and well-being, which is concurrent with cultural stigma and taboos regarding such topics (Chandra-Mouli et al., 2017). Poor outcomes related to adolescent reproductive health and well-being include unsafe abortions resulting in maternal mortality, adolescent pregnancy, and RTI. Despite considerable research on sexual practices and menstruation, the understanding of reproductive health and its implications for a woman's body remains at a preliminary level. Reproductive health issues can lead to nutritional diseases, high prevalence rates of non-communicable diseases (NCDs) and mental disorders, and other nutritional health risks such as overweight and obesity (Azzopardi et al., 2019), which adversely affect outcomes for lifelong health issues, including sexual and reproductive health. Excess weight and abdominal fat are risk factors for menstrual abnormalities (Douchi et al., 2002), ovulatory dysfunction and altered endometrial function (DeUgarte, 2010), miscarriage (Rittenberg et al., 2011), and pregnancy and perinatal complications (Weiss & Ferrand, 2019). Discussions on sexual health, including positive and respectful approaches to sexuality, relationships, and sexual pleasure, are often minimized and ignored (UNESCO, the case for comprehensive sexuality education, 2019). A greater engagement of adolescents with their health is positively associated with the utilization of healthcare and can enhance the effectiveness and sustainability of sexual and reproductive health and rights (SRHR) interventions for adolescents (Sebastian et al., 2014).

Roy (2024) in her doctoral thesis worked on lived experiences of more than 1,000 women and other stakeholders like doctors, counselors, and educationists who work in the domain of empowering adolescent girls health behavior concerning their sexual, reproductive, and overall health to build a social communication model for reproductive health awareness and well-being among adolescent females. She reported implications from her findings which will help effectively communicate with adolescent girls about their health awareness and management. The first and foremost thing she talked about was *the importance of designing culturally relevant communication* for the culturally and socio-demographically diverse groups of adolescent girls by designing toolkits to deliver knowledge through gamified ways. Second, making adolescent girls aware of and *understand the relevance of scientific perspectives of existing cultural traditions* is important. To be able to question the relevance of such traditions will help do away with myths and misconceptions surrounding sexual and reproductive health. Third, there is a need to *address generational information gaps*. Generations have passed with enduring misconceptions and misinformation, particularly regarding female physiology. In her study, only a small proportion of her participants ($n = 629$) possessed a comprehensive knowledge of their own bodies, revealing a significant knowledge gap. Recognizing this gap, the participants felt a profound responsibility to equip future generations with greater awareness and the capacity to take ownership of their physical well-being. The fourth important point is to *establish adolescent-centric communication*. Effective communication necessitates relevance and contextually, as concepts that are not immediately relevant often struggle to gain traction. This challenge extends to conveying future health risks to any demographic. Renfree et al.

(2016) noted the difficulty in communicating such risks effectively. In such scenarios, constructive fear catalyzes or motivates health behavior in unforeseen circumstances (Maddux & Rogers, 1983). Additionally, sharing lived experiences that shed light on future implications can inspire individuals to become self-reliant and self-aware to the best of their abilities (Bruine de Bruin & Bennett, 2020). The last and most important thing Roy (2024) suggests is *empowering agency in reproductive time*. The concepts of tracking and calculating feature prominently in the strategies women employ to manage their biological clocks. This expectation of agency over reproductive time involves both planning and future anticipation. Among the adolescent research participants in the study, this practice of self-awareness acted as a technology of power that regulated individual health behaviors. The agency exercised through the awareness and knowledge has futuristic potential of bringing healthy behavior in adolescent girls for their life trajectory of sexual and reproductive health.

Motherhood: A Complex Reality for Indian Women

Motherhood in India is a revered institution, often defining a woman's identity and conferring upon her a respected status. From a young age, girls are groomed for their eventual roles as mothers, a cornerstone of the family unit (Bhambhani & Inbanathan, 2018). However, as the traditional joint family structure gives way to nuclear families, the onus of child-rearing increasingly falls on women, often compelling them to pause or end their careers. India's maternal healthcare system, coupled with limited awareness of reproductive health, poses additional hurdles for women seeking to balance motherhood with professional aspirations. As family incomes rise, the economic necessity for women to work diminishes, reinforcing traditional roles and sometimes leading to workforce withdrawal. This phenomenon is influenced by sociocultural norms that equate a woman's employment with lower family status.

Respectful maternity care (RMC) is recognized as a universal human right for every childbearing woman within health systems globally. As an integral component of quality of care (QoC), RMC is gaining international recognition as a pivotal element of the maternal and newborn health agenda. Despite this, India's ranking in the gender gap index for healthcare and survival is alarmingly low, standing at 155 out of 156 countries. The recent review by Biswas (2021) on adolescent girls' reproductive health in South Asia underscores the myriad of healthcare challenges faced by Indian adolescent girls, ranging from menstrual health to unsafe abortion. Complementing this, a mixed-method study involving 669 women from tier two and tier three cities in Western India, aged 26–57, revealed a significant gap in knowledge about sexual well-being, which was acquired informally over time (Roy, 2024).

The traditional role of women as caregivers often leads to their health needs being overlooked. Their daily tasks, such as cooking and collecting water, particularly when using wood or kerosene stoves, increase their risk of health issues. Yet access to healthcare is frequently obstructed by a lack of decision-making autonomy and patriarchal barriers that restrict women's mobility (Tiwari et al., 2020).

In the context of sustainable growth, gender equality, and women's empowerment, the provision of maternal and reproductive healthcare, and the awareness and accessibility of such care are paramount. This necessitates a community-level behavior change communication strategy to advocate for more RMC, achievable only with the support of policy makers and welfare organizations.

Giving and Receiving Care: The Ground Reality

The unpaid care work traditionally assigned to Indian women includes childcare and domestic chores, such as cooking, cleaning, and washing. This work limits women's participation in other life spheres and employment opportunities (Chopra et al., 2020). In India and Nepal, women are the primary caregivers in 84% of households, a figure expected to rise to 90% (Patil, 2018). On average, Indian women dedicate six hours daily to unpaid work, with up to 85% of this time spent on household tasks, while Indian men contribute a mere 36 minutes to such work (Ferrant et al., 2014).

A Help Age India survey (2019) found that women predominantly provide care and assistance for the elderly's daily activities. Daughters and daughters-in-law represent 28–68% of elderly family caregivers across 20 Indian cities, offering instrumental support and emotional care. The caregiver burden often leads to frustration, entrapment, and health issues for women (Jamuna, 2003). Perceived social support is closely linked to the caregiver burden experience (Ugargol & Bailey, 2018). Although community members, family, and neighbors can be supportive (Chopra et al., 2020), women in India generally receive little familial support, as men engaging in household tasks face societal disapproval (Ravindran & Baral, 2014).

Women as Caregivers and Care-Receivers: Insights From Value Integrated and Sustainable Models of Eldercare

Funded by the Indian Council for Medical Research and the Swedish Council of Health and Family Care, this mixed-method research aimed to understand the need for eldercare and attitudes toward caregiving services among various stakeholders. The initial phase involved 105 in-depth interviews with eldercare stakeholders and six focused group discussions with rural elderly, revealing some unspoken truths. The subsequent phase examined eldercare organizations and services across six Indian states. The eldercare sector, predominantly staffed by women, is largely unorganized and characterized by low pay, stigma, and high turnover rates. Despite these challenges, older adults showed a preference for female caregivers (Biswas et al., 2020).

Home-based female caregivers encounter significant challenges, including safety concerns, exploitation, and blurred lines of dignity and rights. Interviews highlighted the job's lack of legitimacy and social respect, leading to imbalanced work–life dynamics (Biswas et al., 2020).

The research also identified gender discrepancies in care receiving. Elderly women primarily seek rehabilitative care post-hospitalization or surgery, while men opt for home healthcare, often influenced by financial dependency (Biswas, 2022). The Agewell Foundation's financial assessment (2017) indicates a higher financial dependence among elderly women than men, exacerbating challenges for older women due to declining health and limited coping capacities (Rajan & Balagopal, 2017). Furthermore, even in old age, women are expected to fulfill familial responsibilities, impacting their health and career aspirations.

On-ramping and Off-ramping

Sociocultural factors such as religious beliefs, family structure, social norms, and market changes affect female labor force participation rates (Mehrotra & Sinha, 2017). Goldin (1995) observed that increased family income can lead to women exiting the workforce, a phenomenon known as the income effect. Consequently, educated women from affluent backgrounds may not engage in paid employment but instead contribute to "status generation" within family businesses (Abraham, 2013). This dynamic is influenced by the rising education levels of females.

The concept of "off-ramping" refers to women taking career breaks for caregiving duties, with a significant majority expressing the desire to "on-ramp" or return to work once these responsibilities subside. Yet societal expectations and the stigma attached to maternity leave create barriers, often forcing women to choose between family and career.

Despite these challenges, organizational support and inclusive workplace policies can play a pivotal role in facilitating women's return to work, enhancing their career satisfaction and commitment. The interplay of cultural values and gendered expectations continues to shape Indian women's work–life decisions, highlighting the need for a nuanced understanding of motherhood's impact on their professional journeys.

Migration, Emigration, and Immigration: Bane or Boon

According to the 2011 census data, there were 450 million internal migrants in India, accounting for 37.7% of the total population (Rajan et al., 2020). Among these, nearly 70% were women (Chakraborty, 2020). Migrant work is generally characterized by public health measures, insecurity in employment, poor access to housing, and lack of sanitation facilities (ILO, 2020b).

Although women constitute a large majority of the total internal migrants, they are often disregarded. It is considered migration due to marriage or associational migration (Jones, 2020; Chakraborty, 2020; Rajan et al., 2020). According to the 2011 census data, 69.8% of women migrated due to marriage-related reasons. However, women continue to work even after marriage-related migration and face unique challenges compared to men. The portrayal of women's migration as related only to marriage or other social reasons leads to a general ignorance of the challenges and issues faced by female migrants, at their workplaces. Thus, women migrants struggle to become "invisible" as compared to their male counterparts (ILO, 2020a).

Moreover, women migrants are not identified as workers upon employment. They are considered helpers to their male relatives or spouses, known as the "jodi" system, and they are thus unpaid while males are paid 1.5 labor units for the pair (ILO, 2020a). The caste and class of women are also important determinants of the migration of women. These factors also contribute to the vulnerabilities of women migrants across India. Compared to the upper-class women, women belonging to ST, SC, and OBC were engaged in cyclic, short-term migration predominantly for agriculture, construction, or brick-making work (Mazumdar et al., 2013).

According to the International Labor Organization report, most female migrants to cities like Delhi and Mumbai were domestic laborers. In such work environments, female migrants experience harassment, exploitation, lack of privacy, and deprivation from access to healthcare and other facilities. Due to a lack of formal employers, these women are underpaid or unpaid in some circumstances and become highly vulnerable to bonded labor and human trafficking (ILO, 2020a).

During the COVID-19 crisis, migrant women were among the most affected populations in the country. Research reports that women are more vulnerable as they are considered less productive and possess lower ranks in society. Women have had to experience significant distress due to loss of livelihood, human rights violations, domestic violence, and economic, health, and other spheres (UN, 2020).

Young Indian Women's Immigration: Search for Independence and Dignity

A project titled "Understanding the vulnerabilities of Indian female migrants during COVID-19 pandemic: Rethinking policies for better integration of immigrant women's work lives" was funded by Sashtri Indo Canadian Institute to the author (Biswas & Leach, 2020–2022) to (a) identify the challenges and issues encountered by Indian immigrant women in Canada who are engaged in active work lives, as a consequence of COVID-19 pandemic and lockdown, from psychosocial and intersectional perspectives, and (b) to understand the aspirations and reasons behind emigration for young women from India who are moving to Canada. Biswas and colleagues (2023) studied the obstacles encountered by Skilled Indian Women Immigrants (SIWI) during the COVID-19 pandemic and how these women used their agency to cope with the situation. The researchers suggested examining both pre- and post-migration experiences of female immigrants to gain insight into how they employed their agency in dealing with challenges arising from restrictions and uncertainties related to immigration processes. The study involved first-generation Indian women who had immigrated to Canada, some before and some after border closures, as well as aspiring immigrants. The findings highlighted various difficulties faced by SIWIs, such as job insecurity, unemployment, networking challenges, delays in obtaining residency and visas, access to resources, and adherence to COVID-19 protocols. Mental health issues included feelings of isolation and concerns about financial support. The women employed everyday strategies like skills enhancement, seeking therapy, using digital platforms for connections, accessing government and consultancy services, and utilizing social media networks tailored to Canadian immigrants. The study recommended that universities and colleges provide more support for international students with programs focusing on cultural education and job search training for post-graduation success. It also suggested equal access to settlement services for all immigrant groups and better information dissemination about such services. The study highlighted how SIWIs in Canada and those in India displayed agency by addressing the challenges posed by the pandemic, compounded by migration-related stresses. Despite facing significant hurdles due to the pandemic and migration processes, these women demonstrated resilience by adapting to the circumstances and taking proactive steps to meet their financial, emotional, and social needs. Their agency mainly comprised everyday actions and practical measures within the constraints of the pandemic, reflecting their commitment to their goals despite the difficulties they encountered.

The primary driving forces behind migration and immigration were perceived independence and freedom of choice. Better lifestyle and healthcare also figure out as a significant precursor to emigration motives. Despite the threats and challenges, they expressed their aspirations and ambitions to emigrate to pursue freedom of choice and a safe environment to work and live.

Conclusion

The chapter has identified the drivers of sustainable and equitable growth and development of Indian women, keeping in focus the requirements of SDG 5. It urges for actions by the stakeholders responsible for policies and legislation, the development sector, and the community at large to improve the status of Indian women in terms of their economic growth and development, reducing gender inequality in the larger society, improving healthcare, and creating layers of support systems to reduce the care burden of Indian women. The major learnings from the research work reported here indicate the following implications in this regard.

- Creating awareness among the beneficiaries and target groups about existing policies and strategies for women's empowerment and growth will facilitate the implementation of the programs' communication with the target groups by establishing public–private partnerships, and strengthening the program delivery system will help to reduce inequality.

- Sensitizing the immediate family members, neighbors, kin network, and society at large by advocacy and social marketing about the consequences of inequality would be helpful. It has worked for "Beti Bachao, Beti padhao" (save the girl child, educate the girl child); and Janani Suraksha Yojana (maternal health and safety) programs. Thus, it may work for other issues as well.
- Doing impact assessment surveys for implemented programs, devising a monitoring process to assess the target penetration of the program, and modifying it will be helpful. It has earlier worked with the mandatory Corporate Social Responsibility Act in India to follow the model.
- Introducing women-friendly policies at the workplace like telecommuting, flexi-time, support for child care at the office, encouraging parental leaves for male partners, etc., will help encourage women to continue with their career ambitions and reduce off-ramping.
- Enabling an incapacitating environment at family and work to help women make their own choices, make independent decisions, and respect basic human rights, as well as the rights of women, will accentuate gender equality in society.
- The ranking of Indian women in political empowerment (in position 55 out of 156 countries ranked) shows the impact of policies and legislation implementation. The same may be followed for the educational attainment of women, healthcare, and workforce participation.

A gender-inclusive sustainable development agenda requires an ecosystem addressing the long-term gendered fault lines in India's labor markets and targeted policy measures to enhance women's participation and employment across sectors. Tools of gender inclusion, beneficiary assessments, policy appraisals, and gender budgeting analysis are needed to correct these aberrations in human development, keeping in view the guiding principle of the SDGs agenda—"Leave no one behind," particularly women and girls.

References

Abraham, V. (2013). "Missing labour or consistent" De-feminisation"?. *Economic and Political Weekly*, *48*(31), 99–108.

Alam, N., Roy, S. K., Ahmed, T., & Ahmed, A. M. S. (2010). Nutritional status, dietary intake, and relevant knowledge of adolescent girls in rural Bangladesh. *Journal of Health, Population, and Nutrition*, *28*(1), 86. https://doi.org/10.3329/JHPN.V28I1.4527

Azzopardi, P. S., Hearps, S. J. C., Francis, K. L., Kennedy, E. C., Mokdad, A. H., Kassebaum, N. J., Lim, S., Irvine, C. M. S., Vos, T., Brown, A. D., Dogra, S., Kinner, S. A., Kaoma, N. S., Naguib, M., Reavley, N. J., Requejo, J., Santelli, J. S., Sawyer, S. M., Skirbekk, V., . . . Patton, G. C. (2019). Progress in adolescent health and wellbeing: Tracking 12 headline indicators for 195 countries and territories, 1990–2016. *Lancet (London, England)*, *393*(10176), 1101–1118. https://doi.org/10.1016/S0140-6736(18)32427-9

Barcellos, S. H., Carvalho, L. S., & Lleras-Muney, A. (2014). Child gender and parental investments in India: Are boys and girls treated differently? *American Economic Journal*, *6*(1), 157–189. https://doi.org/10.1257/app.6.1.157

Barhate, B., Hirudayaraj, M., Dirani, K., Barhate, R., & Abadi, M. (2021). Career disruptions of married women in India: An exploratory investigation. *Human Resource Development International*, *24*(4), 401–424.

Bhambhani, C., & Inbanathan, A. (2018). Not a mother, yet a woman: Exploring experiences of women opting out of motherhood in India. *Asian Journal of Women's Studies*, *24*(2), 159–182. https://doi.org/10.1080/12259276.2018.1462932

Biswas, U. N. (2016). *Sex-selective abortion and female feticide-can a public campaign produce effective change: A comparative analysis*. Report submitted to Indian Council of Social Science Research (ICSSR), New Delhi.

Biswas, U. N. (2021, January). Adolescent reproductive health in South Asia: Issues and challenges. In W. Leal Filho, A. Marisa Azul, L. Brandli, A. Lange Salvia, & T. Wall (Eds.), *Gender equality. Encyclopedia of the UN sustainable development goals* (pp. 32–41). Springer. https://doi.org/10.1007/978-3-319-95687-9_47

Biswas, U. N. (2022). Understanding care-receiver's perspective about eldercare services in India. In P. Roy, S. Sanyal, & S. Patel (Eds.), *Elderly in India: A collection of selected writings* (pp. 5–20). Alternote Press. ISBN 978-93-94213-00-5

Biswas, U. N., Dellve, L., Bhattacharjee, A., & Walmesjo, W. (2020). Ageing and values in the developments of home-based eldercare: Perspectives from India and Sweden. *Psychology in Developing Societies (Special Issue on Ageing in Developing Societies)*, *32*(2), 224–253. https://doi.org/10.1177/0971333620937373

Biswas, U. N., & Essau, C. (2012). Violence against women and girls: The case of India. In A. Browne-Miller (Ed.), *Violence and abuse in society: Understanding a global crisis* (Vol. 4, pp. 335–357). Praeger/ABC-CLIO. ISBN 13 9780313382765

Biswas, U. N., & Leach, B. (2020–2022). *Understanding the vulnerabilities of Indian female migrants during COVID 19 pandemic: Rethinking policies for better integration of immigrant women's work lives*. Research report submitted to Shastri Institutional Collaborative Research Grant (SICRG) from Shastri Indo Canadian Institute.

Biswas, U. N., Leach, B., Jijina, P., & Niraula, A. (2023). Lived experiences of Skilled Indian Women Immigrants (SIWI) navigating the COVID-19 pandemic: Immigration trajectories to Canada. *Journal of International Migration and Integration* (Vol. 25, pp. 595–619). www.doi.org/10.1007/s12134-023-01078-w

Bruine de Bruin, W., & Bennett, D. (2020). Relationships between initial COVID-19 risk perceptions and protective health behaviors: A national survey. *American Journal of Preventive Medicine*, *59*(2), 157–167. https://doi.org/10.1016/J.AMEPRE.2020.05.001

Chakraborty, A. (2020). Negotiated agency amidst overlapping vulnerabilities of women migrant workers in South Asia. *Social Change*, *50*(1), 61–76. https://doi.org/10.1177/0049085719901070

Chandana, H., Madhu, B., & Murthy, M. N. (2020). Awareness about cervical cancer among women residing in urban slums of Mysuru city of Karnataka, India: A crosssectional study. *Clinical Epidemiology and Global Health*, *8*(3), 835–839.

Chandra-Mouli, V., Plesons, M., Adebayo, E., Amin, A., Avni, M., Kraft, J. M., Lane, C., Brundage, C. L., Kreinin, T., Bosworth, E., Garcia-Moreno, C., & Malarcher, S. (2017). Implications of the global early adolescent study's formative research findings for action and for research. *Journal of Adolescent Health*, *61*(4), S5–S9. https://doi.org/10.1016/j.jadohealth.2017.07.012

Chopra, D., Saha, A., Nazneen, S., & Krishnan, M. (2020). *Are women not 'working'? Interactions between childcare and women's economic engagement*. IDS Working Paper 533.

Daral, S., Khokhar, A., & Pradhan, S. (2016). Prevalence and determinants of child maltreatment among school-going adolescent girls in a semi-urban area of Delhi, India. *Journal of Tropical Pediatrics*, *62*(3), 227–240.

Das Sharma, A. (2023, March 3). MPW2023: India's female labour force is plunging: Can country's growing economy afford this? *Business Today*.

Desai, S., & Joshi, O. (2019). The paradox of declining female work participation in an era of economic growth. *The Indian Journal of Labour Economics*, *62*(1), 55–71.

DeUgarte, D. A. (2010). Surrogate obesity negatively impacts pregnancy rates in third-party reproduction. *Fertility and Sterility*, 1008–1010.

Dhar, S. (2018). Gender and sustainable development goals (SDGs). *Indian Journal of Gender Studies*, *25*(1), 47–78.

Douchi, T., Kuwahata, R., Yamamoto, S., Oki, T., Yamasaki, H., & Nagata, Y. (2002). Relationship of upper body obesity to menstrual disorders. *Acta Obstetricia et Gynecologica Scandinavica*, *81*(2), 147–150. https://doi.org/10.1080/J.1600-0412.2002.810210.X

Economic Times. (2022). *Indians top as Canada admits 108,000 new immigrants in the first quarter*. Retrieved May 1, 2022, from https://economictimes.indiatimes.com/nri/migrate/indians-top-as-canada-admits-108000-new-immigrant-in-the-firstquarter/articleshow/90587538.cms?utm_source=contentofinterest

Evans, J., Sahgal, N., Salazar, A. M., Staff, K. J., & Corichi, M. (2022, March 2). How Indians view gender roles in families and society. *Pew Research Center*.

Ferrant, G., Pesando, L. M., & Nowacka, K. (2014). *Unpaid care work: The missing link in the analysis of gender gaps in labour outcomes*. OECD Development Center.

Financial Status of Older People in India-An Assessment. (2017). Retrieved May 10, 2024, from https://social.un.org/ageing-working-group/documents/seventh/AgewellFoundationSubmission.pdf

Global Gender Gap Report. (2023). Retrieved May 7, 2024, from www.weforum.org/publications/global-gender-gap-report-2023/in-full/benchmarking-gender-gaps-2023/

Goldin. (1995). *Career and family: College women look to the past*. NBER working paper (w5188).

Gouda, S., & Sekher, T. V. (2014). Factors leading to school dropouts in India: An analysis of national, family health survey-3 data. *IOSR Journal of Research & Method in Education*, *4*(6), 75–83.

Government of India. (1974). *Towards equality: Report of the committee on the status of women in India*. Government of India: Ministry of Education and Social Welfare. http://pldindia.org/wp-content/uploads/2013/04/Towards-Equality-1974-Part-1.pdf

Gupta, R., Nimesh, R., Singal, G. L., Bhalla, P., & Prinja, S. (2018). Effectiveness of India's National Programme to save the girl child: Experience of Beti Bachao Beti Padao (B3P) programme from Haryana State. *Health Policy Plan*, *33*(7), 870–876.

Hajivandi, L., Noroozi, M., Mostafavi, F., & Ekramzadeh, M. (2020). Food habits in overweight and obese adolescent girls with polycystic ovary syndrome (PCOS): A qualitative study in Iran. *BMC Pediatrics*, *20*, 277. https://doi.org/10.1186/s12887-020-02173-y

Haq, R. (2013). Intersectionality of gender and other forms of identity: Dilemmas and challenges facing women in India. *Gender in Management: An International Journal*, *28*(3), 171–184.

HelpAge India Annual Report. (2019–20). Retrieved May 30, 2021, from www.helpageindia.org/wp-content/uploads/2021/05/HelpAge-India-Annual-Report-2019-20.pdf

High Level Committee on the Status on Women. (2015). Report on the status of women in India. *Four volumes and summary report*. MWCD, Government of India. http://wcd.nic.in/documents/hlc-status-women

International Labor Organization. (2020a). *Road map for developing a policy framework for the inclusion of internal migrant workers in India*. Retrieved May 30, 2021, from www.ilo.org/wcmsp5/groups/public/—asia/—ro-bangkok/—sro-new_delhi/documents/publication/wcms_763352.pdf

International Labour Organization. (2020b). *COVID-19: Impact on migrant workers and country response in Malaysia*. Retrieved May 20, 2022, from www.ilo.org/asia/publications/issue-briefs/WCMS_741512/lang%2D%2Den/index.html

Jamuna, D. (2003). Issues of elder care and elder abuse in the Indian context. *Journal of Aging and Social Policy*, *15*(2–3), 125–42.

Jones, G. W. (2020). New patterns of female migration in South Asia. *Asian Population Studies*, *16*,(1), 1–4. https://doi.org/10.1080/17441730.2019.1701802

Joshi, S., Borkotoky, K., Gautam, A., Datta, N., Achyut, P., Nanda, P., & Verma, R. (2020). Poised for a dividend? Changes in the life trajectories of India's young women over the past two decades. *PLoS One*, *15*(12), e0242876. https://doi.org/10.1371/journal.pone.0242876

Kataria, I., Siddiqui, M., Treiman, K., Foley, S., Anand, M., Biswas, S., Shastri, D., Bhatla, N., Radhakrishnan, D., Mamidi, P., & Sankaranarayanan, R. (2022). Awareness, perceptions, and choices of physicians pertaining to human papillomavirus (HPV) vaccination in India: A formative research study. *Vaccine*, *X*, *12*, 100228.

Khanna, G. (2022). The Indian odd: Rising education and declining workforce participation. In *Official conference proceedings of IAFOR\ International conference on Hawaii*.

Li, N. (2022). Women's work in India: Evidence from changes in time use between 1998 and 2019. *World Development*, *161*. https://doi.org/10.1016/j.worlddev.2022.106107

Liang, M., Simelane, S., Fortuny Fillo, G., Chalasani, S., Weny, K., Salazar Canelos, P., Jenkins, L., Moller, A. B., Chandra-Mouli, V., Say, L., Michielsen, K., Engel, D. M. C., & Snow, R. (2019). The state of adolescent sexual and reproductive health. *Journal of Adolescent Health*, *65*(6), S3–S15. https://doi.org/10.1016/J.JADOHEALTH.2019.09.015

Maddux, J. E., & Rogers, R. W. (1983). Protection motivation and self-efficacy: A revised theory of fear appeals and attitude change. *Journal of Experimental Social Psychology*, *19*(5), 469–479. https://doi.org/10.1016/0022-1031(83)90023–9

Mazumdar, I., Neetha, N., & Agnihotri, I. (2013). Migration and gender in India. *Economic and Political Weekly*, 54–64.

Mehrotra, S., & Sinha, S. (2017). Explaining falling female employment during a high growth period. *Economic and Political Weekly*, *52*(6), 54–62.

Mittal, A., & Pokale, A. B. (2021). Catching them young: Impact of educational intervention on cervical cancer knowledge and human papillomavirus vaccine hesitancy in adolescent girls in urban India. *DY Patil Journal of Health Sciences*, *9*(3), 99.

Nagpal, S., & Viswanathan, V. (2023). *What reports on Indian women's falling participation in labour force don't tell you*. https://theprint/what-reports-on-indian-womens-falling-participation-in-labor-force-dont-tell-you/1311436

Patil, A. (2018, March 28). *Why caregiving needs to be "de-feminized."* White Swan Foundation. www.whiteswanfoundation.org/caregiving/how-the-role-of-caring-disproportionately-burdens-women

Rajan, S. I., & Balagopal, G. (2017). Caring India: An introduction. In *Elderly care in India* (pp. 1–36). Springer.

Rajan, S. I., & Morgan, S. P. (2018). Selective versus generalized gender bias in childhood health and nutrition: Evidence from India. *Population and Development Review*, *44*(2), 231–255. https://doi.org/10.1111/padr.12132

Rajan, S. I., Sivakumar, P., & Srinivasan, A. (2020). The COVID-19 pandemic and internal labour migration in India: A 'Crisis of mobility'. *The Indian Journal of Labour Economics*, *63*, 1021–1039. https://doi.org/10.1007/s41027-020-00293-8

Ravindran, B., & Baral, R. (2014). Factors affecting the work attitudes of Indian re-entry women in the IT. *Vikalpa*, *39*(2), 31–42. https://doi.org/10.1177/0256090920140204

Renfree, I., Harrison, D., Marshall, P., Stawarz, K., & Cox, A. (2016, May 7–12). Don't kick the habit: The role of dependency in habit formation apps. In *Conference on Human Factors in Computing Systems—Proceedings* (pp. 2932–2939). https://doi.org/10.1145/2851581.2892495

Rittenberg, V., Sobaleva, S., Ahmad, A., Oteng-Ntim, E., Bolton, V., Khalaf, Y., Braude, P., & El Toukhy, T. (2011). Influence of BMI on risk of miscarriage after single blastocyst transfer. *Human Reproduction*, *26*(10), 2642–2650. https://doi.org/10.1093/HUMREP/DER254

Roy, D. (2024, April). *Social communication model for reproductive health awareness and wellbeing amongst adolescent females* [Unpublished PhD dissertation submitted to Department of Psychology]. The M.S. University of Baroda.

Sawyer, S. M., Afifi, R. A., Bearinger, L. H., Blakemore, S. J., Dick, B., Ezeh, A. C., & Patton, G. C. (2012). Adolescence: A foundation for future health. *The Lancet*, *379*(9826), 1630–1640. https://doi.org/10.1016/S0140-6736(12)60072-5

Sebastian, R. A., Ramos, M. M., Stumbo, S., McGrath, J., & Fairbrother, G. (2014). Measuring youth health engagement: Development of the youth engagement with health services survey. *Journal of Adolescent Health*, *55*(3), 334–340. https://doi.org/10.1016/J.JADOHEALTH.2014.02.008

Sekher, T., & Hatti, N. (2010). *Unwanted daughters: Gender discrimination in modern India*. Rawat Publications.

Tiwari, A., Singh, S. K., Manar, M. K. Mohan, U., & Pandey, K. (2020). Gender equity and equality in Indian healthcare. *Galore International Journal of Health Sciences and Research*, *5*(2), 26–34.

Ugargol, A. P., & Bailey, A. (2018). Family caregiving for older adults: Gendered roles and caregiver burden in emigrant households of Kerala, India. *Asian Population Studies*, *14*(2), 194–210.

UNESCO. (2019). *The case for comprehensive sexuality education*. Global education monitoring report. United Nations. (2020). *Policy brief: The impact of COVID-19 on women*. www.un.org/sexualviolenceinconflict/wp-content/uploads/2020/06/report/policy-brief-the-impact-of-covid-19-on-women/policy-brief-the-impact-of-covid-19-on-women-en-1.pdf

Vidya Bharathi, R., Swetha, S., Neerajaa, J., Varsha Madhavica, J., Dakshina Moorthy Janani, Rekha, S.N., Ramya S., Usha B., (2017). An epidemiological survey: Effect of predisposing factors for PCOS in Indian urban and rural population. *Middle East Fertility Society Journal*, *22*(4), 313–316. https://doi.org/10.1016/j.mefs.2017.05.007

Weiss, H. A., & Ferrand, R. A. (2019). Improving adolescent health: An evidence-based call to action. *The Lancet*, *393*(10176), 1073–1075. https://doi.org/10.1016/S0140-6736(18)32996-9

WHO, Health Information System. (2023). Retrieved May 7, 2024, from https://cdn.who.int/media/docs/default-source/health-information-system/mh-profiles/mh_profile_india.pdf

World Economic Forum (WEF). (2022). *Global gender gap report 2022*. Retrieved June 12, 2023, from www.weforum.org/reports/global-gender-gap-report-2022/in-full/1–6-in-focus-country-performances/

11 Changing Landscape of Social Interactions

Decoding Route to Harmony

Purnima Singh, Girishwar Misra, Preeti Kapur, Arvind Kumar Mishra, and Roomana N. Siddiqui

Social psychologists often argue that motivated by the desire for distinctiveness groups tend to see themselves as unique and different from others. This need for differentiation is crucial in the identity-making process. Distinctiveness is crucial for group identity but can become a 'double-edged sword,' leading to exclusion and othering. However, too much assertion of one's positive distinctiveness may result in 'othering.' Constructing the 'other' is a process through which the 'other' is created in societies by assigning certain values, beliefs, and practices to the other and promoting one's own group's values, beliefs, and practices. This creates boundaries separating 'us' and 'them,' often maintaining social distance and creating barriers to shared spaces. In this context role of the state and leaders play critical role. The state ideally should provide good governance and create conditions for societal harmony. However, political interference and identity politics often create divides. The role of the state and leaders can be ambiguous, with some fostering harmony and others exploiting identity politics for personal gain. Leaders can also play a role in creating specific identities for political gain, which can further widen the divide between social groups. Social life has a high concern for interdependence resulting in coexistence. Coexistence and interdependence are central to the protection and appreciation of shared spaces. Creating social spaces where people can interact, share views, learn from each other, and accommodate differences can build interdependence and promote harmony. It may be noted that despite belonging to different religions, castes, language groups, and regions, people have been living amicably for centuries together. Certain geographical spaces have remained peaceful throughout their known history due to the interplay of interdependence, mutual trust, and the belief in their ability to continue to do so. Interdependence and coexistence are foundational for maintaining peace and harmony, with shared spaces allowing for mutual understanding and respect. This chapter explores the complex dynamics of social identity, distinctiveness, and the construction of the 'Other' in society.

The desire for distinctiveness is indeed a powerful force in shaping group identities and can lead to both positive outcomes, such as a strong sense

DOI: 10.4324/9781003461302-15

of community, and negative consequences, like polarization and othering. The examples of peaceful coexistence in Ram-Rahim Nagar and Malerkotla, highlight the importance of active community involvement and leadership in fostering intergroup harmony. Sufi shrines serve as another example of spaces where diverse groups come together, transcending social categories to find common ground. In essence, while distinctiveness and the construction of the 'Other' can lead to division, the conscious efforts of communities and leaders to build interdependence and shared spaces can counteract these forces, promoting a more harmonious society. It's a delicate balance that requires ongoing attention and nurturing. This exploration of the dynamics of social spaces and intergroup relations highlights the intricate balance between the need for group distinctiveness and the pursuit of communal harmony through shared spaces and interdependence. The concept of functionality in intergroup relations is particularly interesting, as it underscores the fluidity of social dynamics. As you mentioned, what may serve as a bridge in one context could become a barrier in another. This dynamic nature of social relationships is reflective of the 'see-saw relationships' you described, which can oscillate between positive, neutral, and negative states, influencing social cohesion or tension accordingly. The decoding of shared spaces is a critical aspect of fostering a harmonious society. These spaces are born out of mutual respect for cultural identities and diversity, and they serve as a foundation for positive behaviors and emotions like compassion, love, and generosity. The multiplicity of identities within a plural society can indeed enlarge these shared spaces, promoting connectivity and joint activities that are essential for societal harmony. However, there are challenges to maintaining these shared spaces, especially in the face of sociopolitical contestations and conflicts that threaten the pluralistic fabric of society. The role of group identities, both self-constructed and ascribed by others, is central to this discussion. The challenge lies in leveraging the plurality of identities to strengthen shared spaces, rather than allowing them to become rigid and exclusive, leading to an ethnocentric outlook. In conclusion, the appreciation of shared spaces and their significance for harmony requires a nuanced understanding of social reality and a focus on relational units rather than just individuals. This broader perspective allows for a more profound grasp of the dynamic social reality and the potential for fostering coexistence and mutual understanding.

We have seen several kinds of trauma across the world, be it from COVID-19 pandemic, conflicts and wars among nations, intergroup skirmishes between the powerful and less powerful, and many others, all resulting in human suffering and thwarting development processes and peace and prosperity. Social psychologists need to think of ways and means that help humanity overcome the current state of affairs and move toward a social order that is based on the premises of peace and harmony. In the past several years, many changes have happened which have impacted all of us. The major force has been globalization which is often associated with economic integration and the emergence of a borderless global market and has impacted all of us in diverse ways. It has brought sweeping changes in the social, cultural, and political arenas as well as resulted in the emergence of new identities and consolidation of traditional ones. Various contradictory processes of globalization have led to wide-ranging changes in the social fabric impacting social relationships at all levels, within social groups, within nations and across nations. The forces of globalization have led to the merger of some boundaries, but newer boundaries have emerged. The neoliberals advocated that the process of globalization would result in a deteriorated space, but this myth as is apparent has been shattered. Undoubtedly, the boundaries continue to play critical and functional roles at varied levels of societal living. Some of the boundaries have become more relative but gradually more boundaries have emerged. This among other factors has impacted harmony and peace and has changed the landscape of social interactions.

Dynamic Nature of Social Interactions and Relations

The social world is continuously evolving, and the dynamics of social relations are becoming increasingly complex in today's world. Societal realities have become complex and have an important bearing on the nature and formation of our social and relational fabric. The relational world is undergoing rapid transformation. In certain respects, the relational space is shrinking, and the quality of relationships is being compromised and contested. Furthermore, the realization of interconnectedness which was at the core of social relationships is often missed in the increasingly intense articulation of individuality in the fast pace of technology-dominated globalized world today. It may be noted that the relationships at the group and community levels as well as relations between communities and groups are also changing. What we see today are various shades of acceptance and exclusion of each other which is often creating schisms in the social fabric of the society. In most societies, diversities of various kinds are the rule. Living amidst diversities and promoting peace and harmony will facilitate opportunities and secure spaces where diverse groups interact and share their joys and sorrows. As most of us are products of these pluralities, at one or the other point in time, we do share some commonalities in terms of good and bad experiences. Under these circumstances what is the road to harmony is the central question we are focusing on in this chapter. We are doing this in the context of India—a land known for its unity in diversity.

Variable Pattern of Social Interactions: The Indian Landscape

India like many nations in the world is a pluralistic society—constituted by diverse ethnic, religious, and linguistic communities inhabiting varied ecological spaces. Historically, these diverse groups have grown following various paths of cultural evolution and development. These are inscribed in a range of forms of performing arts, architecture, literature, educational institutions, social customs and life rituals, and patterns of intra- and intergroup relationships. Historically communities and social groups have interacted with people of other cultures from within as well as other countries. The influence has brought in a rich tapestry of thinking patterns, customs, and traditions. The coexistence of several communities has led to assimilation, accommodation, and integration of ideas and practices in varying degrees. At the same time, we have seen frequent eruptions of conflicts on account of episodes of discrimination, prejudice, unfounded stereotypes, atrocities, and organized violence toward the weaker and marginalized sections. This situation is further complicated by the fast-expanding social media that sharpens social comparison and fuels the fantasies of a consumer-centric life. In the course of such developments, the personal and social identities and frames of belongingness are being reworked and negotiated. In a significant sense, new boundaries are emerging, and the shared social spaces of today are shrinking, giving way to the promotion of an individualistic (like) framework of functioning. The resulting exclusion goes against the pluralistic spirit of societal living and poses threats to the well-being of society and the nation. Often there is a tendency to overlook or consciously ignore or exclude the existing plural identities and impose a singular classificatory system. This is notable when for example religion or caste is considered. For example, when religion becomes an all-encompassing motivator, it leads to the formation of an exclusive identity. This religious identity then functions more as a barrier rather than a bridge. For boundaries to serve as a bridging function, researchers have to understand what Amartya Sen (2006) refers to as the 'power of the competing identities.' These include not only the commonalities of shared identities but also the many identities that one simultaneously holds. As people crisscross several social boundaries with relative ease, they are likely to have social contacts and develop expanded shared spaces. In simple mathematical terms, it is at the intersection of these boundaries that grounds for shared spaces are born, and it is these shared spaces that may become the building blocks of much sought-after social integration and social cohesion and pave the way for harmony.

Finding the key to achieving harmonious coexistence among various ethnic groups with diverse cultural traditions in multi-ethnic and plural societies is a major problem worldwide.

Indian society is transforming rapidly due to a vast number of influences emanating from the forces within as well as outside the country. We have, in a project, examined how people make sense of these changes as they impact the pattern of social interactions and quality of social life (Singh et al., 2023). We argue that creating shared spaces is a possible route to harmony in plural societies. In the above-mentioned project, we set forth exploring the emerging shared spaces in contemporary Indian society—spaces that provide members from different communities with opportunities to meaningfully engage with each other. Mapping these shared spaces was a daunting task and at the very outset, we could realize that we need to adopt appropriate ways and means to assess and appreciate the shared spaces. This was particularly true when we planned to map the 'bridges and barriers' in social relations. We tried to study the concept of 'bridges' by looking at the diverse strategies and steps of the people, such as sharing, helping, supporting, facilitating, and bonding end. These impinge on a multitude of closely related features of social living—social harmony, coherence, social well-being, and coexistence. In an attempt to understand the 'barriers,' the focus was on the difficulties, anxieties, suspicions, mistrust, etc., that trigger conflicts, violence, discrimination and stereotyping, unproductive differentiations, and clefts in social life. In this chapter, we attempt to present a synoptic picture of this research endeavor and to offer a conceptual articulation of the emerging understanding as a possible way ahead for harmony.

Assessing Intricacies in Social Interactions: Some Methodological Challenges

Given the complexity of the issues involved in the study of shared spaces, it was decided that multiple methodological lenses be adopted. Thus, both inductive and deductive analyses examine aspects of sharing and social well-being, deciphering both the facilitators and impediments in social relations across a variety of social groups and settings among youths from different caste and religious groups. The social ecology is known to be more peaceful as well as conflict-prone social contexts known to attract people from all walks of life and known as centers of coexistence and harmony, textual analysis of newspaper reports, and selected novels all facilitated our understanding. The chief concern throughout was to examine the diverse threads of social experiences that weave together to create these spaces. We have also attempted to delineate the political and historical understanding of sharing and barriers in social relationships across time and space. This allowed identifying new ways of understanding interactions between social groups and provided a holistic view of the phenomenon. Accordingly, a multi-method approach was adopted using diverse data sources which not only enriched the scope of research but also allowed to delve deeper into contextual aspects and understand the social reality better.

The Complex Cycle of Intergroup Relations

Today, the sociopolitical matrix of India is complex yet vibrant. In the last few decades, we have seen rapid sociopolitical and economic changes that have had a multifaceted impact on the social fabric of the nation. On the one hand, these changes have led to rising expectations and aspirations of people, and on the other hand, our inability to create opportunities that will meet aspirations and expectations has resulted in large gaps that we see in society today. We notice challenges at the sociopolitical level which have to be handled if we are interested in creating a harmonious society. We aspire to be at par with the rest of the world and also be world leaders in many spheres but at the same time, our internal contradictions pull us back from realizing our aspirations. Furthermore, as we all can see, the pace of social changes has been demanding newer time and space arrangements which means reorganization of life especially the social space is imminent, but we have not been able to do so. Changing contexts call for the emergence of new identities and the process of contestation in the construction and maintenance of these identities results in differences and possible conflicts. Furthermore, group-based identities, including religious, caste, and regional identities, are impacted and are being consolidated day by day. This consolidation has positive consequences for some groups but has also emboldened forces to create divisions in society. In the last few decades, newer political arrangements that have propped up have led to further disruptions. It might not be an exaggeration if we were to say that Indian society is at the crossroads today and trying to work out various options.

Although there were and are vast differences and disparities in the society, it is astonishing to note that these coexisted in the life world. They tend to occupy the same space and are invariably found to occupy that space with regular frequency. As a nation, we have a strong ability to reconcile the competing demands and are, by and large, accommodative although strains and contradictions do emerge concerning our relationships with other social groups and communities. In turn, we get to see a myriad of shades of acceptance and colors of exclusion. It is also true that despite living amidst such diversities, the overarching value of the age-old dictum '*vasudhaiv kutumbukam*' (the entire world is like a family) prompts us to look for opportunities and spaces where diverse groups interact, share, and reconstruct their joys and sorrows.

Coexistence is the predominant way of social life of the Indian people which has given a syncretic culture. This is the result of centuries of interactions between the various social groups. Living with differences was possible owing to accepting diversity as a part of the deep-seated grand cultural narrative. This narrative was not monolithic or cultural and therefore allowed managing the diversities. Despite social tensions, conflicts, riots, and even instances of lynching resulting in polarization and mistrust, one can also argue that by and large, we live together peacefully and share our joys and sorrows. Peace and conflict are thus inseparable parts of the social order. The cycle of peace and conflict is tautological, and we are embedded in this apparent cycle of contradiction. Plurality plays a dual role in bringing forth discrimination, violence, and conflict, yet it also provides us with opportunities for interactions and social contacts and thereby helps develop expanded shared spaces that bring about peace, harmony, and sharing.

The cycle/s of peace and violence continues periodically, and we witness and are in turn influenced by such episodes. It may also be viewed as a contradiction of sorts as we note a cyclic phenomenon of harmony in everyday social conduct as well as conflict, violence, and discrimination. In this section, we would like to throw light on some of the factors which possibly nurture and provide a foundation of this kind for social relations.

Inequality

A major factor behind several social conflicts is inequality seen in the various realms of our social life. Caste-based inequalities and inequalities emanating due to conflict between majority and minority groups have often been cited as factors leading to violence and conflict. Inequality creates potential conditions which trigger hostility and enmity. Much has been written about the rising inequality in our country and other parts of the world and about the increasing divide between those who acquire and control the social spaces *versus* the disadvantaged ones who are destined to face deprivation and are handicapped in terms of access to resources and freedom to organize their lives. Similarly, we need not spell out the nature of the relationship between inequality and violence as it has been well documented. Different scholars have their take on this relationship between inequality and conflict. An interesting thesis on the relationship between the two has been proposed by Scheidel (2017), a historian, who has presented an argument that violence has been a great leveler of inequality throughout the ages. Without getting into this debate, if we look at the relationship between inequality and violence, we posit that inequality results in various psychological processes such as exclusion, marginalization, deprivation, and others, which create a gap between those who are privileged and those who are not. The consequence of the widening of this gap is the resultant shrinking of shared spaces which might be a potential trigger of social tension.

Shrinking Shared Spaces

In contemporary times, we see that shared spaces are changing. The shared social spaces are shrinking slowly and are paving for the promotion of an individualistic (like) framework of social functioning. Priorities in life and the inclination to share seem to be limited to personal selves and immediate social subgroups. This is being done with a growing utilitarian mindset of 'functionality' involving strategic positioning to celebrate a separated self. Consolidation of social identities (e.g., caste, religion, language, and locality) at various levels is happening at a fast speed. Although for day-to-day interactions, the likelihood of going beyond our social groups is present; these are marked mainly by casual relationships. Our close interactions are by and large confined to our salient groups. Social psychologists have shown that ingroup bias (Hewstone et al., 2002) is a robust phenomenon fostering intergroup ties. A large part of our social interactions is dominated by ingroup bias as has been reported to occur in a variety of settings (Fowler & Kam, 2007; Fu et al., 2012; Rand et al., 2009). However, it may not be the case that in all situations, it leads to negative consequences for social interactions. However, it does have the potential for discrimination as far as outgroups are concerned. This may reduce the shared social spaces and ultimately turn out to be a precursor of conflict. It may also make the boundaries between ingroups and outgroups pronounced leading to the possibility of creating differentiations and barriers in social relationships.

The Salience of Social Categorization

Social categories to which people belong are assuming greater importance in social lives. The process of social categorization results in differentiation between groups which triggers social psychological processes like thinking more positively about the ingroup, favoring them, and derogating the outgroups and often these may become barriers to the harmonious relationships between 'us' and 'them.' Let us look at the process and consequences of social categorization as emerging from the present work more closely.

Rediscovery, Re-Articulation, and Consolidation of Social Identities

We see the trend of increasing consolidation of identities based on caste, region, language, and religion. Associations and organizations based on them are flourishing in our social world. This consolidation becomes problematic when it results in exclusionary and discriminatory behavior toward others. The consolidation takes place not just in social groups but is evident even in the form of the state's response and the role it plays in such consolidations. After independence, the state has been acknowledging community identities and bringing change in terms of provisions for access to resources and intervening in the opportunity structure. As a result, these newer identities created by the state can be noted (Jodhka, 2001). These newer identities have not only created further crevices in society, but more and more social groups are clamoring for these identities by claiming that they too should be given the benefits accruing to such identities. Groups want to have their share of the pie available. Apart from the state-created identities, technological advancements, professional mobility, and migration are also facilitating the articulation of newer identities. A challenge of the 21st century, the processes of identity construction are becoming more nuanced as is there are diverse layers or levels of social identities. They are active and salient in different contexts. We must appreciate that identity construction takes a completely different shape and character when identity is no longer based on a single factor such as caste or religion. In this way, new boundaries get created and newer shared spaces emerge, which in consequence blur the earlier ones.

Accentuating Sense of Relative Deprivation

The existence of diverse groups enjoying different levels of social and economic status has widened the gap between groups which in turn has resulted in varied perceptions of one's status. Those who belong to the marginalized sections of society (e.g., minorities, women, lower castes and classes, and others) feel relatively deprived in comparison to those who enjoy the privileges by being a part of the mainstream. As the term suggests deprivation is not an absolute condition but is always measured relative to some norm and is a result of social comparison. As Thorbecke and Charumilind (2002) have argued deprivation-induced discontent is generated not from inequality per se but from the gap between the expected and achieved degrees of well-being, where the present state of one's ingroup is judged less favorable than that of the outgroup. Relative deprivation and resultant reactions would depend on factors like ingroup identification, the belief that such actions will bring about a change (Klandermans, 1997), and the nature of perceived injustice that underlies relative deprivation, etc. Both lower caste groups, tribal groups, and poor and minority group members experienced relative deprivation. They felt that they were worse off than their higher caste and majority group counterparts who enjoyed the benefits of development. Relative deprivation is also reflected in the simmering discontent expressed by the members of these groups. Since relative deprivation is linked to prejudice and protest behavior, it has the potential to be a trigger for conflict.

Perceptions of Threat

A threat is defined as a situation in which one group has either the capability or intention to inflict a negative outcome on another group (Davis, 2000). Past research has shown that threat perceptions play a key role in shaping intergroup relations (see Riek et al., 2006) and has been identified as an important proximal predictor of prejudice (Stephan & Stephan, 2000). When a group perceives that another group (outgroup) is detrimental to the ingroup, both for real reasons such as competition over resources, territory, or status, or for symbolic reasons, such as identity issues and sacred values, threat may be perceived. Perception of threat is a function of the differentiation between the ingroup and the outgroup and a host of other factors that make these distinctions more salient. The realistic group conflict theory propounds that when two groups compete for scarce resources, the potential success of one group threatens the well-being of the other, thereby resulting in a negative outgroup attitude (Sherif & Sherif, 1969). In many instances, threat seems to be an important barrier in the creation of shared spaces. Power, opportunities, and political support attributed to one group made these perceptions of threat more salient. Stephan and Stephan (2000) in their integrated threat theory have classified threats into four types: realistic threat, symbolic threat, intergroup anxiety and negative stereotypes. Realistic threats include perception of competition, conflicting goals and threats to physical and economic well-being. Symbolic threat pertains to threats arising due to conflict in values, norms, and beliefs between groups. Intergroup anxiety involves feelings of uneasiness and awkwardness in the presence of outgroup members because of uncertainty about how to behave toward them, which makes interaction with outgroups threatening. Finally, negative stereotypes generate threats by creating negative expectations concerning the behavior of outgroup members. Evidence for all four types of threats was found to affect the relationships between the high caste and the lower caste groups and minority and majority groups (Singh et al., 2023).

The Desire for Distinctiveness

We have a strong tendency to see our groups as different and unique in comparison to others. This need for differentiation is important in the identity-making process. Vignoles et al. (2006) posit that the distinctiveness principle requires the perception that one (or one's ingroup) is unique, separate, and positively distinctive from others (or outgroups). Distinctiveness plays a significant role in the construction and consolidation of identity. Attempts to assert distinct identities by groups often get contested resulting at times in polarization within the community as a whole. Distinctiveness provides anchors that hold the group together but also creates barriers in the group member's relationship with other groups. Thus, distinctiveness becomes a double-edged sword. Too much assertion of one's positive distinctiveness may result in othering.

Constructing the 'Other'

The 'other' is created in societies by selecting certain aspects of the other's lives (Tripathi & Singh, 2016). Two processes that help create the other are by assigning certain values, beliefs, and practices to the other and by promoting and recognizing values, beliefs, and practices of one's group resulting in creating boundaries separating 'us' and 'them.' 'They' the other and 'we' are not just different, but we are better than the other because 'we' do not indulge in similar practices. The resultant creation of privileged spaces for 'our' ingroup and the oft exclusion of 'them,' that is, those who we consider as constituting the outgroup. Social distance is often maintained with those representing the 'other' and the boundaries created between self and 'other' are at times less permeable. Othering creates boundaries and barriers to shared spaces as the 'other' is seen as different and assigned a peripheral status. Othering helps maintain ingroup advantage and dominance; therefore, it is preferred.

The Role of the State and Leaders

Ideally, the role of the state is to give good governance and create amiable conditions so that harmony prevails in society. However, we find that this has not been the case and is noticed as creating a divide between the masses through political interference and indulgence in identity politics. Government policies with an implicit agenda of appeasement of the minority and deprived groups were not seen by other groups as those aiding welfare, but instead as those having political motives. Furthermore, new identities given by the state have often led to the negotiation of identities and reorganization of identities resulting in stress/tensions in the social system. If we look at the situation in India, we can see that the state has failed in creating an egalitarian society despite several attempts because of the backhand politics that plagued these attempts. The role of the state in controlling such social conflicts and the emanating violence has been largely criticized by scholars for its use of putative means in the control of violence which is said to be marred by ideological inclinations. Thus, education could be a more important and valid tool for more peaceful interaction and respect for each other than state interventions.

The importance of the role of leaders in maintaining peace and harmony is a matter of discussion. Some leaders like Gandhi were recognized for their role in creating harmony but others were seen as entrepreneurs who attempted to create a specific identity. In our country, we can see how different leaders, have actively tried to create particular identities to be able to take political mileage out of it. Reicher et al. (2005) argue that leaders are active entrepreneurs of social identity. Leaders facilitate creating new identities by providing frames, tactics, and organizational vehicles that are necessary to create a new collective identity (Morris & Staggenborg, 2004). These new identities created by the leaders further widen the divide between the social groups by consolidating only certain kinds of identities.

In the above section, we have talked about the various forces and factors that have aided in amplifying the fissures between the social groups and reducing the social, and psychological spaces between groups. As mentioned in the beginning, the ethos of Indian culture is coexistence; thus, we will now look at the colors of coexistence and interdependence that we have nurtured for ages and which have fashioned and established harmony in our plural society.

Interdependence Resulting in Coexistence

Coexistence and interdependence are central to the protection and appreciation of shared spaces. In this section, we examine the interlinkages of coexistence and interdependence which have kept us together. Creating those social spaces where people can interact, share their views, learn from each other, and appreciate and empathize with each other which slowly builds interdependence. People learn to accommodate for differences and accept them, and this goes a long way in creating harmony and peace.

Islands of Bonding and Sharing

While we have in our midst people belonging to different religions, castes, language groups, and regions, it is also true that they have been living amicably for centuries together. The rich values and traditions of tolerance, perseverance, plurality, and assimilation have helped us to live together. Despite belonging to different geographical areas and varied religious compositions or even in places where one group is dominant, we can identify several geographical spaces which have broadly remained peaceful throughout their known history. Factors that keep such groups together are the interplay of interdependence, mutual trust for each other, and the belief of their ability to continue to do so. There are several places in India where despite conflicts in adjoining areas these places have remained peaceful. Ram-Rahim Nagar near Ahmedabad and Malerkotla in Punjab are examples, where communal flare-ups over the years have been overcome by the mediation of the local masses. We then need to ask what has helped to preserve these islands of sanity? Active interaction and involvement of the members from both social groups have played an important role. Ram-Rahim Nagar has not experienced riots since the Ram-Rahim. The Welfare Committee came into existence in 1974. The Committee is chaired by a Hindu or a Muslim in rotation and members of both religious groups are members of it. The peaceful coexistence of Hindus and Muslims is the accepted norm, and attempts are made toward sustaining it. Several steps have been taken in the past and yet many more are being taken at present, to preserve the harmony and facilitate the development of shared spaces in these two places. Power sharing has been planned in such a way as to allow space for both communities by rotating the chairmanship of the committee. Explicit attempts were made to maintain harmony by adopting appropriate measures such as guarding the region from outsiders, which shows commitment to preserving harmony. In the case of Malerkotla, the prevalent peace among the groups can be attributed to the brave leadership of the Nawab and the vigilance of the kingdom's army, apart from people's effort, which has instilled the value of coexistence.

Sufi shrines or *majars* are other places that are bound by some kind of spiritual beliefs, bringing people from various socio-religious backgrounds together to participate in the rituals and embrace their association with the almighty. These places represent physical spaces where people from different cultural and religious backgrounds go beyond their boundaries of social categories and share their experiences and symbolize social integration between different religious groups, thereby infusing a feeling of communal harmony. Such physical spaces provide opportunities for sociocultural interaction and help in espousing a feeling of brotherhood among the people at the local level. The experience of mutual support and cooperation in matters central to life seems to generate a sense of transcendental awareness. This perhaps reduces the differences fermenting between people and instead; the shared existence helps promote acceptance and mutual respect, while also upholding cohesiveness and creating shared spaces.

Such islands of bonding also exist in rural areas and smaller towns. Varshney (2002) suggested that low levels of communal tension in smaller towns and villages can be seen due to a lack of anonymity and greater routine interaction between Hindus and Muslims in such spaces. This routine interaction helps to appreciate the social position of the other community and also suppresses prejudice, which results in creating communal harmony. Furthermore, considering that rural settings are more collectivistic, hence both sacred values and responsibilities are more important for people, and their interplay facilitates creation of shared spaces. There is mutual interdependence and coexistence between families and groups.

Those social spaces that provide opportunities for interaction and communication like public spaces, markets, and residential settings are important for developing social networks. Besides they extend opportunities to share concerns, joys, and sorrows and help develop relationality. Everyday communication between the members of different communities often goes beyond the boundaries of business and professional matters and nurtures networks that have significance for social well-being. We would like to argue that everyday sociality keeps the channels of communication between the groups open. Such a sociality existing between majority and minority group members does play a role in bridging the differences between them and in turn, promotes harmony.

Whether Functionality?

Throughout the various studies (Singh et al., 2023), evidence has been presented to show that the social relationships between groups in contemporary times are functional and keep on changing according to the context. Our relationships with our group members and other groups keep on changing. It may be noted that the context/situation plays a very major role in determining the quality of social relationships. By saying this, we mean that it could be the case that a factor that may act as a bridge in a given situation, may become a barrier in another. For example, education may be seen as an equalizer and may serve a bridging function between communities, but at the same time, lack of education may be seen to be responsible for the prevalent stereotypes and thus create barriers to shared spaces. Thus, functionality appears to be the core element for guiding intergroup relations and being politically and socially correct seems to be the dominating motive more so among urban dwellers. This emphasis on functionality and dynamicity of intergroup relations results in what one can call 'see-saw relationships' ranging from positive to neutral and at times negative resulting in social tensions of various kinds.

Decoding Shared Spaces

The shared spaces stem from respect for each other's cultural identity, nurturing diversity and invoking a broader unity of purpose toward a shared goal. Sharing and associated forms of positive behaviors and emotions such as compassion, love, and generosity help in creating societies where values of harmony and social cohesion take precedence over conflict, dissension, and violence. We argue that in most plural societies there is a need to understand the complexity of intergroup interactions at various levels. While plurality may be at the root of stereotypical and discriminatory behaviors on the part of advantaged groups toward the less advantaged ones, at the same time it can also form the basis of harmonious relations. Today we see that the boundaries between social groups are more differentiated, and the meanings ascribed to them have also undergone changes. Traditionally the main function of boundaries was to create barriers but in today's time, many boundaries serve the bridging function that enables contact among those residing within these boundaries. The fast-changing geo-political scenario has provided several options—a person can be organized into many groups (based on nation, gender, region, language, profession, activism, political affinity, social status, and so on), and all the resulting social identities are functionally as well as emotionally relevant to those who belong to them. This multiplicity of identities helps enlarge the shared spaces and inculcates bonding and connectivity which lays the edifice for harmony and joint activity in various spheres of life. Today we see that apparent inconsistencies and contradictions abound in many walks of life resulting in a paradoxical situation. Sharing, accommodation, and trust are the backbone for coexistence, while mistrust, fear, and exclusion are the bedrock for conflict and strife, and both are seen in social relationships. While oppression, hatred, mistrust, and fear can be ascertained between social groups, advocates of liberty, humanity, compassion, and harmony are also active. Often such paradoxes exist side by side and have resulted in barriers and boundaries in social relationships at some places and at a specific time, while at other places and at other time points acted as bridges. We are very constrained in our relationships with other groups in some respects while indulgent in others. In general, as has already been pointed out, the intergroup relational world is shrinking. The downside of this is a lack of stability in relationships and dynamic relationships with less affective engagement with others.

In the sociopolitical sphere, at one time, we come across expressions of individual political ideologies and (sub) cultural beliefs; we also notice spaces accommodating expressions and assertions of diverse ethnic, religious, and regional identities. Since these are essential features of a pluralistic design of social life one would expect that sharing, mutual understanding and respect and coexistence are nurtured and sustained. In reality, however, we witness challenges and threats to the pursuit of pluralistic ideological concerns. Contestations, debates, and even violent conflicts between diverse groups in the spheres of religion, region, caste, and language are fast becoming visible. They are leading to disparate identities which often do not go together. Often these proclamations pose a challenge to the very basics of Indian society particularly when the diverse groups assert and attempt to consolidate their own identities at the expense of other groups and communities.

We must also appreciate that group identities and their representation at a given time are embedded in the historical, social, and political processes and contexts. A group's identity entails not only how the group members identify themselves, but it is also equally affected by the identities given by others; that is, identities are constructed both by group members themselves and by others. Thus, a given group may be simultaneously acknowledged with many diverse identities. The experience tells that identity formation may involve building a barrier between one's group and other groups. However, these same identities can become bridges fostering social harmony and mutual facilitation. Today the challenge is to focus on the social diversities and try to identify and decipher the shared spaces and strengthen them. As Amartya Sen (2006) argues, it is this plurality that allows the possibility of shared spaces, but if these choices are denied and a regimented compartmentalization superimposed, then the boundaries become rigid and impenetrable. It is this rigidity or exclusiveness that results in an ethnocentric outlook.

To have an appreciation of shared spaces and their importance for harmony, a more chiseled-out understanding of social reality and appreciation of each other's position ought to be developed. The focus should be on the relational unit and not just the individual. This helps us not only to move away from the narrow focus that psychology has often been blamed for but also to grasp the dynamic social reality better. The responsibility for the creation of harmony is on the groups and communities. The power of group and community needs to be harnessed. Some recent work has shown that social networks and identities have a profound impact on the mental and physical health of people (Jetten et al., 2011). Groups provide social support and a sense of community and enhance feelings of group efficacy which paves the way for well-being. The power of social will, character, and ability to withstand difficulties as well as to bring about social change for the betterment of the world needs to be acknowledged. People like his Holiness Dalal Lama have been talking about detoxing the mind and seeking spiritual development that connects through sharing on an extensive platform. It is this spiritual ethos with its emphasis on understanding and inclusion which will help us to create more shared spaces in the long run. The emerging institutional arrangements and technological innovations must keep the relational nature of reality in view where dialogues and debates between social groups, communities, and nations are encouraged and help in conflict resolution and political and social transformation.

References

Davis, J. W. (2000). *Threats and promises: The pursuit of international influence.* Johns Hopkins University Press.

Fowler, J. H., & Kam, C. D. (2007). Beyond the self: Social identity, altruism and political participation. *Journal of Politics*, *69*, 813–827.

Fu, F., Tarnita, C. E., Christakis, N. A., Wang, L., Rand, D. G., & Nowak, M. A. (2012). Evolution of in-group favoritism. *Scientific Reports*, *2*(1), 460.

Hewstone, M., Rubin, M., & Wills, H. (2002). Intergroup bias. *Annual Review of Psychology*, *53*, 575–604.

Jetten, J., Haslam, C., & Haslam, A. S. (Eds.). (2011). *The social cure: Identity, health and well-being* (1st ed.). Psychology Press. https://doi.org/10.4324/9780203813195

Jodhka, S. S. (2001). *Community and identities: Contemporary discourses on culture and politics in India*. Sage.

Klandermans, B. (1997). *The social psychology of protest*. Wiley.

Morris, A. D., & Staggenborg, S. (2004). Leadership in social movements. In D. A. Snow, S. A. Soule, & H. Kriesi (Eds.), *The Blackwell companion to social movements*. Blackwell Publishing Company.

Rand, D. G., Pfeiffer, T., Dreber, A., Sheketoff, R. W., Wernerfelt, N. C., & Benkler, Y. (2009). Dynamic remodelling of in-group bias during the 2008 presidential election. *Proceedings of the National Academy of Sciences (PNAS)*, *106*, 6187–6191.

Reicher, S., Haslam, S. A., & Hopkins, N. (2005). Social identity and the dynamics of leadership: Leaders and followers as collaborative agents in the transformation of social reality. *The Leadership Quarterly*,*16*, 547–568.

Riek, B. R., Mania, E. W., & Gaertner, S. L. (2006). Intergroup threat and outgroup attitudes: A meta-analytic review. *Personality and Social Psychology Review*, *10*, 336–353.

Scheidel, W. (2017). *The great leveler: Violence and the history of inequality from the stone age to the twenty first century*. Princeton University Press.

Sen, A. (2006). *'Identity and violence', The illusion of destiny*. Allen Lane.

Sherif, M., & Sherif, C. W. (1969). Ingroup and intergroup relations: Experimental analysis. In M. Sherif & C. W. Sherif (Eds.), *Social psychology* (pp. 221–266). Harper & Row.

Singh, P., Misra, G., Kapur, P., Mishra, A. K., & Siddiqui, R. (2023). Towards deciphering shared spaces among religious groups in contemporary Indian society: Some illustrations and challenges. *Social Change*, *53*(4), 469–485. https://doi.org/10.1177/00490857231203413

Stephan, W. G., & Stephan, C. W. (2000). An integrated theory of prejudice. In S. Oskamp (Ed.), *Reducing prejudice and discrimination: The Claremont symposium on applied social psychology* (pp. 23–45). Lawrence Erlbaum Associates, Inc.

Thorbecke, E., & Charumilind, C. (2002). Economic inequality and its socioeconomic impact. *World Development*, *30*(9), 1477–1495.

Tripathi, R. C., & Singh, P. (2016). *Perspectives on violence and othering in India* (1st ed.). Springer.

Varshney, A. (2002). *Ethnic conflict and civil life: Hindus and Muslims in India*. Oxford University Press.

Vignoles, V. L., Regalia, C., Manzi, C., Golledge, J., & Scabini, E. (2006). Beyond self-esteem: Influence of multiple motives on identity construction. *Journal of Personality and Social Psychology*, *90*(2), 308–333.

Part IV

Affective and Cognitive Processes and Change

12 Social Influence Revisited

Vanita Sondhi

In *The Saturated Self* (1991), Gergen claims that constant media exposure leads to a state of "social saturation" in which people are overwhelmed with an ever-expanding range of contacts and knowledge. Smartphones show the most recent news and enticing advertisements, e-commerce platforms send personalized recommendations for the latest fashion trends, a Facebook friend invites you to sign a petition, an Instagram influencer shares healthy eating tips, and Netflix suggests the most recent films. These are just a few examples of how important social media has become in our daily lives. Every message, suggestion, and post is intended to affect our attitudes, beliefs, or behaviors. Pandey (2022, p. 3) defines social influence as the "overt or covert efforts of one or more individuals to change in their own or others' interests, attitudes, beliefs, perceptions, affect, and behaviour of one or more others." The terms "social influence" and "social impact" are used interchangeably throughout the chapter.

Social influence can be investigated on four levels: intrapersonal, interpersonal, intragroup, and intergroup (Doise, 1986). Cognition and social motivation are examples of intrapersonal processes that have a social consequence. For example, a sedentary person may have cognitive dissonance after hearing a persuasive health advertisement, which can be alleviated by practicing healthy habits. The interpersonal level focuses on self and identity; for example, a student may be convinced to join a specific college club because she believes that being a member of this group corresponds with her self-identification and supports her values. The intragroup level analyzes group processes like as norms and group decision-making; for example, a team may establish specific work regulations, and an individual may adapt to these norms to satisfy the group's expectations. Finally, at the intergroup level, social influence refers to interactions between groups. For example, during a sporting event, followers of one team may show extreme loyalty and support for their team while showing hatred for the opposing side. These examples show how almost every discipline of social psychology seeks to understand social influence processes and their consequences. Many definitions of social psychology include a focus on social impact (Allport, 1954).

DOI: 10.4324/9781003461302-17

Most academics agree that social impact approaches prioritize interpersonal and group levels above intraindividual ones (e.g., Wood, 2000; Spears, 2021). In this perspective, self-centered social processes such as social categorization and social identity have gained in prominence. Although the literature focuses on a variety of cognitive processes, they are increasingly being integrated with social activities. The literature on social influence is diverse, encompassing a wide range of phenomena. Due to space limits, the present review is selective rather than exhaustive and is limited to the standard themes of conformity, compliance, and obedience, with an extra discussion of attitude change, persuasion, and self-presentation. This review is therefore only selective and not exhaustive.

The chapter is organized into four sections. It begins with emerging perspectives in social influence, highlighting key phenomena such as conformity, compliance, and submission to authority. This is followed by a discussion on attitude change and persuasion. The next section examines self-presentation as a source of social influence, focusing on how individuals manage the impressions they make on others. The penultimate section addresses the role of social influence within cultural contexts, while the final section provides a summary of the key points discussed.

Perspectives on Social Influence

Symbolic interactionism was among the earliest sociological theories to provide a framework for studying social influence processes. Flattery, a common form of social influence, can be understood via this perspective. According to Goffman's dramaturgical perspective (1959), the flatterer may be understood as actively carrying out a specific social function, analogous to an actor on stage. This front-stage function comprises carefully selecting words, gestures, and displays of appreciation and praise to increase the target's self-esteem and elicit a favorable response. In the backstage area, away from the topic, the flatterer may remove the mask and reveal his or her true intentions or emotions. In this view, social relationships and symbolic communication are significant components of social effect. Other notable sociological theories of symbolic interactionism, such as Cooley's "looking-glass self" (1902), Mead's symbolic interactionism (1934), and Weber's social action theory (1947), highlight these components in different ways.

While sociologists use observational methods to understand the symbols of social influence in wider social and cultural contexts, psychologists began by emphasizing intraindividual processes and frequently employ experimental methods to investigate social influence. Pandey (2022) traces the history of social influence back to numerous classical studies in the field that inspired modern methods to understand social influence processes. In psychology, Norman Triplett (1898) conducted one of the first tests on social impact, demonstrating that people spin a fishing reel faster when they are around others. Muzafer Sherif (1935, 1936) and Solomon Asch (1948, 1951, 1955) conducted conformity studies, whilst Milgram (1963) investigated obedience to authority. This research provided the foundation for our understanding of social impact processes. Moscovici (1976, 1980) transformed the paradigm with his groundbreaking experiments on minority social influence, which proved how a smaller group attempts to influence the beliefs of a larger group.

Another paradigmatic shift occurred during the "crisis" of the 1970s, when contributions, paradigms, techniques, and ethical issues in social psychology were critically examined. This era witnessed the rise of the social cognitive method, which sparked renewed interest in persuasive communication, as seen by Carl Hovland's research at Yale University (e.g., Hovland et al., 1953). Jones and his colleagues carried out several experiments in the 1980s (e.g., Jones & Pittman, 1982) to study the interpersonal influence processes that support self-presentation. Bob Cialdini's 1984 book "Influence" was a watershed moment in social influence research because it distilled past research into essential principles of influence, enabling a new generation of academics to explore these ideas. According to Pandey (2022), important studies in the field in India include Sengupta and Singh's (1926) exploration of social facilitation, Kakar's (1971) analysis of traditional-moral authority, Sinha's (1980) theory of the nurturant taskmaster, and Pandey's (1986) investigation of ingratiation and manipulative tactics. Since these early studies, the field has seen significant alterations, with efforts to incorporate new types of social influence as a result of the rise of social media and digital communication.

Conformance

Sherif (1936) and Asch (1951) conducted pioneering studies on the dynamics of majority influence, which resulted in significant progress in the subject. These and subsequent investigations revealed two major types of influence that explain conformance. Informational influence is the desire to obtain precise knowledge and be correct, whereas normative influence is compliance to achieve favor or avoid social criticism (Deutsch & Gerard, 1955). The social impact theory (Latané, 1981) states that conformity to normative pressures is determined by several key factors, including the strength of the influencing group (its perceived importance), immediacy (both spatial and temporal proximity to the individual), and the number of people exerting influence.

Several government efforts, like as "Swachh Bharat Abhiyan" (2014–present) and "Beti Bachao Beti Padhao" (2015-present), effectively use conformity principles to motivate individuals to match their behaviors with greater society goals. Campbell and colleagues (2010, as cited by Pandey, 2022) mention one social movement aimed at the underprivileged and led by the Indian People's Health Movement's Jan Swasthya Abhiyan. This unit successfully rallied over a million impoverished people to demand better healthcare services, and even the elite, wealthy class supported them. This grassroots campaign convinced the government to prioritize primary care on the public agenda. Any such movement must include an active influence process that begins with educating the public about the issue and progresses to a deeper understanding of the power dynamics, governance structures, and policy decisions that affect their lives, ultimately leading to empowerment and the ability to take informed action (Misra & Pandey, 2010).

However, there is a disadvantage to succumbing to social pressures. Individuals may subscribe to false beauty ideals promoted by the media, which can lead to several mental health issues, including body dissatisfaction and eating disorders. Teenagers who submit to peer pressure may engage in risky behaviors such as drug use, underage drinking, and reckless driving. Citizens under authoritarian regimes may support the official ideology to avoid prosecution, resulting in a lack of political dissent and the perpetuation of severe policies. However, there are those in every community who break well-established rules despite being often penalized. These individuals, who are frequently a minority, play a critical role in challenging the status quo and moving societies forward.

While early studies focused on how the majority could influence the minority, following conformity research revealed that this can be a bidirectional process. Moscovici and his colleagues (e.g., Moscovici et al., 1969) undertook a series of groundbreaking experiments on minority influence that changed the path of the field. Following Moscovici's work, minority influence research has evolved to overcome the "conformity bias" (Moscovici & Faucheux, 1972) by including a wide range of cognitive, social, and contextual factors that yield useful insights. According to Alvaro and Crano (2017), the field has evolved from a "social influence, perception-oriented view to a more dynamic persuasion, attitude-centric orientation" (p. 161).

Cognitive Perspectives. Information processing is included in cognitive-based models, and a key question that arises from this perspective is: What happens when an individual encounters a majority or minority position that differs from one's own? According to the conversion theory (Moscovici, 1980, 1985), under such situations, individuals scrutinize minority ideas more closely since they are unusual and out of the ordinary. This increased scrutiny can lead to private influence, even if it occurs indirectly on peripheral issues rather than explicit fundamental flaws. This is particularly true if the minority remains stable. According to the objective-consensus approach (Mackie, 1987), people expect to agree with the majority because they feel the majority is likely to be correct, as well as to disagree with the minority. When confronted with a divergent majority position, people experience cognitive dissonance and question the majority's reasoning, whereas a divergent minority position is typically absorbed less completely. These and other models have some parallels to existing attitude change models, including Petty and Cacioppo's Elaboration Likelihood Model (1981) and Chaiken's Heuristic-Systematic Model (1987).

Social Identity Perspective. While the cognitive method has provided significant insights into how people understand information from majority versus minority sources, it is also important to recognize the importance of social processes. This enables us to apply our findings more effectively to real-world issues like prejudice, group discrimination, intergroup conflict, and, finally, societal change. According to Tajfel and Turner's (1979) social identification hypothesis, social influence is the product of self-categorization processes in which individuals identify as group members. This identification leads to the formation of group norms that highlight similarities within the ingroup and disparities with the outgroup. Group members then internalize these standards through a process called as depersonalization, which involves aligning the self with the ingroup. Individuals conform because internalized group standards motivate them to behave similarly to their ingroup mates. According to this idea, the distinction between informational and normative impact merges into a unified process: what is normative is seen as instructive about acceptable and appropriate behaviors.

Consistent with this theory, research has shown that minority attitudes have a limited impact when they are linked to social identities perceived as divergent or unconventional by the majority because people are less likely to accept perspectives that threaten their own social identity or ingroup cohesion. This is also consistent with the findings, which show that a minority group's influence has a lower impact on direct measurements than indirect ones (Wood, 2000). Direct measures involve openly examining attitudes toward the core issue, with receivers understanding that their responses are directly tied to the deviant minority source. In these instances, the minority group's influence is frequently lessened because people may consciously or unconsciously adjust their responses to align with the majority or avoid explicitly endorsing the minority opinion, especially if it deviates from the norm. In contrast, indirect measures investigate attitudes toward related topics. Because these tactics do not address the core issue, receivers are frequently unaware that the minority group's viewpoint may influence their decisions. As a result, the minority's influence can be subtle but broad.

Pandey (2022) also highlights the role of social identity in social impact. In India's complex society, ethnic ingroups, such as those based on caste, religion, or indigenous roots, play an important role in influencing social dynamics. These ingroups are not only internally consistent, but they also grow, enhancing their social power (Singh & Siddiqui, 2019). Ethnic organizations regularly participate in lobbying and activism to advance social justice, affirmative action, and resource allocation. Self-categorization theory (Turner, 1991) examines how social categorization processes determine social influence, highlighting that those seen to be similar to them have a greater impact on others. As a result, minorities can wield power if they are perceived to belong to the ingroup. However, these mechanisms have the potential to increase conflict. According to Pérez and Mugny's (1996) conflict-elaboration theory, any form of influence, whether from a majority or minority source, can result in conflict, which is handled through a conflict-elaboration procedure. This elaboration requires giving meaning to competing viewpoints based on the collective work and its relevance to social identity. Understanding how social influence works in different situations necessitates a study of conflict dynamics. Pandey (2022) suggests several approaches to addressing the challenges of reducing conflicts within and between groups, such as superordinate re-categorization (Hogg & Hornsey, 2006), multiple categorizations (Crisp & Hewstone, 2007), relational identity construction (Hogg, 2015), and the adoption of a multicultural framework of intergroup relationships.

Compliance and Submission to Authority

Compliance entails altering behavior in response to requests rather than direct commands from authorities, and compliance tactics are widely used in marketing and advertising, negotiation and conflict resolution, health and wellness, education and training, workplace and organizational behavior, fundraising, political campaigns, and personal relationships. Robert Cialdini, a well-known social psychologist, identified six key principles of compliance in 2006 and later added a seventh (Cialdini, 2021). The reciprocity principle indicates that people are compelled to return favors, yet the commitment and consistency concept shows humans' need to align actions with previous convictions. The social proof principle illustrates how people are heavily influenced by the behaviors of others, especially those they consider to be similar to their own. Compliance methods based on the principle of authority capitalize on people's natural desire to submit to those with legitimate expertise or power. The liking principle indicates that pleasant interpersonal relationships can encourage compliance, but the scarcity concept suggests that a sense of limited availability can instill a sense of urgency.

Cialdini (2021) added a seventh principle to his previous six, referring to it as "unity," which is created by sharing a common identity and can act at both the micro- and macrolevels. This principle is congruent with the emerging literature on social influence, which acknowledges the importance of self-identity. Pandey (2022) gives examples of Indian politicians who frequently employ this strategy in their speeches, which include local issues, cultural references, and regional languages. This approach enables leaders to connect more deeply with their audience by highlighting a shared identity and addressing specific local issues.

Submission to authority requires following direct instructions from recognized authorities, such as parents or teachers. Stanley Milgram, a psychologist at Yale University, conducted one of the most influential experiments on loyalty to authority in the 1960s (see Milgram, 1963). This research was prompted by the Nuremberg War Criminal Trials, in which Nazi war criminals claimed in their defense that they were merely "following orders." In one experiment, participants were instructed to administer more severe electric shocks to a confederate for delivering erroneous responses. Despite their reservations at times, 65% of participants followed the instructions to administer the shock to the end of the scale, which was 450 volts. Milgram's experiments surprised the world, but they also sparked widespread concern about the ethical implications of his methods. Due to ethical reasons, further research was unable to fully repeat the original experiment. However, investigations that either partially duplicated Milgram's original tests or utilized new approaches to investigate loyalty to authority (e.g., Bickman, 1974; Burger, 2009; Meeus & Raaijmakers, 1986) discovered similar levels of adherence to authority.

Agentic Perspective. Milgram (1974) characterized the experiment's findings using the Agentic theory, which states that people typically outsource responsibility for their actions to authoritative authorities. Furthermore, people are more likely to follow orders if they perceive the authority has legitimate power. In everyday life, it is evident that persons in positions of authority frequently exhibit their legal authority by wearing distinctive status symbols such as dress regulations, badges, and unique titles. By making their power and authority visible, these symbols foster the expectation that individuals would obey commands and respect hierarchical organizations. Milgram even claimed that adherence to such social norms has evolutionary advantages since a nonconfrontational technique fosters social cohesion and calm. In traditional cultures like India, where social hierarchies and familial respect are deeply established, how authority is expressed has a significant impact on obedience. According to Pandey (2022), most Indian homes address elders and authority individuals using respectful and relationship-based titles rather than their names. Instead of simply addressing mothers and fathers by their names, terms like "Mata Ji" and "Pita Ji" are used. The usage of polite titles instead of names reflects a cultural emphasis on maintaining hierarchical relationships and developing respect for authority.

Power and Influence. The concept of lawful power has been redefined in light of the social categorization theory of influence (Turner, 1991, as cited by Spears, 2021). According to Spears, Turner's reformulation of power means that true influence is more about how individuals internalize and identify with authority, rather than simply obeying it due to external pressures. Such power is more effective and long-lasting, since it does not require constant monitoring or enforcement. Similarly, Haslam, Reicher, and colleagues (Haslam & Reicher, 2012; Haslam et al., 2014) argue that Milgram's classic obedience studies must be interpreted in terms of group identity. According to their viewpoint, participants in Milgram's studies were not merely following commands out of blind obedience but were influenced by their affiliation with Milgram's scientific goals, and the authority figures in the experiment were recognized as genuine leaders in that context.

Attitude Change and Persuasion

According to Wood (2000), social impact theories of attitudes concentrate on how attitudes are developed through interactions with others, highlighting the social aspects of attitudes. As a result, studies in this field commonly incorporate interactions with other participants to study how these social dynamics affect the self, and they typically focus on two incentives for group conformity: informational and normative (Deutsch & Gerard, 1955). Unlike social influence paradigms, traditional attitudinal and persuasion research usually focuses on topics such as the link between attitudes and behaviors or the effectiveness of persuasive appeals. This traditional approach focuses on intraindividual processes while ignoring the importance of relationships with others (Wood, 2000). This section will focus less on these traditional domains and more on the social influence theories of attitudes. However, these two approaches do not run parallel; rather, they overlap at distinct points. This section will also cover these themes. The emergence and development of dual-process models such as the Elaboration Likelihood Model (Petty & Cacioppo, 1986) and Fazio's MODE model (Fazio, 1990), as well as the development of implicit measurement tools and renewed interest in Moscovici's work on minority influence, marked a new era in attitudinal research (Prislin & Crano, 2008). In recent years, researchers have attempted to investigate social impact processes in attitude modification.

Cognitive Perspective: Dual-Mode Processing Models

Before the onset of this new age in attitudinal research, some researchers, including Carl Hovland and his colleagues (e.g., Hovland et al., 1953), undertook significant studies. While Hovland's method for examining persuasion was novel, it was more focused on identifying the components that impact persuasion than on the underlying mechanisms that explain why persuasion occurs. Dual-mode processing models have substantially altered the field of attitude research and persuasion, addressing previously overlooked issues and giving a comprehensive framework for evaluating attitude and persuasion processes in social impact settings (Wood, 2000). The Elaboration Likelihood Model (Petty & Cacioppo, 1986) and the Heuristic-Systematic Model (Chaiken et al., 1989) are important dual-mode processing models that explain how attitude change occurs in response to the level of message elaboration, which is then determined by the individual's motivation and ability to process the message. Individuals carefully assess and elaborate on message content in central route processing, which involves great desire (e.g., the topic is personally meaningful) or high ability (e.g., the individual has enough time). This leads to long-term attitude changes. In contrast, peripheral route processing occurs when there is a lack of desire (e.g., the issue is not personally significant) or ability (e.g., the person is in a hurry), causing the individual to rely on heuristics such as "majority has accumulated wisdom" to form attitudes without conducting extensive analysis. Attitude shifts generated by peripheral processing are frequently less stable and more susceptible to change.

The self is essential for understanding social influence processes, yet it is typically overlooked in traditional attitudinal and persuasive techniques. However, there has been a shift in emphasis as academics include social identification (Tajfel, 1981, 1982) and social categorization (Turner, 1982, 1991) methodologies into dual processing models. This integration stresses how a common group identity and a drive for self-improvement influence message processing. When people adopt the attitudes of a favored ingroup, they feel validated and engage in heuristic processing (such as "majority has accumulated wisdom"). In contrast, disagreement within the ingroup confuses, driving discussions to reconcile the difference, which might lead to more careful thinking and meticulous processing (Wood, 2000). As a result, cultural background plays an increasingly crucial role in defining social influence. In India, the self is usually considered as interdependent, resulting in people making decisions based on social norms and community expectations. Furthermore, Misra and others' research (e.g., Misra & Mishra, 2022) shows that the self in the Indian context encompasses both the Atman, which represents the spiritual self and the empirical self, which is influenced by social interactions and traditions. Individuals are guided by the Atman toward self-realization and spiritual growth, but social standards and duties (dharma) have a significant impact on behavior.

The ego has also been important in contemporary interpretations of Cognitive Dissonance Theory (Festinger, 1957). While the original theory proposed that when a person has two or more opposing ideas, attitudes, or actions, they suffer internal discomfort or dissonance, subsequent theories have attempted to reinterpret discord in terms of the self. Impression management theory (Tedeschi et al., 1971), for example, posits that the source of dissonance is not actual internal discomfort from holding contradictory opinions, but rather the person's urge to manage how he or she appears to others. Inconsistency between one's attitudes and actions can provide a poor impression, which most individuals attempt to avoid. Individuals typically change their attitudes to match their actions, resulting in a consistent image and a good impression on others. Individuals, according to Steele's self-affirmation hypothesis (1988), have an innate need to maintain a good self-image. Individuals feel dissonance when their self-concept is threatened in one area as a result of beliefs that contradict their behaviors. Individuals will affirm their expertise in another field to reduce cognitive dissonance and restore self-integrity. Resistance to attitude change can also stem from extremely personal mechanisms, such as psychological reactance, in which people reject persuasive attempts to preserve their autonomy (Brehm, 1966).

The approaches discussed above have influenced numerous awareness campaigns throughout the world. Pandey (2022) uses the Clean India Mission (Swachh Bharat) campaign as an example of how some of the aforementioned approaches were successfully combined. The Indian government created the project, which attempts to address the widespread issue of open defecation, particularly among rural poor and urban slum dwellers in India. Several factors contribute to the Clean India Mission's success. The program effectively raises awareness about the health risks connected with open defecation, while simultaneously offering incentives to encourage better sanitation habits. The program also considered the social identities and cultural norms of the many groups it wanted to serve. Coffey et al. (2014) highlighted how deeply rooted social identities and cultural ideas are in India's sanitation practices. In many parts of India, having a toilet at home is regarded as dirty and polluting, whereas pooping outside is associated with cleanliness and strength, particularly among men. Efforts to promote bathroom use and improve sanitation had to be attentive to these values, and attitudes had to be changed so that they were related to greater public health goals while respecting local customs.

Affective Processes

Another area in which considerable disparities exist is the link between affect and social influence. According to Pandey (2022), our emotions and thoughts are not separate entities but rather are inextricably linked in a dynamic and reciprocal relationship. Pandey and Griffitt (1974) discovered that similar perspectives contribute to a pleasant affect, which impacts prosocial behavior. The effects of mood vary with the level of elaboration (Wegener & Petty, 1996). In low-elaboration situations, where people are not completely engaged in information processing, mood influences how they respond to a message through simple associations and heuristic principles. In contrast, in high-elaboration situations, how someone perceives the message may have a substantial impact on their attitude. People strategically control their moods at moderate levels of elaboration; happy people seek knowledge that makes them happy, whereas sad people study a broader range of content in the hopes of mending their mood (Wegener & Petty, 1996). According to the feelings-as-information perspective, positive and negative emotions guide the selection of appropriate processing mechanisms. Positive emotions indicate a safe and positive environment, leading people to employ heuristic strategies rather than lengthy studies. In contrast, negative moods highlight potential problems, prompting people to perform a more thorough and methodical assessment of the content.

The effect of fear-inducing communication, particularly in health communication, has also been studied. According to research, fear appeals function best when there is a strong perceived threat and a wide range of available coping mechanisms. Witte's Extended Parallel Process Model (1992, 1998) proposes that when people sense a high level of threat but lack coping abilities, they may respond with fear control, resulting in protective reflexes and message rejection. Research has delved deeper into the role of fear on message perception, incorporating these findings into broader theories of mood and social influence (Wood, 2000).

Self-Presentation

Self-presentation, often known as impression management, refers to the use of tactics to influence how others view oneself. While some presentations may use exaggeration, the majority are not dishonest. Believability is critical;

if projected images are seen as incorrect, they will be interpreted as deceptive (Schlenker & Weigold, 1992). People commonly use one of their many identities to convey specific images to others (Schlenker, 1980).

Jones and Pittman's Framework

While Goffman's work focused on self-presentation and the dynamics of social interaction, Jones and Pittman's (1982) theory examines the motivational, cognitive, and moral factors that drive self-presentation. The primary motive for strategic self-presentation is the actor's desire for more power to the goal. The actor aims to alter the target's perceptions of his or her dispositions in such a way that the actor benefits from the alteration. The relationship between the actor's power drive and self-presentational behaviors is mediated by cognitive processes. The actor evaluates the availability of cognitive resources in a particular interactional situation to determine the chances of generating the desired impression on the target. However, moral constraints influence the actor's self-presentational behaviors. There may be conflicts between the actor's desire for self-consistency, authenticity, and integrity with the benefits obtained through strategic impression management. Finally, the actor's self-presentation tactics are influenced by a complex interaction of motivational, cognitive, and moral factors. These strategies are further divided into five broad categories based on the specific attribution the actor seeks to elicit from the target: ingratiation, self-promotion, exemplification, supplication, and intimidation (Jones & Pittman, 1982).

Ingratiation and Its Dynamics

Ingratiation has been identified as a prevalent self-presentation method (Jones & Pittman, 1982; Pandey, 1986). Individuals make deliberate efforts to gain favor and be perceived as more pleasant, such as through flattery. The literature describes four major ingratiation tactics: other enhancement, conformity, favor-rendering, and self-presentation (Jones & Wortman, 1973), and the use of these strategies is influenced by factors such as incentive value, subjective probability, and perceived legitimacy. While ingratiation can increase an actor's likability and early success, it can also have negative consequences if used excessively (Higgins et al., 2003). Gordon's (1996) meta-analysis, which included several pioneering Pandey studies (e.g., Bohra & Pandey, 1984; Pandey & Singh, 1987), emphasized that ingratiation frequently improves likability more than competency and that the effectiveness of ingratiation is determined by the perspective from which it is evaluated.

In the 1980s, Pandey and his colleagues (e.g., Bohra & Pandey, 1984; Pandey & Kakkar, 1982; Pandey & Singh, 1986, 1987) conducted groundbreaking research on ingratiation strategies in India. They proposed that the majority of Indian society is marked by a hierarchical structure, a rigid caste system, a high power distance, and a scarcity mindset, which may result in ingratiation processes that differ significantly from those in the West. Approval, conformity, acquiescence, and praise are some of the social persuasion techniques used in this setting. Furthermore, a scarcity mindset caused by the perception of limited opportunities may lead people to adopt unethical social influence methods, such as manipulation (Pandey, 2022). However, modernity has caused a gradual shift in these hierarchical systems, with a greater emphasis on participative tactics (Kaasa & Minkov, 2020, as cited in Pandey, 2022).

Pandey's ingratiation paradigm focuses on actors, targets, bystanders, and conditions. The common ingratiatory strategies used in the Indian context include name-dropping, where individuals invoke the names of prestigious individuals to gain favor and are related to the phenomenon of basking in reflected glory; situation-specific behavior, where people adjust their conduct to align with the expectations of the target individual or group; and instrumental dependency, where one portrays reliance on the target's resources or support to elicit a sense of obligation.

The actor's characteristics have a significant impact on the type, timing, and context of ingratiation strategies performed. According to Bohra and Pandey's (1984) research, actors use ingratiation more with authoritative characters like bosses than with friends or strangers. Personality traits of actors, such as Machiavellianism, which incorporates dishonesty and self-interest, contribute to ingratiatory behavior. Individuals with these characteristics frequently use manipulative tactics, such as praise and thought conformity, to gain authority and access to scarce resources, especially when it helps them achieve their goals (Pandey, 1981, 1986; Pandey & Rastogi, 1979; Tripathi, 1981, cited by Pandey, 2022). Machiavellianism is not restricted to current situations, as historical books such as Niccolò Machiavelli's "The Prince," Kautilya's "Arthasastra," and "The Book of Lord Shang" show similar administration techniques throughout periods of political struggle (Pandey, 2022).

How do such ingratiating tactics influence the target's perception and response? Targets who are ingratiated commonly experience self-enhancement and overwhelming favorable affect toward the ingratiating actor, leading in increased assessments of the actor's beauty, productivity, and potential for success (Pandey & Kakkar, 1982). According to Clore and Byrne's (1974, referenced by Pandey, 2022) reinforcement-affect model, positive interactions with ingratiators may impair the target's objective assessment, resulting in incorrect views and preferring undeserving individuals. However, the target's personality traits, such as Machiavellianism, can reduce the effectiveness of ingratiation by increasing their ability to recognize and reject manipulative strategies (Tripathi, 1981).

Authoritarianism is a significant personality feature of the target in India due to the country's hierarchical social structure (Lewis, 1962; Pandey, 2022). Authoritarianism is also closely related to Machiavellianism, which has been examined earlier. Individuals with authoritarian inclinations are submissive to those in positions of authority while dominating others in lower positions. They create an environment in which ingratiation becomes a common method for obtaining favor and holding positions. In such cases, authoritarian leaders demand compliance from their subordinates while encouraging ingratiation. Subordinates use ingratiation to gain favor and rewards, bolstering the leader's authority and sustaining the flattery-dominance cycle (Pandey, 1986).

The Indian concept of authoritarianism differs significantly from Western concepts. In addition to authority and control, Indian authoritarian leaders value asceticism, a Brahminic worldview (Nandy, 1967), and Gandhian values of social equality and nonviolence (Nandy & Kakar, 1980). Sinha (1980) categorizes Indian authoritarianism into two types: behavioral representation, which is defined by rigorous, disciplined behavior, and psychodynamic dispositions, which are defined by underlying characteristics such as neuroticism and paranoia.

Kakar (1971, as cited in Pandey, 2022) emphasized the importance of familial authority and traditional values in Indian family structures, particularly the moral need to respect elders. He describes leadership figures as either strong or loving, frequently using emotional manipulation, such as guilt, to gain agreement. Sinha's Nurturant-Task Leadership paradigm (1980) highlights both of these characteristics. This notion highlights how an organization's authoritarian leaders nurture their subordinates, creating a balance between task completion and personal growth. These concepts contrast with Western perceptions, which usually highlight features associated with authoritarianism and fascism (Adorno et al., 1950).

Another important consideration in self-presentation scenarios is the bystanders' perspective as they see the interactions between the ingratiator and the target. They create opinions on both despite not being personally involved. Bystanders' reactions to ingratiation (such as approbation or disapproval) provide immediate feedback to both the performer and the target. According to studies, these sentiments are frequently unfavorable toward both the target and the ingratiator, while there may be instances of good impressions of the target or even mixed feelings (e.g., Pandey, 2022; Pandey & Bohra, 1986; Pandey & Kakkar, 1982). One possible explanation for the negative perceptions is because a bystander's ego or social image ("face") is not directly involved in the conversation, making it easier for the bystander to question the ingratiator's actions (Pandey & Bohra, 1986). Furthermore, viewers who see the target get preferential treatment as a result of ingratiation, may perceive this as unfair, particularly if they believe they are as deserving. This idea of injustice can lead to feelings of envy and other undesirable emotions for both the target and the flatterer. However, viewers may take praise as genuine, especially if they believe the target merits it. Mixed feelings, on the other hand, can be created by two processes: explicit good attitudes (if the flattery is genuine) and implicit negative attitudes (due to feelings of jealousy and impatience) (Pandey, 2022).

Ingratiatory tactics have been widely used throughout history, not just in modern times. Stengel (2000) investigates this evolution from ancient Egypt to modern American politics, revealing how ingratiation has been used throughout history. Pandey (2022) provides a thorough historical examination of ingratiation in the Indian context, including its portrayal in Indian mythology, historical practices, and traditional strategies. Pandey's examples, including Lord Krishna's persuasion tactics in the Mahabharata, the role of professional flatterers ("Bhants"), royal jesters, and the traditions of "Nazrana" and "Dastoors," demonstrate how ingratiation has become institutionalized and culturally acceptable. On the other hand, Chanakya Neeti cautioned against employing flattery for personal benefit and instead advocated for astute and genuine leadership. Thus, Pandey indicates that the use of flattery and social influence varies even within the same cultural environment, emphasizing the importance of gaining a deeper understanding of social influence. According to the study, unlike in the West, authoritative leaders in India are generally respected, and influencing them by socially acceptable tactics such as flattery and gift-giving is considered normal, if not crucial. Excessive flattery, however, is frowned upon, even in India, where it is derogatorily referred to as "Chamchagiri" (Pandey, 2022). This tendency is associated with the "slime effect," which stresses the risks of overusing self- and other-enhancement tactics (Vonk, 1998).

Social Influence in Cultural Context

Throughout the chapter, including the preceding section, research findings have demonstrated that cultural settings determine social influence and can fluctuate substantially even over time (Pandey, 2022). However, research on various forms of social influence has mostly been conducted from a Western perspective. Individual autonomy, personal responsibility, free choice, and direct communication are examples of Western values that may fail to capture the complexities of social influence in collectivistic or non-western cultures where values such as group harmony, hierarchical relationships, and indirect communication are more prevalent. This section will go deeper into the problems at hand.

Conformity may be regarded as a sign of weakness in Western countries that emphasize individualism, and people are more likely to react when they perceive their identity or independence is threatened. Nonconformity is occasionally rewarded in such circumstances. In contrast, in collectivistic cultures such as India, individuals are encouraged to align their behaviors and attitudes with group norms to maintain unity and avoid conflict. According to Markus and Kitayama (1991), in collectivistic communities, conformity acts as a type of "social glue," helping to maintain social cohesiveness. Bond and Smith (1996) conducted 133 tests in 17 nations using the Asch paradigm and discovered that individuals in collectivist cultures were more likely to conform to group norms than those in individualistic cultures. From 1952 to the 1980s, U.S. participants demonstrated a decline in conformity, showing that cultural norms promoting independence and autonomy can influence conformity levels. Furthermore, young teenagers were more susceptible to peer influence.

There have also been attempts to study Robert Cialdini's theories on social impact across cultures. According to studies, free choice, which is a more important value in individualistic cultures than in collectivistic cultures, influences the commitment principle. This could be because the desire to appear consistent with their freely chosen actions reinforces their commitment (Iyengar & Brockner, 2001). Other research indicates that the concept of social proof is more effective in collectivistic cultures such as Poland, but commitment and consistency are more effective in individualistic countries such as America (Cialdini et al., 2001). Morris et al. (2001) discovered that power was the most effective means of persuasion in the United States, whereas formal status was more essential in Germany. In Spain, friendship and formal standing were equally important, whereas in Hong Kong, power and official position were more crucial.

Obedience to authority must be understood in context. Some studies have indicated that Milgram's expectations about respect to authority are broadly consistent across cultures (Blass, 2012). However, Milgram's classic study (1963) and its interpretation may reflect a Western bias toward destructive compliance. The definition of obedience may differ between cultures. In Indian households, for example, obedience is highly valued since it indicates respect for elders, promotes family unity, and is reinforced as a moral obligation by religious teachings (Kakar, 1971, cited by Pandey, 2022). It highlights the value of familial authority and conventional moral principles in Indian society, where obeying elders is a moral need. Kakar finds that authoritarian figures frequently use emotional manipulation, such as guilt, to compel conformity, reflecting a cultural emphasis on internal moral standards and personal accountability. If obeying an elderly family member results in a poor decision, the family is more likely to blame situational conditions or share group responsibility than the person. Several studies have demonstrated that non-Western participants give more situational reasons for misbehavior than Westerners (Tang et al., 2014). Pandey (2022) also emphasizes that people from WEIRD (Western, Educated, Industrialized, Rich, and Democratic) societies are more likely to make the fundamental attribution error, which is to attribute someone's obedience to their dispositions, such as being submissive, conformist, or lacking moral courage, rather than considering the situational pressures that may influence their behavior. In contrast, Western civilizations value individual autonomy and frequently question obedience. When obeying an authoritative person has negative implications, the individual is more inclined to face them. Thus, the moral implications of disobeying may differ dramatically between the two cultural contexts.

The assessment of social influence must be culturally relevant. Srivastava and Pandey (1998) developed the Social Influence Scale, which covers 12 qualities of influence classified into three categories: hard, rational, and soft influence. The scale has demonstrated good reliability and validity in identifying major influence qualities. Certain social influence methods are more commonly used in India than in the West. These methods include appeals to ethnic identity, intimidation, disparagement, ingratiation, and coalition building (Srivastava & Pandey, 1998).

Final Remarks

Social influence is central to the study of social psychology, permeating theory, practice, and everyday life. This chapter examines classic forms of social influence such as conformity, compliance, and obedience, as well as attitude adjustment, persuasion, and self-presentation. Due to space limits, some topics, such as social impact in leadership and organizational contexts, were left out. Furthermore, critical phenomena such as groupthink, group polarization, and social facilitation are overlooked for similar reasons. The chapter concentrates on social influence at the interpersonal and group levels, rather than the intraindividual. It accomplishes this by assessing numerous frameworks and ideas aimed at better understanding the impacts of social influence by finding relevant antecedents and moderators. Social processes such as social classification and social identity have been highlighted throughout the chapter. Social influence cannot be fully understood without considering the cultural and social contexts in which it occurs, and future research should focus more on this component. Although the chapter has examined several forms of social influence, its relevance to broader societal challenges such as social movements and social transformation warrants further examination. Collectively, social influence is a tremendous force for raising awareness, preparing people, and persuading them to take important action (Pandey, 2022). However, much of the existing research on the minority effect relies on experimental methods, with a focus on cognitive mechanisms and individual-level investigations. Prislin (2022) is harshly critical of this approach since it ignores numerous key issues about the broader dynamics of social transformation. Cultural standards, sociopolitical settings, economic factors, and media portrayals all contribute to minority opinion acceptability. Such larger difficulties may not be amenable to lab experimentation, needing a more collaborative approach.

It is vital to understand social impact in a variety of settings, including online platforms. In the digital age, social influence is influenced by the rapid transfer of knowledge, anonymity, and less formal standards seen on social media. These variables can highlight strong points of view, allow for comparisons of other points of view, and enable immediate reactions, enabling public opinion to shift rapidly. Social influence techniques must constantly evolve to keep up with the changing nature of human interactions. To quote Pandey (2022, p. 214): "The process of globalisation, national-international migrations, changing rural-urban communities and families, and emerging new organisations with minimum face-to-face contacts are going through continuous cycles of changes requiring innovative communication, social interactions, and mutually influencing."

In conclusion, social influence approaches prioritize interpersonal and group levels over the intraindividual level. Self-centered social processes like social categorization and social identification have grown in importance. The literature on social impact covers a wide range of phenomena, but this chapter focuses on themes of conformity, compliance, and obedience, as well as attitude modification, persuasion, and self-presentation. Dual-process models, such as the Elaboration Likelihood Model, explain how attitude change occurs based on the level of message elaboration. Social identity perspective emphasizes the role of social processes and group identity in social influence. Ingratiation is a common self-presentation strategy, and its effectiveness depends on factors such as the actor's traits, the target's personality, and bystanders' perceptions. Social influence is influenced by cultural contexts, with conformity being more prevalent in collectivistic cultures. Overall, social influence is a complex and multifaceted phenomenon influenced by various factors and operates at different levels.

References

Adorno, T. W., Frenkel-Brunswik, E., Levinson, D. J., & Sanford, R. N. (1950). *The authoritarian personality* (p. 228). Harper and Row.

Allport, G. W. (1954). *The nature of prejudice*. Addison-Wesley.

Alvaro, E. M., & Crano, W. D. (2017). Reflections on Gabriel Mugny's contributions to attitude-centric theory and research on minority influence. *International Review of Social Psychology*, *30*(1), 161–171. https://doi.org/10.5334/irsp.25

Asch, S. E. (1948). The doctrine of suggestion, prestige and imitation in social psychology. *Psychological Review*, *55*(5), 250–276. https://doi.org/10.1037/h0057270

Asch, S. E. (1951). Effects of group pressure upon the modification and distortion of judgments. In H. Guetzkow (Ed.), *Groups, leadership and men; research in human relations* (pp. 177–190). Carnegie Press.

Asch, S. E. (1955). Opinions and social pressures. *Scientific American*, *193*(5), 31–35.

Bickman, L. (1974). The social power of a uniform. *Journal of Applied Social Psychology*, *4*(4), 47–61.

Blass, T. (2012). A cross-cultural comparison of studies of obedience using the Milgram paradigm: A review. *Social and Personality Psychology Compass*, *6*(2), 196–205. https://doi.org/10.1111/j.1751-9004.2011.00417.x

Bohra, K. A., & Pandey, J. (1984). Ingratiation toward strangers, friends, and bosses. *The Journal of Social Psychology*, *122*, 217–222.

Bond, R., & Smith, P. B. (1996). Culture and conformity: A meta-analysis of studies using Asch's (1952b, 1956) line judgment task. *Psychological Bulletin*, *119*(1), 111–137. https://doi.org/10.1037/0033-2909.119.1.111

Brehm, J. W. (1966). *A theory of psychological reactance*. Academic Press.

Burger, J. M. (2009). Replicating Milgram: Would people still obey today? *American Psychologist*, *64*, 1–11.

Campbell, C., Cornish, F., Gibbs, A., & Scott, K. (2010). Heading the push from below: How do social movements persuade the rich to listen to the poor? *Journal of Health Psychology*, *15*(7), 962–971.

Chaiken, S. (1987). The heuristic model of persuasion. In M. P. Zanna, J. M. Olson, & C. P. Herman (Eds.), *Social influence: The Ontario symposium* (Vol. 5, pp. 3–39). Lawrence Erlbaum Associates, Inc.

Chaiken, S., Liberman, A., & Eagly, A. H. (1989). Heuristic and systematic information processing within and beyond the persuasion context. In J. S. Uleman & J. A. Bargh (Eds.), *Unintended thought* (pp. 212–252). Guilford Press.

Cialdini, R. (1984). *Influence: The psychology of persuasion.* HarperCollins.

Cialdini, R. B. (2021). *Influence, new and expanded: The psychology of persuasion.* HarperCollins.

Cialdini, R. B., Wosinska, W., Barrett, D. W., Butner, J., & Górnik-Durose, M. (2001). The differential impact of two social influence principles on individualists and collectivists in Poland and the United States. In W. Wosinska, R. B. Cialdini, D. W. Barrett, & J. Reykowski (Eds.), *The practice of social influence in multiple cultures* (pp. 33–50). Lawrence Erlbaum Associates Publishers.

Clore, G. L., & Byrne, D. (1974). A reinforcement affect model of attraction. In T. L. Huston (Ed.), *Perspectives on interpersonal attraction* (pp. 143–170). Academic Press.

Coffey, D., Gupta, A., Hathi, P., Khurana, N., Spears, D., Srivastav, N., & Vyas, S. (2014). Revealed preference for open defecation. *Economic & Political Weekly*, *49*(38), 43.

Cooley, C. H. (1902). *Human nature and the social order.* Scribner's Sons.

Crisp, R. J., & Hewstone, M. (2007). Multiple social categorization. In M. P. Zanna (Ed.), *Advances in experimental social psychology* (Vol. 39, pp. 163–254). Academic.

Deutsch, M., & Gerard, H. B. (1955). A study of normative and informational social influences upon individual judgment. *Journal of Abnormal and Social Psychology*, *51*, 629–636.

Doise, W. (1986). *Levels of explanation in social psychology.* Cambridge University Press.

Fazio, R. H. (1990). Multiple processes by which attitudes guide behavior: The MODE model as an integrative framework. *Advances in Experimental Social Psychology*, *23*, 75–109.

Festinger, L. (1957). *A theory of cognitive dissonance.* Row Peterson.

Gergen, K. J. (1991). *The saturated self: Dilemmas of identity in contemporary life.* Basic Books.

Goffman, E. (1959). *The presentation of self in everyday life.* Anchor Books.

Gordon, R. A. (1996). Impact of ingratiation on judgments and evaluations: A meta-analytic investigation. *Journal of Personality and Social Psychology*, *71*(1), 54–70.

Government of India. (2014). *Swachh Bharat Abhiyan (Clean India Mission).* Ministry of Urban Development. https://mohua.gov.in/cms/swachh-bharat-mission.php#:~:text=The%20Swachh%20Bharat%20Mission%20%2D%20Urban,statutory%20towns%20in%20the%20country

Government of India. (2015). *Beti Bachao Beti Padhao.* Ministry of Women and Child Development. https://wcd.nic.in/bbbp-schemes

Haslam, S. A., & Reicher, S. D. (2012). Contesting the "nature" of conformity: What Milgram and Zimbardo's studies really show. *PLOS Biology*, *10*(11), e1001426.

Haslam, S. A., Reicher, S. D., & Birney, M. E. (2014). Nothing by mere authority: Evidence that in an experimental analogue of the Milgram paradigm participants are motivated not by orders but by appeals to science. *Journal of Social Issues*, *70*, 473–488.

Higgins, C. A., Judge, T. A., & Ferris, G. R. (2003). Influence tactics and work outcomes: A meta-analysis. *Journal of Organizational Behavior*, *24*(1), 89–106.

Hogg, M. A. (2015). Constructive leadership across groups: How leaders can combat prejudice and conflict between subgroups. *Advances in Group Processes*, *32*, 177–207.
Hogg, M. A., & Hornsey, M. J. (2006). Self-concept threat and multiple categorization within groups. In R. J. Crisp & M. Hewstone (Eds.), *Multiple social categorization: Processes, models, and applications* (pp. 112–136). Psychology Press.
Hovland, C. L., Janis, I. L., & Kelley, H. H. (1953). *Communicator and persuasion*. Yale University Press.
Iyengar, S. S., & Brockner, J. (2001). Cultural differences in self and the impact of personal and social influences. In W. Wosinska, R. B. Cialdini, D. W. Barrett, & J. Reykowski (Eds.), *The practice of social influence in multiple cultures* (pp. 13–32). Lawrence Erlbaum Associates Publishers.
Jones, E. E., & Pittman, T. S. (1982). Toward a general theory of strategic self-presentation. In J. Suls (Ed.), *Psychological perspectives on the self* (Vol. 1, pp. 231–262). Erlbaum.
Jones, E. E., & Wortman, C. B. (1973). *Ingratiation: An attributional approach*. General Learning Press.
Kaasa, A., & Minkov, M. (2020). Are the world's National cultures becoming more similar? *Journal of Cross-Cultural Psychology*, *51*(7–8), 531–550.
Kakar, S. (1971). The theme of authority in social relations in India. *The Journal of Social Psychology*, *84*, 93–101.
Latané, B. (1981). The psychology of social impact. *American Psychologist*, *36*(4), 343–356.
Lewis, O. (1962). *Village life in Northern India*. Vintage.
Mackie, D. M. (1987). Systematic and nonsystematic processing of majority and minority persuasive communications. *Journal of Personality and Social Psychology*, *53*(1), 41–52.
Markus, H. R., & Kitayama, S. (1991). Culture and the self: Implications for cognition, emotion, and motivation. *Psychological Review*, *98*, 224–253.
Mead, G. H. (1934). *Mind, self, and society: From the standpoint of a social behaviorist*. University of Chicago Press.
Meeus, W. H., & Raaijmakers, Q. A. (1986). Administrative obedience: Carrying out orders to use psychological-administrative violence. *European Journal of Social Psychology*, *16*(4), 311–324. https://doi.org/10.1002/ejsp.2420160402
Milgram, S. (1963). Behavioral study of obedience. *The Journal of Abnormal and Social Psychology*, *67*(4), 371–378. https://doi.org/10.1037/h0040525
Milgram, S. (1974). *Obedience to authority: An experimental view*. Harper and Row.
Misra, G., & Mishra, I. (2022). Selfhood and pathways to well-being: Some Indian perspectives. *Mind and Society*, *11*(03), 9–16. https://doi.org/10.56011/mind-mri-113-20222
Misra, G., & Pandey, J. (2010). Psychology and societal development. In P. Martin, F. Cheung, M. Kyrios, L. Littlefield, M. Knowles, B. Overmier, & J. Maria Prieto (Eds.), *IAAP handbook of applied psychology* (pp. 588–602). Wiley-Blackwell
Morris, M. W., Podolny, J. M., & Ariel, S. (2001). Culture, norms and obligations: Cross-national differences in patterns of interpersonal norms and felt obligations toward coworkers. In W. Wosinska, R. B. Cialdini, D. W. Barrett, & J. Reykowski (Eds.), *The practice of social influence in multiple cultures* (pp. 97–123). Lawrence Erlbaum Associates Publishers.
Moscovici, S. (1976). *Social influence and social change*. Academic Press.
Moscovici, S. (1980). Toward a theory of conversion behavior. In L. Berkowitz (Ed.), *Advances in experimental social psychology* (Vol. 13, pp. 209–239). Academic Press.
Moscovici, S. (1985). Social influence and conformity. In G. Lindzey & E. Aronson (Eds.), *Handbook of social psychology* (3rd ed., Vol. 2, pp. 347–412). Random House.

Moscovici, S., & Faucheux, C. (1972). Social influence, conformity bias, and the study of active minorities. In L. Berkowitz (Ed.), *Advances in experimental social psychology* (Vol. 6, pp. 149–202). Academic Press.
Moscovici, S., Lage, E., & Naffrechoux, M. (1969). Influence of a consistent minority on the responses of a majority in a color perception task. *Sociometry*, *32*, 365–379.
Nandy, A. (1967). Adorno in India: Revisiting the psychology of fascism. *Indian Journal of Psychology*, *51*, 168–178.
Nandy, A., & Kakar, S. (1980). Culture and personality. In U. Pareek (Ed.), *A survey of research in psychology: 1971–1976*, Part 1, (pp. 136–167). Popular Prakashan.
Pandey, J. (1981). Ingratiation as social behavior. In J. Pandey (Ed.), *Perspectives on experimental social psychology in India* (pp. 157–188). Concept.
Pandey, J. (1986). Socio-cultural perspective on ingratiation. In B. Maher & W. Maher (Eds.), *Progress in experimental personality research* (Vol. 14, pp. 205–229). Academic Press.
Pandey, J. (2022). *Nature and dynamics of social influence: Interpersonal and organizational context*. Springer.
Pandey, J., & Bohra, K. A. (1986). Attraction and evaluation as the function of ingratiating style of a person. *Social Behavior and Personality*, *14*(1), 23–28.
Pandey, J., & Griffitt, W. (1974). Attraction and helping. *Bulletin of the Psychonomic Society*, *3*(2), 123–124.
Pandey, J., & Kakkar, S. (1982). Supervisor's affect, attraction, and positive evaluation as a function of other enhancement. *Psychological Reports*, *50*, 479–486.
Pandey, J., & Rastogi, R. (1979). Machiavellianism and ingratiation. *The Journal of Social Psychology*, *108*, 221–225.
Pandey, J., & Singh, A. K. (1986). Attribution and evaluation of manipulative social behaviour. *The Journal of Social Psychology*, *126*(6), 735–744.
Pandey, J., & Singh, P. (1987). Effects of Machiavellianism, other enhancement and power position on affect, power feeling, and evaluation of ingratiator. *Journal of Psychology*, *121*(3), 287–300.
Pérez, J. A., & Mugny, G. (1996). The conflict elaboration theory of social influence. In E. H. Witte & J. H. Davis (Eds.), *Understanding group behavior* (Vol. 2, pp. 191–210). Lawrence Erlbaum.
Petty, R. E., & Cacioppo, J. T. (1986). *The elaboration likelihood model of persuasion*. Springer.
Prislin, R. (2022). Minority influence: An agenda for study of social change. *Frontiers in Psychology*, *13*, 911654.
Prislin, R., & Crano, W. D. (2008). Attitudes and attitude change: The fourth peak. In W. D. Crano & R. Prislin (Eds.), *Attitudes and attitude change* (pp. 3–15). Psychology Press.
Schlenker, B. R. (1980). *Impression management: The self-concept, social identity, and interpersonal relationships*. Brooks.
Schlenker, B. R., & Weigold, M. F. (1992). Interpersonal processes involving impression regulation and management. *Annual Review of Psychology*, *43*, 133–168.
Sengupta, N. N., & Singh, C. P. N. (1926). Mental work in isolation and in group. *Indian Journal of Psychology*, *1*, 106–110.
Sherif, M. (1935). A study of some social factors in perception. *Archives of Psychology (Columbia University)*, *187*, 60.
Sherif, M. (1936). *The psychology of social norms*. Harper.
Singh, P., & Siddiqui, R. N. (2019). Identity discourse: From negotiations to harmony in plural societies. In G. Misra (Ed.), *ICSSR research surveys and explorations: Psychology, Vol. 3, Individual and the social: Processes and issues* (pp. 248–282). Oxford University Press.
Sinha, J. B. P. (1980). *The nurturant task leader*. Concept Publishing Company.

Spears, R. (2021). Social influence and group identity. In S. T. Fiske, & D. L. Schacter (Eds.), *Annual Review of Psychology* (Vol. 72, pp. 367–390). Annual Reviews. https://doi.org/10.1146/annurev-psych-070620-111818

Srivastava, S., & Pandey, J. (1998). *Social influence scale (SIS)*. Centre of Behavioral and Cognitive Sciences & Department of Psychology, University of Allahabad, Allahabad. https://cbcs.ac.in/people/faculty/jpandey/

Steele, C. M. (1988). The psychology of self-affirmation: Sustaining the integrity of the self. In L. Berkowitz (Ed.), *Advances in experimental social psychology* (Vol. 21, pp. 261–302). Academic Press.

Stengel, R. (2000). *You're too kind: A brief history of flattery*. Simon & Schuster.

Tajfel, H. (1981). *Human groups and social categories: Studies in social psychology*. Cambridge University Press.

Tajfel, H. (1982). Social psychology of intergroup relations. *Annual Review of Psychology*, *33*, 1–39.

Tajfel, H., & Turner, J. C. (1979). An integrative theory of intergroup conflict. In W. G. Austin & S. Worchel (Eds.), *The social psychology of intergroup relations* (pp. 33–47). Brooks/Cole.

Tang, Y., Newman, L. S., & Huang, L. (2014). How people react to social-psychological accounts of wrongdoing: The moderating effects of culture. *Journal of Cross-Cultural Psychology*, *45*(5), 752–763. https://doi.org/10.1177/0022022114527343

Tedeschi, J. T., Bonoma, T. V., & Brown, R. C., Jr. (1971). A paradigm for the study of coercive power. *Journal of Conflict Resolution*, *15*(2), 197–223.

Tripathi, R. C. (1981). Machiavellianism and social manipulation. In J. Pandey (Ed.), *Perspectives on experimental social psychology*. Concept.

Triplett, N. (1898). The dynamogenic factors in pacemaking and competition. *The American Journal of Psychology*, *9*(4), 507–533.

Turner, J. C. (1982). Towards a cognitive redefinition of the social group. In H. Tajfel (Ed.), *Social identity and intergroup relations* (pp. 15–40). Cambridge University Press.

Turner, J. C. (1991). *Social influence*. Brooks/Cole.

Vonk, R. (1998). The slime effect: Suspicion and dislike of likeable behaviour toward superiors. *Journal of Personality and Social Psychology*, *74*(4), 849–864.

Weber, M. (1947). *The theory of social and economic organization* (A. M. Henderson & T. Parsons, Trans.). Oxford University Press. (Original work published 1920).

Wegener, D., & Petty, R. (1996). Effects of mood on persuasion processes: Enhancing, reducing, and biasing scrutiny of attitude-relevant information. In L. L. Martin & A. Tesser (Eds.), *Striving and feeling: Interactions among goals, affect, and self-regulation* (pp. 329–362). Erlbaum.

Witte, K. (1992). Putting the fear back into fear appeals: The extended parallel process model. *Communication Monographs*, *59*(4), 329–349.

Witte, K. (1998). Fear as motivator, fear as inhibitor: Using the extended parallel process model to explain fear appeal successes and failures. In P. A. Andersen, & L. K. Guerrero (Eds.), *Handbook of communication and emotion: Research, theory, applications, and contexts* (pp. 423–450). Academic Press.

Wood, W. (2000). Attitude change: Persuasion and social influence. *Annual Review of Psychology*, *51*(1), 539–570. https://doi.org/10.1146/annurev.psych.51.1.539

13 Science, Technology, Art of Leadership, and Organizational Change

Issues and Implications

Anup K. Singh

Humans are distinctly social and creative by nature. They work in groups and influence one another. Thus, they lead as well as led by others. As creative beings, they come out with new ideas and create new realities. In the process, they manage organization-wide change and lead their fellow beings to embrace the change as smoothly and as quickly as possible. Hence, leadership and organizational change management have been the hallmarks of human civilizations. There are prominent religious, military, and political leaders, such as Ram, Krishna, Chandragupta, Ashok, Akbar, and Gandhi who changed the course of humanity. They inspire and galvanize the masses even today.

Scholars have been pondering over and authoring on leadership. However, leadership literature till the World War II has be arm chair brooding in different nations. Systematic study of leadership and organizational change was missing. Around the World War II, the American society experienced massive economic growth and development. It witnessed rapid growth of research in the different fields of inquiry, including social sciences. Among others, management studies flourished in American universities and research institutions. Leadership and organizational change are among the most researched, studied, and authored topics. Literature on these subjects continues to burgeon. However, the literature is fraught with controversies, contradictions, and confusion. Often, both researchers and practitioners are at a loss to explicate what to do and how to do to effectively confront leadership and change management challenges. This piece explores the nature of leadership, discusses various issues involved in its theory and practice, and finally examines conceptual, theoretical, methodological, and practical implications of themes related to leadership and organizational change.

Fallacious Dichotomy of Leader and Manager

In leadership literature, many make a difference between a leader and a manager. For them, leaders are from a different tribe. For example, Bennis (1989) states that leaders innovate, while managers administer; leaders inspire, while managers control; leaders have a long-term view, while managers have

DOI: 10.4324/9781003461302-18

a short-term view; and most interestingly, leaders do the right things, while managers do things right. This approach unwittingly assumes that leaders do not do the work of a manager. It also implicates that managers can't be leaders. At another level, this approach gives a message that all managers must strive to be leaders and underplay their managerial roles. Being managers, therefore, becomes a less worthy goal.

The hidden assumption behind such an approach is that leaders are superior to managers. All managers should become leaders and as a corollary, all educational institutions must develop leaders. So, we are in a quaint situation. Hardly any educational institution—of any size and shape—intends to develop managers and professionals. They envision to produce leaders, even better "world class leader." The irony, however, is that the future leaders have no work experience, nor they have experienced complex leadership dynamics. When the future leaders are confronted with the reality of the corporate world, they scramble and sometimes fail to adapt to their roles.

The glorification and mystification of leadership have created substantial problems for individuals and organizations. Managers do display influence, thus leadership. But they are not leaders always. Managers can be quite influential in one area, while they can be quite mediocre or ineffective in another. They may demonstrate certain strengths at certain points of time, whereas they may have some foibles other times. Hence, the distinction between the leader and the manager is at best fallacious and illusory. It does not help either researchers or practitioners. Leadership is a dynamic and complex social influence process that works downward, upward, and in a lateral direction. People in different roles do display leadership sometimes, while they follow others in different situations.

Dynamic Nature of Leadership

Leadership is a perennial phenomenon. Nevertheless, its nature has been changing over centuries. The leadership practiced in the agrarian age differs from the leadership applied in the industrial age. Similarly, leadership in the knowledge age is significantly different as compared to leadership in the agrarian and industrial ages. The content and dynamics of leadership have changed over the course of time, but only a few researchers have taken the notice of temporal dimension of leadership (Hall & Janman, 2010; Kellerman, 2012). With the changing times, personal behaviors, power dynamics, expectations of followers, tasks, technologies, etc., vary. As a result, the theories, models, and approaches to leadership also change—the old ones giving the way to the new ones. This is why leadership can be explained, but it can't be predicted. This is why new models and approaches are being proposed in spite of the prevalence of a plethora of literature on leadership. And this trend shall continue in the future.

Figure 13.1 illustrates the central role of time in determining not only leader behaviors and follower characteristics but also nature and dynamics

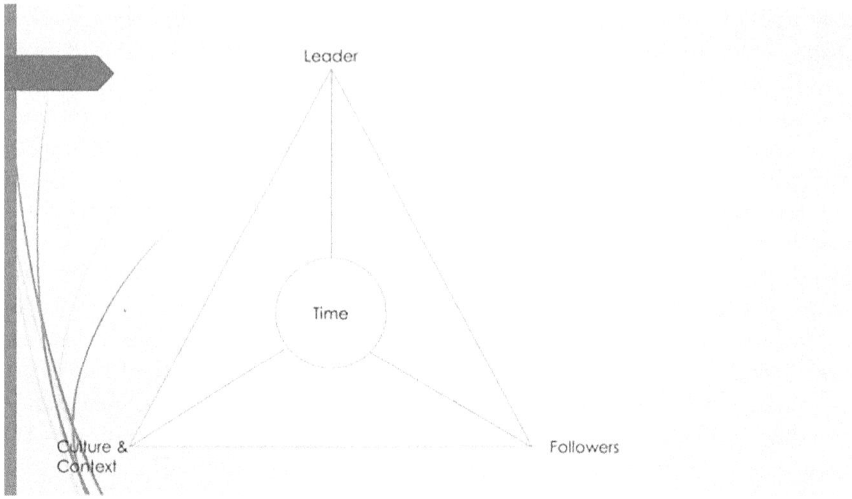

Figure 13.1 Time as a Determiner of Leadership Behaviors, Follower Characteristics, Culture, and Context

of culture and context. Although culture is relatively enduring, it also undergoes subtle changes with the changing times. Norms, values, assumptions, and beliefs—the various constituents of culture—are primed to change over decades. In the same vein, context—nature of tasks, technology, methods, and standards—changes with time. Moreover, leader, followers, and contexts interact dynamically and unpredictably to produce leadership impact.

Evolution of Leadership in India: India has experienced a massive transformation since gaining independence in 1947. Various generations have passed through these times, and they have displayed different leadership behaviors. This transformation has been the mirror of today's new India. Generations are explained through a set of phases people born in. They are divided in Baby Boomers (1946–1964), Gen X (1965–1979), Gen Y (1980–1995), and Gen Z, also called as I Gen (1996–2007). The four generations have played important role in transforming India. She has experienced an exponential growth curve with these different generations. Behavioral norms, values, standards, and work environments have changed and affected individual behavior significantly. We need different theories to understand and explain the behavior of people belonging to different generations. A strait-jacket, fixed approach across periods is ineffectual.

In the first two decades of independence, most social psychologists believed that Indians have leadership problems. They do not have sufficient need for achievement; hence, they are less entrepreneurial and leadership deficient. It was also thought that Indians suffer from dependency syndrome. As a corollary, they are better followers than leaders. However, it was not clear that if all shall be followers, who shall lead.

In the 1970s and 1980s, the Indian industrial scenario was punctuated with the dominance of public sector organizations, owned by central and state governments. The trade unions were quite powerful, and managers were in defensive positions. Managers were encouraged to adopt participatory leadership style. On the other hand, the private sector was characterized by family businesses. License raj was the regulatory mechanism, and competition was conspicuous by its absence. Contrary to the public sector organizations, the private sector organizations viewed trade unions as enemies and made all out attempts to make them enfeebled. Managers followed centralized and authoritarian style.

In the 1990s and the first decade of the 21st century, Indian businesses faced liberalization and globalization. The service industry took a dominant position. IT and ITES organizations became the prime movers of the economy. Financial services also expanded speedily. New media and entertainment organizations came into existence and provided a large number of jobs to the youth. The dynamics of leadership were as diametrically different as compared to their old economy companies. The power distance between the leader and the follower reduced. Teamwork, co-design, and co-creation increased. Respect for authority is reduced. The followers were expected to be more result-oriented and service-minded, using initiative, creativity, and proactivity.

The same trend is continuing for the last one decade. Rather, it is much more accentuated. The followers have many more options in the labor market. Their professional commitment is more as compared to organizational commitment. In addition, the gender ratio is changing in organizations, resulting in subtle differences in organizational influence. As a consequence of globalization, several multinational organizations have entered the Indian industry. They are able to attract talent. In a talent war, Indian companies are also changing their practices to attract talent and to retain them.

In summary, leadership dynamics have been changing over the last seven decades. Indian organizations have changed in products/services, outlook, culture, and management practices. It is but natural that leadership behavior changes have accompanied those changes. And it would so happen in the future.

Culture, Context, and Leadership: Culture is a paramount factor of the leadership–followership process. As pointed out earlier, leadership research has essentially been an American research tradition. Almost 80% of research literature on leadership emanates from the United States. Hence, leadership literature is embedded in American culture. It offers some insights and implications for leadership in other cultures. However, cultures differ on certain critical dimensions and that make a significant impact on the leadership process. At conceptual level, it may seem that American theories apply to all cultures. Nevertheless, at behavioral level, leaders across cultures differ in their leadership behaviors and values (Singh, 1998).

For example, researchers have pointed out that cultures differ on power distance. The Western world has low power distance. On the other hand,

Indian culture is characterized by high power distance. As a result, subordinates in India are not quite comfortable is sharing their independent views with their superior, lest he gets annoyed. Indian managers face several system constraints; therefore, they evolve various ways to be creative in their functioning. Some call it *jugaad*. In contrast, the principles of quality management emphasize adherence to systems. Similarly, Indian followers tend to display the need for approval from their leader. Those leaders who are quite independent and provide autonomy to their subordinates without caring for the need for approval and assurance from the leader may not be effective.

In a subcontinent like India, there exist several subcultures. Sinha has described numerous cultural clusters, affecting the behaviors of managers differentially.

Context is the king. The context can be macro, meso, or micro. The macro-context is usually at industry and organizational levels. The effective leader in the IT industry may not be successful in the manufacturing industry and vice versa. I know one leader who transformed a power producing organization and was considered a charismatic figure. Later, he headed a trading organization. He was ineffectual in the new organization. It was the context that made all the difference in leadership impact. Likewise, a leader who was effective in a small banking organization could not do well in a large banking organization. Tasks differ in terms of autonomy, variety, identity, and feedback. There may be a mismatch between leader behaviors and task characteristics. Hence, some managers are suited for certain tasks, while other managers fit well with others.

The network of a leader also matters. Sometimes, the network of an individual is more important in determining outcomes than individual behaviors. Network members often ensure that their members succeed so that the network remains vibrant. The network can consist of professional members, schoolmates, community members, regional clique, etc. In any case, a good network is the booster to leader effectiveness. Social support and undermining in a group context may help or hinder leader success by increasing or reducing stress and well-being of the leader.

Follower Characteristics: Follower characteristics and group dynamics play a significant role in determining leader success. As a leader moves from one context to another, followers change and consequently group dynamics vary. Effective and collaborative followers can enhance the effectiveness of a leader. Conversely, competent but non-collaborative followers can be a major source of leader failure. The leader–member exchange theory has recognized the role of follower characteristics in affecting leader effectiveness. There is a two-way relationship in determining success. The leaders and the followers evaluate each other. The variety of characteristics of the leader and the follower creates the basis of exchange which can be successful or unsuccessful. Rockstuhl and associates (2012) reported that leader–member exchange is more strongly related to organizational citizenship behavior, justice perceptions, job satisfaction, turnover intentions, and leader trust in Western cultures as compared to Asian cultures.

Science of Leadership

The emergence of the Renaissance and the industrial revolution in Europe gave birth to scientific temperament. In turn, the revealed truth was questioned, and people were encouraged to explore truth through a rational and systematic process. The scientific method stresses on empirical approach and verification of facts. It was a great success with the physical sciences. For example, the theory of gravity was an eye opener for people at large. The scientific method works very well to understand and theorize the deterministic system.

The scientific method is applied to other fields of study, like natural sciences, where it is partially successful. Natural systems, like a living organism, do not follow the immutable theory of gravity. A living organism is a complex system, and it displays randomness and Stochastics in its functioning. Principles and methods developed for inanimate objects have their limitations for understanding when applied to animate beings.

The scientific method is severely restricted when it is applied to even more complex social system, like a human group. The human group has complex dynamics and interacts quite extensively with its environment. Each human group is unique because its internal dynamics are unique, its external environment is unique and the way internal system interacts with the external environment is also unique.

Behavioral sciences, including leadership research, have predominantly used the scientific method to explain and predict human behavior. It has not helped them much. Leadership research came out with one theory after another. The great leader theory was followed up trait theory that in turn had its own lacunae. Later, various leadership style theories were proposed. They also suffered from several conceptual, theoretical, and practical flaws and were not accepted fully by both the academe and the practicing world. As a result, a host of leadership contingency models appeared. These models took both leadership styles and situations and their interactions into consideration. However, their contexts were restricted and they had poor external validity.

Then, a spate of big theories emerged. One of them is transformational leadership. Another such approach is charismatic leadership theory. Later, Level 5 leadership became popular. The sum and substance of the matter is that leadership has become a highly contested field. New theories are constantly evolving, claiming validity and practicability. However, hopes and claims are belied sooner than later.

The moot point is this—is there a science of leadership? The answer is a big NO. Leadership is not a science. In spite of almost one century of leadership research, there is not a single theory that comprehensively explains the leadership phenomenon, not it predicts the success of a leader in a specific context. In the future, there will be several theories of leadership. Humans are fascinated by the leadership phenomenon. They want to understand it and apply it for their betterment. But success is likely to elude them.

Does it mean that there is nothing like influence? Nope, the influence is pervasive in human affairs. It is easily seen in social, political, spiritual, and business domains. There are broader patterns of the influence process. So does music have a soothing impact on people. Musical compositions have broader patterns. The musicians display certain patterns in their exposition. The effectiveness of music is contingent upon the musician, the listeners, genre, culture, and time. But there is no science behind music. Likewise, leadership is an influence process and shows varied patterns in different periods and in different contexts. Making a science out of leadership is a futile exercise.

Technology of Leadership

There is a large leadership development industry spread throughout the world, especially in the United States. The stakeholders in the industry are corporate managers, authors, researchers, publishers, trainers, coaches, consultants, etc. The industry has been growing consistently. Even many universities claim that they are actively engaged in developing leaders. These players depend on research on leadership and associated areas.

A dominant leadership sub-industry is publishing. Some senior managers have documented their leadership experiences and recommended a set of practices that will make young managers more effective (Ashby & Miles, 2002; George, 2003; Haksar, 1993; Khandelwal, 2018; Khorakiwala, 2017; Thomas, 1992). Some of these books are best sellers. Even several Indian top managers have written their autobiographies and proposed certain principles of leadership. Likewise, journalists and authors have written biographies of successful leaders. Generally, these are hagiographies of the protagonists. Moreover, they also draw leadership lessons from them. Then, there are dedicated books on leadership and its development, authored by so-called management gurus, consultants, and professors (London, 2002). The plot of these books has been often simple. First, these books point out that there is a serious leadership crisis, resulting in poor organizational performance. Then, an alternative leadership model is proposed, considered to be well-researched and validated. Besides, supportive case studies are shared to establish the practice of the proposed leadership model (Iyer, 2013). Finally, the books outline the various ways through which individuals and organizations can become more productive (Carter et al., 2005).

A bigger leadership sub-industry is training and development. A large number of corporate, government, and not-for-profit sector managers—junior, middle, and senior—are trained in the leadership field (Parks, 2005). The duration of such training programs may differ from three days to three weeks. These may be classroom training, outbound training, field visits, or a mix of them. Each training program follows one leadership model or a couple of leadership models. They use a set of development practices, like paper and pencil tests, feedback, simulations, exercises, cases, movies, videos. These programs are expensive. However, their impact on individuals and organizations is dubious at best. Many managers term them as "paid holidays," "international tourism" and "loyalty rewards." Some of the participants of leadership programs are sent to leading international b-schools and leadership development agencies. Again, cross-cultural issues impact the usefulness of leadership training.

Leadership coaching is a new trend that is picking up fast. The idea behind leadership coaching is leaders are unable to understand their leadership issues and fail to develop personal effectiveness plans and corporate success strategies. Hence, life and leadership coaches are required to help them identify their personal challenges, strengths, foibles, and business dilemmas. Once they are recognized, the next step is to develop an action plan for self-improvement, interpersonal effectiveness, team building and business transformation. They are often documented and revisited from time to time. Then, leaders implement the action plans under the supervision of the coach. Sometimes the coach may be a retired business leader. At other times, the coach is a trained psychologist or NLP (Neuro-Linguistic Programming) expert. Many large companies hire leadership coaches to help their managers become effective.

Spiritual gurus and management experts interested in religion have also entered the leadership development industry. There are numerous books on the religious scripture and management, explaining how a manager can strengthen his character and enhance his outcomes learning the lessons from them (Banerjee, 1988; Chakraborty, 1987; Chatterjee, 2012: Narayanan & Krishnan, 2003). Mixing religion and leadership produces a unique product: It is highly liked and desired by managers at large, but its applicability in the real world is low. In addition, there is hardly any empirical research to support the claims. There is a wide audience for it, but its impact on practice remains little.

The technology of leadership development suffers from several lacunas. First, as there is no science of leadership, there cannot be a technology of leadership. Any technology is based on certain solid principles of science. A technologist uses those principles to solve a practical problem. In the absence of such principle, there may be snake oil technology without any impact. It is another matter that snake oil can be packaged beautifully and can be sold intelligently in the market. Second, leadership development technologies are so diverse and they subscribe to so many approaches (McCauley & Velsor, 2004). For example, someone uses literature to teach leadership, while another expert applies movies to develop leadership. Similarly, a behavioral scientist may practice the human process lab, while another organizational behavior expert may opt for outbound training for converting managers into leaders. Some use literature and storytelling for leadership development (Singh, 2003). The duration of leadership training programs varies dramatically, say from three days to three weeks. Is there any scientific principle behind it? No, it all depends on the paying capacity of the client. Third, leadership development interventions can leave their scars on a few participants.

For example, human process labs, 360-degree feedback, and leadership coaching may not suit some participants. A participant may suffer from the psychological trauma of high disclosure and high intensity intervention for quite some time. Kellerman, 2012) laments on the leadership industry and conclusively states, "As a whole the leadership industry is self-satisfied, self-perpetuating and poorly policed; that leadership programmes tend to proliferate without objectives assessment; that leadership as an area of intellectual inquiry remains thin" (p. 169). Pfeffer (2016), questioning leadership development industry, states that there is a wide gap between normative and descriptive aspects of leadership. What is written or prescribed by authors and consultants does not work in reality. His thesis is that five ideal attributes of leadership, that is, modesty, authenticity, truthfulness, trustworthiness, and concern for the well-being of other, do not exist in reality. Rather, they can be detrimental to effective leadership. He comments, "The leadership industry is so obsessively focussed on the normative—what leaders should do and how things ought to be—that it has largely ignored asking the fundamental question of what actually is true and going on and why" (pp. 23–24).

Does it mean that the industry development industry would decline? Most probably not. Leadership has been so much valued and branded in the last century that everyone wants to be a leader without its critical understanding. Large organizations sponsor internal and external development programs as a leap of faith. These organizations wish to achieve two objectives. They wish to give a message to their employees that they care for them. In addition, they sincerely want them to contribute more toward organizational objectives. The demand side of the leadership industry is strong. The supply side is innovating contiguously and offering new tools and techniques vigorously. Therefore, there shall not be any decrease in the leadership industry, but there shall also not be any benefit. Fads without fundamentals shall continue to flourish.

Art of Leadership

We have already discussed that power and influence are pervasive elements of social and organizational life. People regularly use power and influence in their dealings. However, their effectiveness may vary owing to a host of factors. An individual may be influential in one context, whereas he can be mediocre in another. People use power and influence tactics, but there is no science behind it. People develop their ways and skills of influence that may suit their contexts and circumstances (Bothwell, 1983). They try the various ways to influence and hone them to fit their temperament and tasks. The expression of power and influence is unique to each individual. One can be inspired by the leadership mode of a successful person. But mimicking his leadership mode may lead to failure.

People take time to understand their power and influence tactics. They analyze with which aspect of a tactic they are comfortable and with which they are not. They continuously receive feedback on their behaviors and modify them to match their comfort level and situational demands. Leadership is best learned by doing on tasks and by self-empowerment (Singh, 1998). As each individual is unique, thus different; similarly, each manager in his leadership role is unique and different. The leadership uniqueness is determined by personality, life experiences, context, culture, industry, and social network. When there is a match between leadership mode and situational and organizational demand, an individual succeeds.

As an individual grows over time through self-efforts, leadership behaviors may also change for better or worse. There is no one best leadership mode. It all depends on the context. In other words, if an individual is able to exhibit leadership mode that meets the needs of the context, he becomes effective.

Every individual has certain leadership strengths and foibles. We are humans and this is our fundamental nature. We cannot have only gifts. Therefore, while gifts are to be preserved and enhanced, liabilities must be managed. The best person to do it is the individual himself. He may read, consult experts, and undergo certain learning experiences. But what he does is the most important level of leadership development. Just as musical fluency depends on talent and Riyaz, leadership effectiveness is contingent upon personal competencies, self-management efforts, and lifelong learning.

In the art of leadership, sense making acquires greater salience. The leader does not have a linear, rigid, and fixed view of reality. For him, organizational reality is complex and in flux. He cannot take it for granted and respond to it in pre-defined ways. In such a situation, he explores the context, task, and people and makes a sense out of them. They extract cues from their context to decide what information is relevant for their action. This is how they make meaning out of their context and enact on their environment (Weick, 1979).

The leader also uses reflexivity to improve his action. He regularly bends back and examines his action. Reflexivity mediates between a leader's context and his action. It is an ongoing process. A leader then has to continuously enhance his self-knowledge. That, in turn, helps him become more reflexive. Furthermore, a leader can be more creative in his actions by bending back and looking forward in a spiral fashion.

When we conceive leadership as art, the role of flexibility and adaptability increases in managing situations. As a leader makes sense and displays reflexivity, he has to be flexible and adaptable in his response. He learns from each leadership encounter and in the process, he grows. Over a period, he grows in his responses. He developed a rich and varied repertoire of actions. It helps him not only in dealing with varied situations but also in managing new situations as he tries various responses and identifies the appropriate response to the situation. Flexibility and adaptability make a leader effective externally. At the same time, they facilitate his internal renewal continuously. A leader impacts managerial situations. In turn, managerial experiences also affect him and grow him as a person. The more challenging and demanding the managerial situations are, better are managerial experiences and their impact on a leader is deeper.

An important tradition in the art of leadership research is to treat a leader as an artist. It is a powerful metaphor to understand leadership. Leadership as art approach (Ladkin & Taylor, 2010) emphasizes that it deals with the realities that are unstable, unknowable, and unpredictable. Furthermore, the approach focuses on the adaptive dimension of leadership. Its tool is sense making. Leaders should stay with senses longer to maximize data from the reality to be more effective, rather than be driven by logic and models. Furthermore, leaders need to work with contradictions and paradoxes, just as artists work with both light and shadow elements of their chosen form.

In a nutshell, it is plausible and desirable to treat leadership as an art. Scientific and technological approaches to leadership have not improved our understanding of leadership knowledge. The art of leadership emphasizes the centrality of a leader. Psychological processes like sense making, reflexivity, and self-renewal play in enhancing leader effectiveness. Besides, this approach helps a leader manage variable, uncertain, ambiguous, and complex reality.

Leadership and Organizational Change

The 21st century is tumultuous and fast changing. The Industrial Revolution 4.0, dynamic geopolitics, the COVID-19 pandemic, emergence of new industries, and sociocultural changes shall influence the future functioning of organizations. Changes take place at the micro- and macrolevels. Top managers are responsible for initiating and managing big changes, popularly known as transformative change. Organization-wide changes are strategic in nature, touching almost all aspects of the organization—product/service, manufacturing, logistics, personnel, finance, sales and distribution, etc. They are generally aimed at a quantum jump in overall performance.

Leadership literature sheds light on organization-wide change propelled through charismatic and transformational leadership. Charismatic leader shares a compelling vision of the future, galvanizes organizational members around the vision, generates high level of enthusiasm among the followers, and finally gets extraordinary performance from them (Conger, 1989; Conger & Kanungo, 1998). However, a charismatic leader has a dark side as well. The charismatic leader can motivate his followers in the wrong direction, resulting in massive losses. Else, organizational change can be effective in the short-term; however, its long-term consequences can be deleterious.

Another major conceptualization of leadership at the top level is developed by Burns (1978) who states that there are two types of leadership: transactional leadership and transformational leadership. Unlike transactional leader, transformational leader appeals to the followers' values and purpose. He has a powerful vision of the future and organizational change. He reframes the critical issues and convinces his followers that they can achieve the set goals. Like a charismatic leader, a transformational leader is often controversial and has a dark side (Tourish, 2013). There is a plethora of literature on transformational leadership. Many books are authored on top successful CEOs. These are written on them by management trainers and consultants who have worked for them. The motive need not be mentioned. Many works are based on already published pieces, thus their validity is a suspect. Finally, charismatic and transformational leadership models have deep roots in political leadership, and their applicability for organizational leadership is limited. Nevertheless, the transformational leadership industry is in a full swing. Leading IIMs, ISB, and MDI in India offer training programs in this area.

Desperate situations and crises often create nurturing grounds for charismatic and transformational leaders. People look for top managers who can rescue them and lead them to a secure future. Every transformational leader makes a promise, leading to a big hope. However, promise may or may not result in performance. Furthermore, long-term consequences of rapid performance remain unknown. Quick fixes often can lead to more fractures.

Concluding Comments

Power and influence are the dominant social phenomenon. Individuals use power and influence to achieve personal and organizational objectives. Nevertheless, they are also influenced by those whom they try to influence. It is never a one-way process. Rather, it is bidirectional. As goals, leaders, and followers change across situations and over periods, there is no fixed way of leading. In other words, leadership exists, but it is quite dynamic and variable. The search for leadership science, hence, is a futile endeavor. As a corollary, the technology of leadership development is at best a nascent technology.

An alternative way to explain leadership is the art of power and influence. As an artist crafts his artifact through sense making, adaptability, flexibility, and reflexivity, a leader can navigate through relationships and tasks using the same processes. He does not use the best way of influencing. On the contrary, he adapts to the context and learns the new ways of doing things in the process. For him, every managerial situation is a new work of art where he has to explore, to think afresh, to believe his gut feeling, and to go for iterations of leadership actions. He has to put his signature on the task, aligning it with follower characteristics, contextual necessity, and historical demands.

References

Ashby, M. D., & Miles, S. A. (Eds.). (2002). *Leaders talk leadership: Top executives speak their minds*. Oxford University Press.

Banerjee, R. P. (1988). *Mother leadership*. Wheeler Publishing.

Bennis, W. G. (1989). *On becoming a leader*. Addison-Wesley.

Bothwell, L. (1983). *The art of leadership: Skill-building techniques that produce results; How to be a successful leader at work and in your personal life*. Prentice Hall Press.

Burns, J. M. (1978). *Leadership*. Harper and Row.

Carter, L., Ulrich, D., & Goldsmith, M. (Eds.). (2005). *Best practices in leadership development and organisation change: How the best companies ensure meaningful change and sustainable development*. John Wiley & Sons.
Chakraborty, S. K. (1987). *Managerial effectiveness and quality of work life: Indian insights*. Tata McGraw Hill.
Chatterjee, D. (2012). *Timeless leadership: 18 leadership sutras from the Bhagavad Gita*. John Wiley & Sons.
Conger, J. A. (1989). *The charismatic leader*. Jossey-Bass.
Conger, J. A., & Kanungo, R. N. (1998). *Charismatic leadership in organisations*. Sage.
George, B. (2003). *Authentic leadership: Rediscovering the secrets to creating lasting value*. Jossey-Bass.
Haksar, A. N. (1993). *Bite the bullet: Thirty-four years with ITC*. Viking.
Hall, T., & Janman, K. (2010). *The leadership illusion: The importance of context and connections*. Palgrave Macmillan.
Iyer, P. (2013). *The secret of leadership: Stories to awaken, inspire and unleash the leader within*. Portfolio.
Kellerman, B. (2012). *The end of leadership*. Harper Business.
Khandelwal, A. K. (2018). *CEO: Chess master or gardner*. Oxford University Press.
Khorakiwala, H. (2017). *Odyssey of courage: The story of an Indian multinational*. New Rupa Publications.
Ladkin, D., & Taylor, S. S. (2010). Leadership as art: Variations on a theme. *Leadership*, *6*(3), 235–241.
London, M. (2002). *Leadership development: Paths to self-insight and professional growth*. Lawrence Erlbaum.
McCauley, C. D., & Velsor, E. V. (Eds.). (2004). *Handbook of leadership development* (2nd ed.). Jossey-Bass.
Narayanan, J., & Krishnan, V. R. (2003). Impact of Sattva and Rajas Gunas on transformational leadership and Karma-Yoga. *Journal of Indian Psychology*, *21*(2), 1–11.
Parks, S. D. (2005). *Leadership can be taught: A bold approach for a complex world*. Harvard Business School Press.
Pfeffer, J. (2016). *Leadership BS: Fixing workplaces and careers one truth at a time*. Harper Business.
Rockstuhl, T., Dulebohn, J. H., Ang, S., & Shore, L. M. (2012). Leader–member exchange (LMX) and culture: A meta-analysis of correlates of LMX across 23 countries. *Journal of Applied Psychology*, *97*(6), 1097.
Singh, A. K. (1998). Management of transformation. *Prestige Journal of Management and Research*, *2*(2).
Singh, S. P. (2003). *Leading: Lessons from literature*. Response Books.
Thomas, T. (1992). *To challenge and to change*. Viking.
Tourish, D. (2013). *The dark side of transformatinal leadership: A critical perspective*. Routledge.
Weick, K. E. (1979). *The social psychology of organizing* (2nd ed.). Addison-Wesley.

14 Emerging Perspectives on Social Decision-Making

Nishtha Jain and Purnima Singh

Decisions are an integral part of life, shaping our actions and consequences in every sphere of life, from mundane daily choices to critical life-changing decisions. Such decisions often involve combining diverse kinds of information, considering or disregarding the emotional significance of the issues involved and drawing inferences under conditions of insufficient information. Also, the decisions also vary in their perceived scope of influence. Thus some decisions connect more with a single person while others intrinsically relate to collectives like family or community. According to the Oxford Dictionary, a decision is "a choice or judgement that you make after thinking and talking about what is the best thing to do." Eisenfuhr (2011) has stated that "decision-making is a process of choosing from several alternatives to achieve the desired result" (p. 7). These definitions raise several questions: What is the best thing or the desired outcome? How do we create a choice set, and from where do these numerous alternatives emerge? How do people make decisions in regular situations? Decision research is a broad interdisciplinary field founded on philosophy, statistics, and economics (Mcfall, 2015). Several disciplines, including cognitive psychology, medical informatics, business management, and political science, have developed a variety of decision-making methodologies and models for use in a variety of scenarios. Here, we analyze the various theories and models, arguing for a greater emphasis on the social and cultural background, which has previously received little attention. The majority of decision-making theories are divided into two categories: normative (how individuals should make decisions?) and descriptive (how individuals make decisions?). Here, the emphasis is on the latter approach. The majority of decision research has been conducted using experimental methods. Most lab investigations present participants with a decision dilemma that neatly divides two possibilities or alternatives. The participants are asked to compare the two options and then make a selection. Most decisions, however, do not occur in a social and cultural vacuum; they are rooted in, and frequently constrained by the social and cultural environment. We offer an overview of how decision-making research has transitioned from optimality to errors and biases, and how it must eventually become more context-specific.

DOI: 10.4324/9781003461302-19

From Classical Rationality to Real Context

The classical rational choice theory (Falzer, 2004) suggests that individuals make self-interested decisions based on cost–benefit analysis. This normative framework made several assumptions about human behavior and the nature of choices: choice alternatives are known; individuals have complete and transitive preferences (if A over B and B over C, then A over C); and individuals have complete knowledge of the risks and uncertainty associated with choice options (Falzer, 2004). These normative models of decision-making established the concept of "optimal" decisions made by a "rational" agent. Though these ideas were later harshly criticized for their limited applicability in social settings and failure to explain complicated human behavior, they were crucial in laying the groundwork for descriptive theories.

In his key study, Simon (1955) observed the expansion of the term "rationality" in traditional economics theory, which equates an "economic man" with a "rational man." His concept of bounded rationality acknowledges that our decision-making power is restricted. We do not always optimize; rather, we are satisfied. Simon's critique of classical economic theory attacked the idea of an all-knowing, fully rational decision-maker. He established the concept of "bounded rationality," which acknowledges that real-world decisions are limited by information, cognitive capacity, and time. Instead of optimizing, people frequently "satisfice" by selecting the first acceptable alternative that fits their demands (Simon, 1956). Furthermore, Kahneman and Tversky's prospect theory (1979) transformed decision-making research. They emphasized that decisions are influenced by observation, judgment, and emotion, rather than being simply intellectual. Prospect theory introduces the concept of reference points, in which outcomes are compared to a neutral reference (often zero). Loss aversion is important because losses have a greater influence on us than profits do.

Kahneman and Tversky's Prospect Theory emphasizes that our rationality is limited. We have biases and deviations from strict reason. It is important to remember that further contextualized research is required. Decisions are not made in isolation; they are shaped by cultural, social, and historical factors. Understanding these contextual nuances allows us to improve our understanding of decision-making processes. To summarize, decision-making is a multifaceted process that incorporates cognitive, emotional, and social components. The classical models prioritized optimality and assumed rational agents. However, real-world decisions are messier. The social and cultural context yields huge impact on our choices. We acquire a better grasp of decision-making processes by taking into account context-specific elements. Thus, decision-making involves a combination of cognition, emotion, and social environment. The next sections demonstrate the breadth of human decisions and the intricate interaction of circumstances that shape them.

Heuristics and Biases

In the 1970s, researchers focused on the phenomenology of error in decision-making, resulting in the "heuristics and biases approach" (Kahneman, 1991). With a strong critique of the normative understanding of decision-making and rationality, Simon's belief that human capability is limited and subject to error, and Kahneman and Tversky's emphasis on uncertain and risky conditions that give rise to heuristics such as loss aversion, the researchers were tasked with explaining decision-making in the real world (Gigerenzer & Gaissmaier, 2011; Kahneman, 1991). Tversky and Kahneman conducted major research on the numerous types of heuristics and systematic errors that influence decision-making under dangerous and uncertain conditions. They argued that by employing these heuristics, humans might lower their cognitive effort when making predictions about difficult decisions with little or incomplete information.

Fast and Frugal Reasoning

Gigerenzer and colleagues (Gigerenzer & Gaissmaier, 2011; Gigerenzer & Goldstein, 1996) argue that heuristics are errors. Instead, they see heuristics as adaptive methods that assist people in making more efficient decisions. Their findings highlight that heuristics are not inherently inferior to complicated decision-making processes. In reality, they can be intelligent and effective.

Nudge Theory

Thaler and Sunstein's (2008) nudge theory focuses on influencing people's choices to make better decisions. They differentiate between "humans" (actual decision-makers influenced by psychological and contextual factors) and "icons" (imaginary rational agents) (Thaler & Sunstein, 2008). Nudges change conduct in predictable ways without removing options or dramatically affecting incentives. The principle underpinning nudge theory is "libertarian paternalism," which seeks to assist individuals in making informed decisions while maintaining their freedom. Nudge theory has practical implications in a variety of fields, including consumer behavior, governmental decisions, company management, healthcare, and AI algorithms (Kosters & Van der Heijden, 2015). The development of a "Nudge Unit" by the U.S. government indicates its practical application (Sunstein, 2014). To summarize, understanding decision-making entails recognizing the interplay of heuristics, context, and nudges. As we continue our exploration, let us acknowledge the importance of these notions in determining our decisions.

Dual Processes in Decision-Making

The dual-process theory of decision-making gained popularity with Kahneman's (2011) seminal book, *Thinking, Fast, and Slow*. System 1 (intuitive, automatic) and System 2 (reflective, intentional) have different functions in determining our decisions and choices. Much of Kahneman's research focuses on System 1, where heuristic judgments frequently result in biases and errors (Kahneman, 2011). Epstein (1994) and Damasio (1994) highlighted the importance of emotions in dual-process theories. The experience system (related to emotions) functions naturally and influences subsequent processing. Damasio's (1996) somatic marker hypothesis explains how emotions influence decision-making at both the conscious and unconscious levels.

Slovic et al. (2002) introduced the affect heuristic, in which people identify items with affective tags (good or negative). In complex judgments requiring limited mental resources, people frequently rely on emotions rather than concrete evidence. The affect heuristic explains a variety of phenomena, including celebrity name changes and public health initiatives (Slovic et al., 2002).

Naturalistic Decision-Making

It investigates how people make decisions in real-world dynamic settings (Klein, 1989). Naturalistic Decision-Making (NDM) recognizes the constraints of time, information, and complexity. Klein's work has been significant in improving our understanding of decision-making in practical settings. Klein (2008) argued that for decades, decision researchers have demonstrated how individuals do not make decisions, how their choices are suboptimal, how there is no systematic review of options, how people rely on heuristics rather than rational or analytical procedures, and so on. NDM scholars understand that decision-making is frequently nonlinear, intuitive, and impacted by a variety of factors, including experience, expertise, emotions, and environmental restrictions (Klein, 2008, 2017). Thus, decision-making is a multidimensional process impacted by cognition, emotions, and external demands.

Socially and Culturally Rooted Decision-Making

Despite the interdisciplinary literature, fundamental concerns about real-world decision contexts remain unaddressed. Norms, social identity, and moral concerns are frequently disregarded in decision-making studies. It is especially intriguing because most main decision theories, including heuristics and biases, fast and frugal techniques, and nudge theory, among others, frequently emphasize "context," the limits and constraints of human reasoning, the proclivity for errors, and the significance of emotions. However, what this context indicates is uncertain.

In this regard, context can be visualized at three different levels: micro, meso, and macro. Individualistic elements such as views, attitudes, and personality influence the decision-making process at the microlevel, whilst group-level factors such as family, neighborhood, ethnicity, and others can have a substantial impact at the meso-level (Jaspal et al., 2016). At the macrolevel, societal structures and institutions such as infrastructure, laws, and literacy, among others, gain importance (Jaspal et al., 2016). In this context, Glatzer et al. (2020) argued against overemphasizing evidence-based decision-making and instead defined three decision-making criteria that are relevant to making real-world decisions: first, "capabilities, confidence, self-efficacy, emotions, frames of reference, and degree of expertise, also influence decision-making" (Glatzer et al., 2020, p. 371); second, decision-specific criteria are based on clinical data, including "performance status, age, presence of comorbidities, cancer stage, biomarkers, or expected treatment toxicity" (Glatzer et al., 2020, p. 371); and third, contextual issues, such as "patient's socioeconomic status, the health-care system, treatment costs, or influence from the pharmaceutical industry" (Glatzer et al., 2020, p. 371).

Salek et al. (2023) conducted a scoping review that yielded 79 papers from both low- and upper-middle-income nations. They updated Glatzer et al.'s (2020) list of variables to include additional considerations for low-resource countries. Contextual factors included healthcare access, resource availability, health literacy, community impact, desire for traditional treatments, and culture/religion, among others.

Some researchers have underlined the need to investigate the effect of cultural and religious beliefs, such as the notion of karma and fatalism.

The widely accepted Indian doctrine of karma conceptualizes cosmic equilibrium through a system of actions, reactions, and reincarnations (Agrawal & Dalal, 1993). It holds that an individual's current circumstances and life events are caused by his or her previous acts in former lifetimes. Thus, good activities will have a positive consequence, and vice versa. This school of thinking offers an internal locus of control because the individual's activities are responsible for both his or her well-being and suffering (Agrawal and Dalal, 1993). Fatalism is the view or attitude that life events are influenced by external causes such as fate, luck, destiny, or God (Choi, 2012). There is little research on the role of such elements in decision-making (Martina et al., 2022; Kohli & Dalal, 1998).

The literature on the likely involvement of norms, social identity, moral impingements, and other factors in making key judgments is severely inadequate (Burns & Roszkowska, 2016; Kohli & Dalal, 1998). For example, in a study of 306 people, Jain and Singh (2024a) investigated how decision-making style and financial status affected trust in doctors, patient agency, emotional discomfort, and responsibility attribution. They discovered that when given the condition that treatment significantly reduced quality of life and failed to remove cancer, participants assigned large levels of decision responsibility to chance, luck, or God, regardless of decision-making style or financial situation.

Some recent studies have emphasized the importance of studying people's lived experiences in real-world contexts. For example, Jain and Singh (2024b) interviewed 25 doctors to learn about their thoughts on the types of key decisions they face in cancer therapy, as well as the process of conducting them. It was discovered that doctors were primarily faced with first, treatment-modality dilemmas, in which choosing between multiple treatment modalities was difficult due to ambiguous data and a lack of patient agency; second, resource allocation dilemmas arising from contextual constraints, such as bed limitations, high treatment costs, and a patient's low financial capacity; and third, communicating the illness to patients and family carers. Furthermore, the doctor's decision-making process included technical and communication considerations. Medical data, investigations, commonly used research, references to well-acknowledged treatment guidelines, and team meetings all influenced the decisions taken by doctors. These decisions were then conveyed to patients and family members who were caretakers. These two processes were frequently repetitive, and the final treatment decisions were made. The doctors stated that they frequently adapted their recommendations to the contextual reality of each patient.

In another study, Jain and Singh (2024c) interviewed cancer patients (n =20) and family carers (n = 27) to learn about the real-life essential decisions they face throughout cancer treatment, the process of making such decisions, and the emotional implications of doing so. It was discovered that both stakeholders relied extensively on doctors' advice and suggestions while making treatment decisions. As a result, the majority of their key decisions concerned logistics and finances rather than substantial treatment challenges. The two stakeholders found it more challenging to make minor, day-to-day decisions like managing funds, arranging transportation, addressing domestic obligations, determining childcare arrangements, picking hospitals or testing centers, and negotiating bureaucratic impediments. Some individuals, however, had to make crucial decisions such as whether to continue treatment or opt for palliative care. Family carers played an important role in the decision-making process, whereas patients were typically passive.

Both studies (Jain & Singh, 2024b, 2024c) revealed that contextual factors, relationships, trust in doctors, the role of cultural beliefs, the financial burden of cancer, and other related factors all contributed to a decision environment in which patients and family carers valued paternalistic decision-making, relied on doctors for decisions, and had limited patient agency. For example, a combination of great trust in doctors, financial stress, belief in God and destiny, and the debilitating impact of cancer therapy frequently left patients and family carers with few options and little control over the decision-making process. However, by focusing on isolated outcomes and ideal choices, key decision-making theories such as heuristics and biases sometimes neglect the intricate interaction of contextual elements that influence decision trajectories (Patel et al., 2002; Weiss & Shanteau, 2021).

Conclusion

The choice study literature largely fails to explain how the social context shapes and influences decisions, and how they, in turn, have the potential to impact others and the emerging social reality. Recent research suggests investigating lived experiences in authentic real-life settings. This examination of contextualized choice research and the various aspects that influence key decisions is both enlightening and thought-provoking. Researchers are increasingly emphasizing the need to study decisions in their larger social, cultural, and institutional contexts. Social conventions, money resources, and complex considerations other than immediate situational elements all impact choices. The role of cultural and religious beliefs requires additional investigation. The study of decision-making necessitates that we be alert to the complexity that underpins key decisions.

References

Agrawal, M., & Dalal, A. K. (1993). Beliefs about the world and recovery from myocardial infarction. *Journal of Social Psychology*, *133*(3), 385–394. https://doi.org/10.1080/00224545.1993.9712157

Burns, T., & Roszkowska, E. (2016). Rational choice theory: Toward a psychological, social, and material contextualization of human choice behavior. *Theoretical Economics Letters*, *6*, 195–207. https://doi.org/10.4236/tel.2016.62022

Choi, M. (2012). Fatalism. *Encyclopedia of Immigrant Health*, 688–688. https://doi.org/10.1007/978-1-4419-5659-0_284

Damasio, A. R. (1994). *Descartes' error : Emotion, reason, and the human brain.* G.P. Putnam. https://search.library.wisc.edu/catalog/999764511802121

Damasio, A. R. (1996). The somatic marker hypothesis and the possible functions of the prefrontal cortex. *Philosophical Transactions: Biological Sciences*, *351*(1346), 1413–1420. https://doi.org/https://doi.org/10.1098/rstb.1996.0125

Eisenfuhr, F. (2011). *Decision making*. Springer.

Epstein, S. (1994). Integration of the cognitive and the psychodynamic unconscious. *American Psychologist*, *49*(8), 709–724. https://doi.org/10.1037//0003-066X.49.8.709

Falzer, P. R. (2004). Cognitive schema and naturalistic decision making in evidence-based practices. *Journal of Biomedical Informatics*, *37*(2), 86–98. https://doi.org/10.1016/J.JBI.2004.02.002

Gigerenzer, G., & Gaissmaier, W. (2011). Heuristic decision-making. *Annual Review of Psychology*, *62*(1), 451–482. https://doi.org/10.1146/ANNUREV-PSYCH-120709-145346

Gigerenzer, G., & Goldstein, D. G. (1996). Reasoning the fast and frugal way: Models of bounded rationality. *Psychological Review*, *103*(4), 650–669. https://doi.org/10.1037/0033-295X.103.4.650

Glatzer, M., Panje, C. M., Sirén, C., Cihoric, N., & Putora, P. M. (2020). Decision-making criteria in oncology. *Oncology*, *98*(6), 370–378. https://doi.org/10.1159/000492272

Jain, N., & Singh, P. (2024a). Exploring the influence of decision-making style and financial status of cancer patients on varied cultural aspects of decision process. *Psychology and Developing Societies*, *36*(1). https://doi.org/10.1177/09713336241233715
Jain, N., & Singh, P. (2024b, July 1–July 5). Understanding the complexity of the Decision Process for Doctors in the treatment of cancer. In *Paper Presented at 17th international conference on naturalistic decision-making*, Auckland University of Technology, Auckland, New Zealand.
Jain, N., & Singh, P. (2024c). *Understanding the decision process in the treatment of cancer* [Doctoral dissertation]. Department of Humanities and Social Sciences, Indian Institute of Technology, Delhi.
Jaspal, R., Carriere, K., & Moghaddam, F. (2016). Bridging micro, meso and macro processes in social psychology. In J. Valsiner, G. Marsico, N. Chaudhary, T. Sato & V. Dazzani (Eds.), *Psychology as a science of human being: The Yokohama Manifesto*. Springer.
Kahneman, D. (1991). Judgment and decision making: A personal view. *Psychological Science*, *2*(3), 142–145. www.cs.cmu.edu/~jhm/Readings/kahneman-1991.pdf
Kahneman, D. (2011). *Thinking, fast and slow*. Farrar, Straus, and Giroux.
Kahneman, D., & Tversky, A. (1979). Prospect theory: An analysis of decision under risk. *Econometrica*, *47*(2), 263–292. https://doi.org/10.2307/1914185
Klein, G. (1989). Recognition-primed decisions. In W. B. Rouse (Ed.), *Advances in man-machine research* (Vol. 5, pp. 47–92). JAI Press.
Klein, G. (2008). Naturalistic decision making. *Human Factors*, *50*(3), 456–460. https://doi.org/10.1518/001872008X288385
Klein, G. (2017). *Sources of power: How people make decisions*. The MIT Press. https://doi.org/10.7551/MITPRESS/11307.001.0001
Kohli, N., & Dalal, A. K. (1998). Culture as a factor in causal understanding of illness: A study of cancer patients. *Psychology and Developing Societies*, *10*(2), 115–129. https://doi.org/10.1177/097133369801000202
Kosters, M., & Van der Heijden, J. (2015). From mechanism to virtue: Evaluating nudge theory. *Evaluation*, *21*(3), 276–291. https://doi.org/10.1177/1356389015590218
Martina, D., Kustanti, C. Y., Dewantari, R., Sutandyo, N., Putranto, R., Shatri, H., Effendy, C., van der Heide, A., van der Rijt, C. C. D., & Rietjens, J. A. C. (2022). Advance care planning for patients with cancer and family caregivers in Indonesia: A qualitative study. *BMC Palliative Care*, *21*(1), 204. https://doi.org/10.1186/s12904-022-01086-0
Mcfall, J. P. (2015). Rational, normative, descriptive, prescriptive, or choice behavior? The search for integrative metatheory of decision making. *Behavioral Development Bulletin*, *20*(1), 45–49. https://doi.org/10.1037/h0101039
Patel, V. L., Kaufman, D. R., & Arocha, J. F. (2002). Emerging paradigms of cognition in medical decision-making. *Journal of Biomedical Informatics*, *35*(1), 52–75. https://doi.org/10.1016/S1532-0464(02)00009-6
Salek, M., Silverstein, A., Tilly, A., Gassant, P. Y., Gunasekera, S., Hordofa, D. F., Hesson, D., Duffy, C., Malik, N., McNeil, M., Force, L. M., Bhakta, N., Rodin, D., & Kaye, E. C. (2023). Factors influencing treatment decision-making for cancer patients in low- and middle-income countries: A scoping review. *Cancer Medicine*, 1–20. https://doi.org/10.1002/CAM4.6375
Simon, H. A. (1955). A behavioural model of rational choice. *Quarterly Journal of Economics*, *69*(1), 99–118. https://doi.org/10.2307/1884852
Simon, H. A. (1956). Rational choice and the structure of the environment. *Psychological Review*, *63*(2), 129–138. https://doi.org/10.1037/H00427699
Slovic, P., Finucane, M., Peters, E., & MacGregor, D. G. (2002). The Affect Heuristic. In T. Gilovich, D. Griffin, & D. Kahneman (Eds.), *Heuristics and biases: The psychology of intuitive judgment* (pp. 397–420). Cambridge University Press. https://doi.org/10.1017/CBO9780511808098.025

Sunstein, C. R. (2014). Nudging: A very short guide. *Journal of Consumer Policy*, *37*, 583. http://nrs.harvard.edu/urn-3:HUL.InstRepos:16205305

Thaler, R. H., & Sunstein, C. R. (2008). *Nudge: Improving decisions about health, wealth, and happiness*. Yale University Press. https://doi.org/10.1016/s1477-3880(15)30073-6

Weiss, D. J., & Shanteau, J. (2021). The futility of decision-making research. *Studies in History and Philosophy of Science Part A*, *90*, 10–14. https://doi.org/10.1016/J.SHPSA.2021.08.018

Epilogue

Visible and Invisible: Some Reflections on Developments in Social Psychology in India

Girishwar Misra, Purnima Singh, and Pallavi Ramanathan

Historical Background and Influences

India is home to a rich history of social psychology. About 20 years ago, in 2005, Pandey and Singh presented an account of the origins, development, present state, and prospects of social psychology in India. They argued that several factors have contributed to the development of scientific social psychology in modern India. These include the country's deep philosophical heritage, changes in the field's research priorities, news stories, and pressing social and political concerns. Many reviews (Dalal & Misra, 2001; Misra, 1990; Sinha, 1981, 1993, 1998) and six rounds of Indian Council of Social Science Research (ICSSR) surveys (Mitra, 1972; Misra, 2010, 2019; Pandey, 1988, 2000, 2001, 2004; Pareek, 1980, 1981) have addressed the growth of the field, outlined research trends, and criticized the unplanned nature of this expansion, arguing that it has not led to programmatic research. Notwithstanding these caveats, the majority of past reviews acknowledged the swift development of social psychology. Pandey and Singh (2005) sought to review and identify the major developments in the field of social psychology in India, as well as certain overarching themes that interested these researchers. They suggested that "national concerns slowly influenced social psychological research to be relevant for development" (p. 243) after independence, when the country encountered multiple development challenges. When talking about the goal of social psychology research, Pandey and Singh (2005) contended that "the fundamental push for social psychological research in developing nations arises from the conspicuous character of societal problems" (p. 248). They also asserted that the sociopolitical context in India often determines what captures the attention of social psychologists. They stated that "cultural diversity, plurality, human rights issues, social and distributive justice, child labour, gender discrimination and violence against women, and enhancing social capital are all critical concerns in democratic and civil societies" (p. 248). Regardless of whether the issues were related to the political and social climate, the question of the applicability of the research toward comprehending the policy and social milieu persists.

DOI: 10.4324/9781003461302-20

As a nation, India is a society with a diverse and inclusive social structure. It has a unique caste structure, several thousand dialects, many religions, four of which were founded in India, and a wide range of regional variations across its length and width. All these factors contribute to the country's capacity to coexist and prosper. The country's unique socio-political-legal terrain is reshaping its social, economic, and legal systems at a dizzying rate, especially in the last several decades, and the economy is rising at a quick pace. This chapter aims to examine the relationship between social psychology and India's social issues in the new globalized era. More specifically it explores the visible contributions of social psychology research and identifies and addresses the invisible themes that have thus far been neglected and escaped the attention of researchers. Additionally, the chapter aims to evaluate and demonstrate the gap between social psychology research and policy by utilizing a few cases and pinpoints the distance between research and societal issues as its cause.

India's Sociopolitical Landscape

Despite the country's fast transformation, India's social structures have maintained their "continuity and vitality" and "resilience in the face of change" (Stern, 2003). Impressive progress in space and information technology, a thriving economy, and a marked decline in poverty are all signs of India's vitality. On the other hand, the country's complicated sociopolitical matrix includes issues like increasing inequality, regional tensions, unemployment, and more. In this chapter, we also make an effort to chart important events, the level of complexity caused by the social fabric of the country, and how social psychology research has helped to unravel and analyze these events.

The importance of theory formulation and application was just as great in Indian tradition as it was in religion and philosophy, which had tight relationships with one another (Misra & Singh, 2024a). This chapter, however, aims to describe the importance of drawing a connection between cultural and social contexts and empirical research. Most social psychologists have a narrow view of social reality and tend to take an isolated approach, which makes it hard for them to comprehend and explain the complexities of social reality. Their worldview is narrow, and they hardly interact with cognate academic disciplines. As academics, they struggle to make sense of the interconnected web of factors that comprise social reality, including but not limited to individual, group level, structural, cultural, and environmental factors. An additional concern associated with publishing in books and journals and supposedly expanding the body of disciplinary knowledge base is noted. The editors and reviewers often urge writers to emphasize theoretical contributions or knowledge generation. While this is critical, it might lead to the development of ideas and perspectives that aren't always relevant to a given culture. This is because these ideas and perspectives are often shaped by a different cultural ethos. Studies conducted in nations with large populations, like India, fall under this category. Several researchers have drawn attention to this trend (e.g., Arnett, 2009; Heine & Norenzayan, 2006; Sears, 1986; Triandis, 1994; Uskul et al., 2024). Since the researcher's social reality might be at odds with the borrowed theory and methods from different settings, it is important to think carefully about whether this will help the researcher understand their environment and society. Indeed, when we embrace a theoretical framework that was developed by another researcher, we begin to perceive the world through that lens. Even if there are similarities, local and cultural differences may add another level of uncertainty; that perspective might be alien to the sociocultural setting where the empirical study is carried out. Indeed, social reality is complex, multifaceted, and hard to characterize using a borrowed theoretical framework.

Academics seldom consider how well they grasp the nuances of cultural background and social reality. By highlighting how a particular research study adds to theory, we utilize theory to bolster both ourselves and our research. We hold the view that all ideas and theories are universally applicable everywhere. This, however, is far from the truth. Take the case of self and class as articulated by Stephens et al. (2014) as an illustration. They postulated that, as a result of their experiences, middle-class people learn to see themselves as somewhat separate from society, whereas people from lower socioeconomic backgrounds learn to see themselves as strongly interwoven with both. According to Stephens et al. (2014), people can adapt to their unique social-class contexts by developing culture-specific selves and engaging in congruent behaviors. Indian civilization, for example, is largely collectivistic and so promotes interdependence; nonetheless, Stephens et al.'s (2014) study cannot be utilized to comprehend the reality of social-class situations in other societies. Additionally, in the Indian cultural context, several ways of thinking about one's own identity have developed. Rather than slavishly accepting dominant self-concept theories, these results highlight the significance of contextualizing them in the distinctive sociocultural milieu of a country.

Social Reality and Cultural Context

According to several researchers, the bulk of psychological concepts in most parts of the world have been brought in from other countries (Henrich et al., 2010; Pillay, 2017; Uskul et al., 2024). It is amply clear that "researcher assumptions, intuitions, and introspections arise from a particular cultural milieu and set of experiences that may not generalise to most of the world" (Apicella et al., 2020; Uskul et al., 2024). This leads to a distinct form of "topic blindness" when researchers ignore the pressing social issues in their society in favor of Western-popular themes. For instance, in research on justice, most researchers have solely concentrated on distributive, procedural, and interactional justice, while completely disregarding the role that contextual variables play in shaping both the opinions and feelings around these concepts. Justice is perceived and constructed in large part by structural factors like caste and class in India, which impact self-concept and feelings of relative or historical deprivation. There are many other cases like this where, despite their worldwide prominence, psychologists have failed to address under-represented groups and have adhered to a flawed scientific paradigm, as Moghaddam (2022) has forcefully illustrated in his book *How Psychologists Failed*. The cognitive revolution has centered on causal explanations of behavior, but Moghaddam (2022) argues that we should shift our attention to normative frameworks and intentionality instead. For instance, caste is a strong underlying component that shapes thoughts, feelings, and behaviors. Some of these effects may be detrimental to individuals from lower caste groups. Complex and nonlinear conceptual methods are necessary to understand how members of these and other marginalized groups perceive and react to the advantages and disadvantages of others. As Singh (2021) has argued, situatedness in nature is a welcome perspective that prioritizes coexistence and communion over dominance and manipulation. To understand the Indian people in their indigenous social and cultural context, researchers must first disentangle the knots of their intricately linked social fabric. The interpretive potential of social psychology research can only be enhanced, by actively engaging with these features of social reality.

It is crucial to connect with context, issue, and culture to avoid generalizing psychological findings across diverse communities with distinct ecologies, languages, belief systems, and social behaviors (Norenzayan & Heine, 2005). It is also important to note that social, cultural, political, and economic normative systems have a far bigger influence on theory-building than what the prevailing causal-reductionist paradigms allow. The scientific techniques impose still another layer of restriction on hypotheses. The greater sociocultural context necessitates a more holistic approach to data interpretation and a more comprehensive toolbox for tapping into social reality.

The Challenge of Positivist Paradigm

The dominant approach to knowledge production in academic social psychology has tended to follow the positivist paradigm. To this end, the hypotheticodeductive approach to conceptualization and quantitative methodology constituted the main frame strategy of knowledge production. It is also noted that the complexities of the elements that comprise social reality cannot be explored very easily via positivist methods. For example, we classify people into "majority" and "minority" groups. However, even if one is part of the majority, one may not enjoy much in the way of social support and might even live in an isolated place. Thus, it is possible that the larger environment, not merely their membership in the majority or minority group, influences their worldview, emotional experiences, and cognitive orientation The vast majority of the researchers continued to engage with the creation of various forms of direct and indirect verbal measures (e.g., scales, tests, questionnaires, inventories) involving different degrees of procedural sophistication. They provided simple ways for operationalization of concepts and making them researchable in the positivist tradition. This was based on the assumption that a person's endorsement of verbal measures was a dependable representation of the psychological experience corresponding to the psychological state/trait/disposition being tapped by the measure. A smaller group of researchers left to pursue qualitative methods, first-person methods, or naturalistic observation which have scope for deductive ways to approach knowledge creation.

The fact that the response to verbal items was an outcome of introspection, reflection, and reporting by the participating subject did not receive attention or perhaps treated as error variance common to everyone to a common degree or extent. The verbal response of (dis)agreement with a given value of the scale was treated on face value. The resulting value was treated like an objective physical value and subjected to a physical object-like treatment. This became the standard procedure or script of research and was so strongly entrenched in the minds of people that no one thought to question it. There was no dialogue between the measures used, analysis, and interpretation and social reality. There was only an abstract understanding of the reality on the part of the researcher which they considered to be the reality. The weight of numbers and statistical analysis often makes one believe the validity of conclusions drawn; and at that time, methodological sophistication was at a premium and concepts were subservient to them. The publication practices made conformity to ritualistic methodological nuances a precondition of knowledge generation. The context of discovery became less important than the context of justification. Although this approach has been very productive in some sense, it has added a lot of ambiguity and duplication of concepts. This situation has been responsible for pseudo assurance of knowledge creation.

The social sciences in modern India have been heavily influenced by Euro-American tradition since the British colonial period, leading to a lack of indigenous perspectives and superficial research on Indian society. After independence, social sciences in India continued to be taught and researched in their Western form. The application of Western theories to Indian society has resulted in confusion and a disconnect between India's cultural heritage and contemporary reality. The dilemma about choice of research paradigm is very critical for the direction of research. The situation in the growth of social psychology in India can be gauged by the developmental trajectory of scholars. Here we would like to refer to the self-reflections by two reputed Indian social psychologists who in their exemplary careers have earnestly pursued social psychology. The first is Professor JBP Sinha; a very senior social psychologist (birth: 1936) who holds a PhD from Ohio State University, USA. He deciphered three somewhat overlapping phases in his academic career. The first phase involved a "*struggle to outgrow the alien framework by conducting research that addressed the most salient socio-cultural issues in the Indian context with the methods that seemed to be the most appropriate.*" In the second phase of the next 15 years, he tried "*to claim a legitimate space for my research on the international landscape.*" He found the encounters "*enriching and yet frustrating.*" He realized that he could at best be an Indian cultural psychologist. In the third phase, therefore, he "*returned to focus on organisational behaviour deeply embedded in the Indian societal culture inheriting psycho-philosophical thoughts from the ancient time.*" Since then, he has been conducting research "*through multi-authored, multi-centred and multi-methods research, how the ancient Indian wisdom has filtered through contemporary experiences to create an inclusive Indian mindset that manifests in social and organisational behaviour.*" The second is Professor Ramadhar Singh (birth: 1945), who has a PhD from Purdue University, USA. He was nominated to become a part of the Heritage Wall of Fame of the Society for Personality and Social Psychology. In an autobiographical note, Singh (2022) has mentioned that his "accomplishments came from applying, extending, and modifying three research paradigms originally developed in the USA: the attraction paradigm of Donn Byrne, the information integration theory of Norman Anderson, and the social-functionalist models of Philip Tetlock." During his entire career, he meticulously extended this work across cultures and groups in several countries. With unwavering commitment, Singh pursued a theory-driven research program devoted to testing hypotheses. Convinced of the potential of a physicalistic and positivistic methodological paradigm he persistently explored the empirical boundaries of the chosen paradigms as per the game of science. These two models of scholarship illustrate the consequences of the varied deployment of reflexivity that has resulted in diverse academic outcomes. Another concern is the degree of policy relevance of research which is quite low. Tripathi and Sinha (2014) have examined the role of psychology in the domain of social policy. Despite psychologists' worries, very little progress has been made. Psychologists often tend to concentrate on the finer details, whereas policy makers are more concerned with the big picture. There is very little dialogue between the policy-making process as a whole and the research that has been undertaken. Additionally, the applicability of our research methodology to policy in non-Western cultural settings may be questioned due to its foundation in Euro-American concepts. What matters most to policy makers is how the information or conclusions may be used to affect policy, not whatever theory we support or propose.

Following an analysis of the visible (i.e., what we read in books and journals) and a critique of researchers' fixation on Western-developed theory, we now move to discuss some key concerns of social psychology scholars and how they relate to and contribute to our understanding of the invisible (i.e., real-world social issues). Social conflicts, education, and health are just a few of the current issues that are being discussed; however, we know this is a limited explication.

Relationships Between Groups and Social Conflicts

Indian society has always cherished the principle of unity in diversity. No matter how diverse our nation is in terms of geography, language, religion, and caste, we remain united as a people. The pre-Western tradition of tolerance in Indian society is notable. At the same time, social tensions have also existed, as part of self-definition. After roughly two centuries of British colonial rule, the Indian freedom struggle culminated in the partition of the country into two, and subsequently three countries. British diplomatic policy was chiefly involved in the creation of Hindustan and Pakistan. Partition led to large-scale bloodshed and migration across the border. It is estimated that over one million people died, and millions were put through psychological, social, and financial torture. A maelstrom of murder, hatred, and exile happened in 1946–1948. An influential UNESCO program centered on the bloodshed of the partition and resulted in the 1953 book *In the Minds of Men* (Murphy, 1953). The horror of Partition is still fresh in people's minds. Interestingly, the whole approach emphasized the psychologization of social reality and a kind of reductionism from social to individual. This led to a misconstrued appraisal of the problem and this approach extended to other areas too, resulting in a shift in focus to individual prejudices and stereotypes.

Identity Studies

Previous ICSSR reviews have reported on a range of prejudices and preconceptions, and it persists as a common research theme. Of course, it has extended to include identity concerns. The idea of identity has a rich and interesting history in India, where it has recently gained a lot of attention. There are many ways to study identity, but there is a distinct divide between studies that center on group identification, or more specifically, how people feel about themselves about other people, and studies that center on individual identity, which deal with concepts like the self and personal identity. The studies that focus on group identity deal with concepts like social identity. Feelings were the focal point of Indian identity studies following independence. Using the social distance scale, Adinarayan (1953) compared pre- and post-independence racial and communal attitudes among Indians. During this period, the identity theory of Erikson (1950) gained significant attention. Attending to psychosocial development, especially the concept of "identity crisis," led to an abundance of studies in this area. Even in India, the psychoanalytic method of understanding one's identity gained traction; for instance, Sudhir Kakar (1968) examined Erikson's work through an Indian lens, concentrating on Hinduism. While retaining a psychoanalytic and psycho-cultural stance, Nandy (1970) offered another viewpoint on the subject of national identity and nationalism. Personality and sense of self were central to identity studies throughout this period. Both identity studies and social psychology as a whole were in the formative stages in the 1970s and 1980s. An important evolution during this period was the social identity theory (Tajfel & Turner, 1979; Turner et al., 1987); the identity theory developed concurrently (see, e.g., Burke, 1980; McCall & Simmons, 1978). Later, scholars from India began using social identity or identity theory, drawing heavily from the psychoanalytic canon (Agrawal, 1978). There was interest in cross-cultural research in India during this decade. Nandy (1976) made significant inroads into questions of sexual orientation and gender identity. In their 1985 study on social identity, Ghosh and Huq compared Bangladeshis to Indians. Along with this, Paranjpe (1985) investigated similarities between prejudice theory and Indian psychology by delving into the concept of Vedanta and self-realization, another facet of identity, following the global trend of the time in analyzing prejudice. In addition, Tripathi and Srivastava (1981) used intergroup behavior and relative deprivation to understand Hindu-Muslim relations in India. Lacking an in-depth examination of the Indian context, the majority of these studies tested prejudices and perceptions against a backdrop of various Western-developed theories. The Norm Violation theory (DeRidder & Tripathi, 1992) sought to capture the complexities of the social setting and gave a new direction to identity studies. Other studies conducted around this time examined Hindu-Muslim relations (e.g., Ghosh & Kumar, 1991). The effort to "indigenise" mental processes was another notable trend. An important example of this is Paranjpe's (1998) volume on self and identity processes. Researching Indian identity is challenging due to the wide range of factors that contribute to it. Analyzing the complex processes by which Indians construct their social identities in the face of multiple pressures is an enormous undertaking (Kapur & Misra, 2011).

Research in the field of identity in Indian psychology has been moving in recent years toward a more contextualized and specific understanding of the concept. As an example, the research by (Vahali, 2009) and Ramanathan and Singh (2021, 2024) on Tibetan refugees in India. They have deployed a highly contextualized perspective on refugee identity. This anthology delves into how leadership and intergroup interactions have shaped and are shaping the identities of Tibetan refugees. It is believed that the identities of Tibetan refugees are significantly impacted by the social, political, historical, and geographical circumstances. These studies show that researchers are moving away from trying to generalize identity processes and instead looking at them in their specific circumstances. The research conducted by Jogdand and colleagues on the topic of caste and humiliation (Jogdand, 2024; Sharma & Jogdand, 2024) sheds light on a specific form of emotional humiliation that Dalits in India continue to face within the framework of identity politics. Perhaps contextualized research is the way to go to be more applicable to policy and to build indigenous theoretical frameworks while departing from Euro-Western theoretical paradigms.

Health and Wellness

The relevance of both mental and physical health was brought to light by the COVID-19 pandemic which led to a shift toward viewing health as a multifaceted concept that includes not just the body and mind but also the environment in which we live. Both individual and societal factors contribute to one's health and happiness (Dalal & Misra, 2011). But in this modern age of ever-evolving technology and the unavoidable threat of pandemics, the boundaries of health psychology need to be re-examined. Novel approaches to comprehending health practices in the digital age are required due to the increasing prevalence of health communication on social media platforms. During the COVID-19 epidemic, for instance, Jain et al. (2021) analyzed more than 4,000 tweets sent by Indian political personalities regarding health. The tweets, they found, were mostly upbeat and addressed topics, including crisis management, strengthening followers' trust and resilience, managing reputation, and actions taken to deal with the situation. Sodi et al. (2021) highlighted the pandemic's modern dangers and vulnerabilities; "understanding uncertainty helps reduce vulnerability, as it may allow us to plan things better, mitigate some of the risks, and adapt more successfully" (Sodi et al., 2021, p. 235). The pandemic highlighted the importance of taking a more contextualized and action-oriented approach to health psychology (see Hariharan, 2022; Kapur et al., 2022). Research in the field of health psychology has taken a more contextualized approach. As Shamanna (2022) argued, "the key to the development of implementation research strategies is evolving and developing the right research questions and answering them in a local context" (p. 54). For instance, Jain and Singh (2024) looked at the relationship between cancer patients' financial situation, decision-making style (paternalistic vs. shared), and whether they decided to undergo cancer treatment. No matter the participants' decision-making style or financial circumstances, they all put a lot of faith in chance, luck, or God when told that therapy would drastically lower quality of life without eradicating cancer. With infrastructure and resource constraints and millions of people to consider, it is crucial to understand the social and cultural context and issues of well-being and health. More attention needs to be paid to social well-being which is key to harmony as well as an important aspect of overall well-being and development. In today's turbulent times with wars in many parts of the world and internal strife in many nations, there are significant challenges to social well-being. People with marginalized or historically devalued identities face specific challenges that can affect their mental health and well-being like systemic disadvantages, limited access to opportunities, unfair treatment in various aspects of life, education, employment, and so on (Singh, 2024). Thus, well-being is a complex combination of individuals' physical, mental, emotional, and social conditions and research needs a more nuanced analysis which is currently missing. We also need to acknowledge that in today's globalized era, many phenomena like climate change and the aftermath of COVID-19 are becoming more global issues than local as they impact humanity equally in parts of the world with local overtones. This adds another layer of complexity.

Challenges in the Educational Sector

While anecdotal evidence suggests that education can help level the playing field, important questions about fairness and access to education persist. With this in view, let us examine some emerging approaches which expand our approach to social reality. A novel way of looking at educational disparity was introduced by Nair et al. (2018). Following the broad parameters of the "Capabilities Approach" (Sen, 1980; Nussbaum, 2005) requires a multivariate evaluation of accessibility, equity, and quality. When thinking about "lack of access" as a mental and physical threat, human rights discourses often bring up Sen's groundbreaking work on a Human Development Index that takes into account factors like gender, education, food security, and health. Enrollment has increased during 2005 across the country, and education is mandatory up to the eighth grade (13–14 years old) in India. Enrollment in India's rural sector has increased from 11 million in 2005–2006 to 22 million in 2020–2021, with a particular focus on grade 8 children. The ASER 2023 study states that out of the 14- to 18-year-old demographic, 53% are still enrolled in school, with 72% of those students attending public schools. Astoundingly, for a school in rural India, 60% of the students can express themselves in simple English. New technology and policies have brought about significant changes in the last decade, with positive trends in classrooms as a result.

School enrollment and infrastructure, education financing, education policy and curriculum, and digitalizing the classroom are the four main areas that have witnessed changes in the education sector since 2014. These changes have been noted in both urban and rural locations. From 2014 to 2022, the percentage of students enrolled in school rose from 96.7% to 98.4. However, there has been inconsistent progress in school infrastructure; while 75% of schools have access to drinking water and restrooms, just 7% have computers (ASER, 2023). Students in rural and tribal areas were impacted when schools with low enrollment were shuttered (Deeksha & Subramaniam, 2022). Finally, digitizing the classroom is a major focus of National Education Policy 2020 (NEP 2020). The trend of using digital tools in the classroom has been continuing strong for over a decade, but many governments and ed-tech businesses have hastened their adoption due to COVID-19. Public e-learning systems like as Diksha, SWAYAM, E-pathshala, and Manodarpan are being developed by the government to foster digital inclusion (Department of School Education and Literacy, 2021). The problems caused by the digital divide in rural and urban areas' educational systems are discussed in the section that follows.

The percentage of Indians with internet access was 45% in January 2021, according to a report by Digital in India (Kemp, 2021). This enormous growth has exacerbated the digital gap since many people in urban slums, rural areas, and semi-rural areas have not benefited from it. The digital gap differs in magnitude depending on factors such as gender, age, location (urban vs. semi-rural), and caste (in India), according to the NFHS 2019–21. Despite progress, semi-rural men and women are less accessible than those living in cities. There are three tiers of the digital divide, according to Wei et al. (2011): the digital access tier, the digital capacity tier, and the digital result tier. A lack of availability of digital technology in both households and educational institutions is known as the digital access gap. People still don't have the technical know-how to make use of digital technologies, even though they're readily available. The fact that some groups (such as women, girls, the impoverished, and the socially excluded) have not reaped the same benefits from technological progress is highlighted by digital outcome disparities. The NEP recognizes, as stated by Kasturirangan (2019), that the urban poor, tribals, and various caste-based groups are excluded by the present digital breakthroughs. The availability of information and communication technology has been an obstacle to encouraging individuals in semi-rural areas to acquire digital literacy skills, even if initiatives like the Prime Minister's Village Digital Literacy Mission have been implemented. Giving people access to technology and digital training is key to closing the digital divide. Investing in teacher professional development, particularly in digital pedagogy and training in new technology, is crucial if India is to achieve its ambitious aim of becoming a digital nation. Blended learning was accelerated by the pandemic, which compelled ed-tech companies and the government to create digital learning materials platforms and tools (e.g., Diksha, SWAYAM, E-pathshala, Manodarpan).

Salient Thematic Trends

To identify particular research trends, we next examine thematic areas as published in two important Indian journals in critical psychology, *Psychological Studies and Psychology in Developing Societies*. The special issues released by these journals highlight recent research on special issues of Psychology and Developing Societies have been published since 2009, each edited by a different group of psychologists from different parts of the globe and with different areas of expertise. Justice and Diversity were the subject of the 2009 special issue (Singh), and future issues centered on marginalization more generally. For instance, in 2010, 2011, and 2020, special issues were devoted to issues such as poverty (Tripathi), disability (Dalal), and ageing (Kohli & Kar). In 2015, the issue was devoted to issues such as social exclusion and mental health (Thapa & Kumar), and in 2019, the issue was devoted to collective victimhood (Tripathi & Kumar). The environmental aspect has also received attention, with issues centered on the behavioral aspects of limited resource situations and the psychological underpinnings of sustainable development (Tripathi, 2017; Tripathi & Pande, 2022). New Confucian psychology (Liu, 2021), cultural healing for Indigenous people (Liu et al., 2014), and the theory, method, and practice of Indian psychology (Bhawuk & Srinivas, 2010) were some of the special issues that eventually centered on discussing psychological processes in specific communities. Polli Hagenaars's most recent special issue (2023) concludes the process of contextual specificity in psychology by addressing the decolonization of psychology in developing nations.

In a similar vein, *Psychological Studies* has released no less than eight special issues since 2011, with striking similarities between them all that point to these themes as central to the field of psychology. Both the 2011 (Eds & Banerjee) and 2019 (Eds Maheshwari & Mascolo) special issues have dealt with questions of identity and self, suggesting a fairly consistent trend. Also published in 2018 was a special issue on spirituality, edited by Oman, Duggal, and Misra, which focused on the topic's relevance in an Indian context. Issues on children's viewpoints and voices (Konantambigi, 2023) and the psychology of well-being in the margins (Bernardo & Mateo, 2022) are examples of how this journal has prioritized giving a platform to under-represented voices. A special edition of the journal devoted to the psychology of uncertainty was released during the outbreak (Sodi & Han, 2021). Contributions

Table E.1 Thematic issues published in *Psychology and Developing Societies*

S. No.	*Theme*	*Editor(s)*	*Year*
1.	Justice and Diversity	Purnima Singh	2009
2.	The Poor in Developing Societies	R. C. Tripathi	2010
3.	Theory, Method and Practice of Indian Psychology	Dharm P. S. Bhawuk and E. S. Srinivas	2010
4.	Disability in the Developing World	Ajit K Dalal	2011
5.	Cultural Healing for Indigenous People: Challenging Institutions and Building Self-Determination	James H. Liu, Keri Lawson-Te Aho, and Arama Rata	2014
6.	Social Exclusion and Mental Health	Komila Thapa, Rashmi Kumar	2015
7.	Psychosocial Bases of Sustainable Development	R. C. Tripathi	2017
8.	Collective Victimhood and its Consequences	R. C. Tripathi and Rashmi Kumar	2019
9.	Ageing in Developing Societies	Neena Kohli and Bhoomika R. Kar	2020
10.	Prospects for a New Confucian Psychology of the 21st Century: Theoretical Considerations and Empirical Studies	James H. Liu	2021
11.	Behaviour in Scarce Resource Environments	R. C. Tripathi and Namita Pande	2022
12.	Theory development, application, and contribution to societal development: A journey in the scientific discovery process	Uichol Kim and R. C. Tripathi	2023
13.	Decolonising Psychology in Developing Societies	Polli Hagenaars	2023

Table E.2 Thematic issues published in *Psychological Studies*

S. No.	*Name of Issue*	*Editor(s)*	*Year of Publishing*
1.	Contemporary Perspectives on Self and Identity	Girishwar Misra and Robin Banerjee	2011
2.	Kenneth J. Gergen and Social Constructionism	Girishwar Misra and Anand Prakash	2012
3.	Issue on Positive Psychology with a Target article titled Positive Psychology and Indian Psychology: In Need for Mutual Reinforcement by K. Ramakrishna Rao	Girishwar Misra	2014
4.	Spirituality and Psychology: Emerging Perspectives	Doug Oman, Chetna Duggal and Girishwar Misra	2018
5.	Rethinking Self and Identity in a Changing World	Surabhika Maheshwari and Michael Mascolo	2019
6.	Psychology of Uncertainty and Vulnerabilities COVID-19 Pandemic Related	Tholene Sodi and Buxin Han	2021
7.	Psychology of Well-being in the Margins: South Asian and Southeast Asian Research	Allan B.I. Bernardo and Nino Jose Mateo	2022
8.	Socialisation in Contemporary India: Perspectives and Voices of Child	Rajani M. Konantambigi	2023
9.	Special Issue with target article on Durganand Sinha, decolonising psychology in India (2024b)	Girishwar Misra and Purnima Singh	2024b

to the special issues have also sought to offer commentary on seminal and consequential journals and their current status. A few examples include an issue on positive psychology (Misra), Misra and Prakash's (2012) Social Constructionism and Kenneth J. Gergen. Rao (Misra, 2014), and another one focusing on the decolonizing psychology of India by Durganand Sinha. Both the final remark and the one published in Psychology and Developing Societies are identical, suggesting that the two journals collaborate on the same goal of discussing psychology in South Asia, with a focus on India.

Some Emerging Concerns

In India, social psychology has a long history, and its primary focus has been on themes such as cultural pluralism, gender discrimination, social and distributive justice, and the creation of social capital. The eco-social and political climate of the country, which includes its four major religions, caste system, many languages, and regional variances, is a factor that adds to the country's reputation for both unity and variety. The country, on the other hand, is experiencing a complicated sociopolitical matrix as a result of rising inequality, mounting conflicts, and high unemployment rates. To gain a more in-depth understanding of the social contextual components and how they interact with one another, researchers need to broaden their perspectives and become more fully involved in the topics that are currently being discussed. Academic research methodologies frequently adhere to mainstream Western theories, ignoring the complexity of social reality and cultural context, leading to a phenomenon known as "topic blindness."

Understanding individuals in the context of their social and cultural environments necessitates adopting a perspective that places a higher value on coexisting and sharing with other people than on exerting influence on them. To be successful in overcoming the obstacles that have been faced by social psychology research in India, it is necessary to have a toolbox of approaches that is more inclusive and to have a more comprehensive approach to analyzing data within the larger sociocultural context. Applied social psychology has made minimal progress due to adherence to the Euro-American paradigm, which may call into question the relevance of research to policy in different cultural contexts. This is even though psychological understanding is extremely important in the process of producing social policy. It must be noted that India is currently experiencing the emergence of social disputes, problems related to intergroup dynamics, and identity challenges. It is believed that a shift in focus toward identity processes in individual contexts would be more relevant to the process of policy-making and the development of indigenous theoretical frameworks. The abandonment of Euro-Western theoretical frameworks and the investigation of identity at the microlevel through more contextualized research are both necessary steps in the process of addressing the social issues that are plaguing India.

In response to the COVID-19 pandemic, health psychology has adopted a more contextualized approach. This is because the epidemic has brought attention to the significance of both psychological and physical well-being. Several studies have demonstrated that the financial position of cancer patients has an impact on the treatment options and decision-making styles that they choose, stressing the necessity of adopting a more contextualized approach.

Education is another vital domain of social life. Even though India's public schools have seen tremendous expansion since 2005, there are still difficulties to be faced in terms of access and equity. According to the Capabilities Approach, it is important to conduct a comprehensive evaluation of accessibility, equity, and equality. To address the increasing burden due to the population explosion, attention is being paid to the use of virtual classes. With only 45% of Indians having internet connectivity in January 2021, the digital divide in educational possibilities between urban and rural areas is a serious concern. The fact that only 37.6 million Indian students were able to continue their education through the use of internet resources or through television and radio programs during the pandemic is illustrative of the digital gap that exists within the country.

Indigenous research is gaining more and more recognition, and it is essential to have a solid understanding of the contextual and cultural aspects involved. *Psychological Studies* (Springer) and *Psychology* and *Developing Societies* (Sage) are two important Indian journals that concentrate on key topics in psychology and address psychological challenges that are prevalent in South Asian countries, particularly in India. More engagement with the issues and a broader perspective, rather than the present myopic approach, are necessary for researchers to achieve a more thorough understanding of the social contextual factors and their interconnections. Social psychology has fuzzy boundaries with cognate disciplines like sociology, and social work as well as other areas of psychology which often creates dilemmas about what is to be included and what is not to be included. The reality is that human emotions, cognitions, and behavior do not occur in a vacuum and do not make sense without the understanding of sociocultural factors. Social constructivism posits that knowledge is a human product, which is socially and culturally constructed actively and not something that can be discovered (Ernest, 1999; Vygotsky, 1978). Since there are social origins of mind and behavior; social psychology becomes the cusp of understanding which is rather neglected by researchers. Since human behavior is enacted in the social and cultural context, it is important to realize the social framing of behavior which is generally missed. We have not explored the essential sociality of human behavior and relationality and thus, this chapter argues that psychology ought to be strengthened by supporting social psychology. Also if we want to create a global social psychology responding to the realities of the globalized era, an interesting possibility is to develop strong indigenous social psychologies not just from India but from other majority world countries, which could then (Yeh, 2020) be integrated to form a global psychology. Sundararajan and colleagues (2020) in an interesting edited book by scholars have envisioned a Global psychology from Indigenous perspectives. It echoes the realization of JBP Sinha (1997):

> I do not have the need to carry the cross of someone's theory or approach; nor do I have resources to try mine in some other cultures. My hunch is that even if I try, I will be imposing my emic under the delusion of realizing an etic. May be the best I can do is to try to be a cultural rather than cross-cultural psychologist. May be the route to universal science of psychology is through many indigenous psychologies forming overarching patterns.
>
> (Sinha, 1997, p. 83)

Concluding Comments

India has a rich history in social psychology, focusing on topics such as cultural pluralism, gender bias, social equity, and social capital formation. On the other hand, the sociopolitical landscape is experiencing several issues, such as rising levels of inequality and violence, as well as high rates of unemployment. Researchers need to broaden their perspectives and engage with contemporary issues to gain a deeper understanding of social contextual factors. The dominance of Western theories in Indian social psychology has led to "topic blindness" and a disregard for cultural context. To overcome this, researchers should use a wider range of methods and examine data within the sociocultural framework. The applicability of research findings to policy-making in diverse cultural contexts is a concern. The COVID-19 pandemic has highlighted the importance of tailored strategies in health psychology, as it affects both psychological and physical well-being. Education is also a significant field, but there are challenges in terms of availability and fairness, particularly the digital gap between urban and rural communities.

Recognition of Indigenous research is increasing, and understanding the cultural and contextual elements is crucial. Indian journals like Psychological Studies and Psychology and Developing Societies address important psychological issues in South Asian countries. To surmount the challenges faced by the discipline, it is necessary to employ a broader range of methods and conduct a thorough examination of data within the sociocultural framework.

The preponderance of the Euro-American paradigm in India has been a significant factor in the minimal progress that has been made in the field of social psychology. As Pandey (2021) has noted, "the discipline has not reached near autochthonization" (p. 311). Upon examining the expansion of psychology in India, Mishra and Padalia (2021) note that the field exhibits a paradoxical combination of expansion and crisis. Although there has been substantial progress, there is currently an ongoing battle for relevance, aspiration, and identity. Mishra and Padalia (2021) advocate firmly for the cultivation of critical consciousness among scholars and the active pursuit of alternative visions for human existence. These observations raise concerns regarding the applicability of research findings to policy-making in diverse cultural contexts. In order to effectively address social challenges in India, it is crucial to give priority to the processes of identity in individual contexts and utilize a research methodology that considers the particular context of the problem.

In general, it is imperative to fortify social psychology by emphasizing its relationship with social and cultural factors. It is crucial to acknowledge the social framing of behavior and the social origins of mind and behavior. It would be possible to contribute to the development of a global social psychology that is responsive to the realities of the globalized period by developing robust indigenous social psychologies from India and other nations that account for the majority of the world's population.

References

Adinarayan, S. P. (1953). Before and after independence a study of racial and communal attitudes in India. *British Journal of Psychology General Section*, *44*(2), 108–115. 10.1111/j.2044-8295.1953.tb01186.x

Agrawal, P. (1978). A cross-cultural study of self-image: Indian, American, Australian, and Irish adolescents. *Journal of Youth and Adolescence*, *7*, 107–116.

Apicella, C., Norenzayan, A., & Henrich, J. (2020). Beyond WEIRD: A review of the last decade and a look ahead to the global laboratory of the future. *Evolution and Human Behavior*, *41*(5), 319–329.

Arnett, J. J. (2009). The neglected 95%, a challenge to psychology's philosophy of science. *American Psychologist*, *64*, 571–574.

ASER. (2023). *Annual status of education report (rural)—ASER (2023)*. PRATHAM. https://asercentre.org/wp-content/uploads/2022/12/ASER-2023-Main-Findings_Final-22.2.24–1.pdf

Bernardo, A. B. I., & Mateo, N. J. (Eds.). (2022). Psychology of well-being in the margins: South Asian and Southeast Asian research [Special Issue]. *Psychological Studies*, *67*(3).

Bhawuk, D. P. S., & Srinivas, E. S. (Eds.). (2010). Theory, method and practice of Indian psychology [Special Issue]. *Psychology and Developing Societies*, *22*(1).

Burke, P. J. (1980). The self: Measurement requirements from an interactionist perspective. *Social Psychology Quarterly*, *43*, 18–29.

Dalal, A. K. (Ed.). (2011). Disability in the developing world [Special Issue]. *Psychology and Developing Societies*, *23*(2).

Dalal, A. K., & Misra, G. (2001). Social psychology in India: Evolution and emerging trends. In A. K. Dalal & G. Misra (Eds.), *New directions in Indian psychology: Social psychology* (pp. 19–52). Sage.

Dalal, A. K., & Misra, G. (2011). Psychology of health and well-being: Emergence and development. *New Directions in Health Psychology*, 1–45.

Deeksha & Subramaniam. (2022, July 6). *India's mass closure of schools is leaving lakhs of students stranded*. Scroll.in. https://scroll.in/article/1027639/indias-mass-closure-of-schools-is-leaving-lakhs-of-students-stranded

DeRidder, R., & Tripathi, R. C. (Eds.). (1992). *Norm violation and intergroup relations*. Clarendon Press/Oxford University Press.

Erikson, E. H. (1950). *Childhood and society*. W W Norton & Co.

Ernest, P. (1999). *Social constructivism as a philosophy of mathematics: Radical constructivism rehabilitated*.

Ghosh, E. S., & Kumar, R. (1991). Hindu-Muslim intergroup relations in India: Applying socio-psychological perspectives. *Psychology and Developing Societies*, *3*(1), 93–112.

Hagenaars, P. (Ed.) (2023). Decolonising psychology in developing societies [Special Issue]. *Psychology and Developing Societies*, *35*(1).

Hariharan, M. (2022). Evidence-based health care: Contributions of health psychology. In *Health psychology* (pp. 3–24). Routledge India.

Heine, S. J., & Norenzayan, A. (2006). Toward a psychological science for a cultural species. *Perspectives on Psychological Science*, *1*(3), 251–269.

Henrich, J., Heine, S. J., & Norenzayan, A. (2010). The weirdest people in the world?. *Behavioral and Brain Sciences*, *33*(2–3), 61–83.

Jain, N., Malviya, P., Singh, P., & Mukherjee, S. (2021). Twitter mediated sociopolitical communication during the COVID-19 pandemic crisis in India. *Frontiers in psychology*, *12*, 784907.

Jain, N., & Singh, P. (2024). Exploring the influence of decisionmaking style and financial status of cancer patients on varied cultural aspects of decision process. *Psychology and Developing Societies*, *36*(1), 91–124.

Jogdand, Y. (2024). Laying the ground for a critical psychology of caste. *CASTE/A Global Journal on Social Exclusion*, *5*(2), 49–72.
Kakar, S. (1968). The human life cycle: The traditional Hindu view and the psychology of Erik Erikson. *Philosophy East and West*, *18*(3), 127–136.
Kapur, P., & Misra, G. (2011). Being human the Sikh way: Some psychological reflections. *Foundations of Indian Psychology*, *1*, 251–268.
Kapur, P., Misra, G., & Verma, N. K. (2022). *Psychological perspectives, identity, religion and well-being: Empirical findings from India.* Springer.
Kasturirangan, K. (2019). *National education policy (draft) India.* www.education.gov.in/sites/upload_files/mhrd/files/Draft_NEP_2019_EN_Revised.pdf
Kemp, S. (2021, February 11). Digital 2021: India. *Digital in India: All the statistics you need in 2021—DataReportal—Global digital insights.* https://datareportal.com/reports/digital-2021-india
Kim, U., & Tripathi, R. C. (Eds.). (2023). Theory development, application and contribution to societal development: A journey in the scientific discovery process [Special Issue]. *Psychology and Developing Societies*, *35*(2).
Kohli, N., & Kar, B. R. (Eds.). (2020). Ageing in developing societies [Special Issue]. *Psychology and Developing Societies*, *32*(2).
Konantambigi, R. M. (2023). Socialisation in contemporary India: Perspectives and voices of children and adolescents [Special Section]. *Psychological Studies*, *68*.
Liu, J. H. (Ed.) (2021). Prospects for a new Confucian psychology of the 21st century: Theoretical considerations and empirical studies [Special Issue]. *Psychology and Developing Societies*, *33*(1).
Liu, J. H., Lawson-Te Aho, K., & Rata, A. (Eds.). (2014). Cultural healing for indigenous people: Challenging institutions and building self-determination [Special Issue]. *Psychology and Developing Societies*, *26*(2).
Maheshwari, S., & Mascolo, M. (Eds.). (2019). Rethinking self and identity in a changing world [Special Issue]. *Psychological Studies*, *64*(3).
McCall, G., & Simmons, J. (1978). *Identities and interactions* (Revised ed.). Free Press.
Mishra, A. K., & Padalia, D. (2021). Re-envisioning psychology: A critical history of psychology in India. In G. Misra, N. Sanyal, & Sonali De (Eds.), *Psychology in modern India historical, methodological, and future perspectives* (pp. 163–202). Springer.
Misra, G. (Ed.). (1990). *Applied social psychology in India.* Sage Publications.
Misra, G. (Ed.). (2010). *Psychology in India. Volume IV: Theoretical and methodological developments (ICSSR survey of advances in research).* Pearson.
Misra, G. (Ed.) (2014). Special issue on positive psychology with a target article entitled positive psychology and Indian Psychology: In need for mutual reinforcement by K. Ramakrishna Rao [Special Issue]. *Psychological Studies*, *59*(2).
Misra, G. (Ed.). (2019). *Psychology: ICSSR research surveys and explorations.* Oxford University Press.
Misra, G., & Banerjee, R. (Eds.). (2011). Contemporary perspectives on self and identity. [Special Issue]. *Psychological Studies*, *56*(1).
Misra, G., & Prakash, A. (Eds.). (2012). Kenneth J. Gergen and social constructionism [Special Issue]. *Psychological Studies*, *57*(2).
Misra, G., & Singh, P. (2024a). Beyond decolonization: Moving towards a viable alternative. *Psychological Studies*, *69*(Suppl 1), 1–10.
Misra, G., & Singh, P. (Eds.). (2024b). Some reflections on integration of modern psychology with Indian thought [Special Issue]. *Psychological Studies*, *69*(1).
Mitra, S. K. (1972). Psychological research in India. In SK Mitra (Ed.) *A survey of research in psychology* (pp. xvii–xxxiii). Popular Prakashan.
Moghaddam, F. M. (2022). *How psychologists failed.* Cambridge University Press.

Murphy, G. (1953). *In the minds of men*. Basic Books.
Nair, R. B., Singh, P., & Upadhyay, V. (2018). *Capabilities approach to education: Access, equity, and quality*. ICSSR.
Nandy, A. (1970). The culture of Indian politics: A stock taking. *The Journal of Asian Studies*, *30*(1), 57–79.
Nandy, A. (1976). Woman versus womanliness in India: An essay in social and political psychology. *Psychoanalytic Review*, *63*(2), 301.
Norenzayan, A., & Heine, S. J. (2005). Psychological universals: What are they and how can we know?. *Psychological Bulletin*, *131*(5), 763.
Nussbaum, M. (2005). Capabilities as fundamental entitlements. *Capabilities Equality Basic Issues and Problems*, *18*.
Oman, D., Duggal, C. Misra, G. (Eds.). (2018). Spirituality and psychology: Emerging perspectives [Special Issue]. *Psychological Studies*, *63*(2).
Pandey, J. (1988). *Psychology in India: The state of the art* (Vol. 1–3). Sage.
Pandey, J. (2000). *Psychology in India revisited—developments in the discipline: Physiological foundation and human cognition* (Vol. 1). Sage.
Pandey, J. (2001). *Psychology in India revisited—developments in the discipline: Personality and health psychology* (Vol. 2). Sage.
Pandey, J. (2004). *Psychology in India revisited—developments in the discipline: Applied social and organizational psychology* (Vol. 3). Sage.
Pandey, J. (2021). Hundred years of social psychology in India. In G. Misra, N. Sanyal, & S. De (Eds.), *Psychology in modern India historical, methodological, and future perspectives* (pp. 301–315). Springer.
Pandey, J., & Singh, P. (2005). Social psychology in India: Social roots and development. *International Journal of Psychology*, *40*, 239–253. https://doi.org/10.1080/00207590444000186
Paranjpe, A. C. (1985). The identity theory of prejudice. *Journal of Asian and African studies*, *20*(3–4), 232–245.
Paranjpe, A. C. (1998). *Self and identity in modern psychology and Indian thought*. Plenum.
Pareek, U. (1980). *A survey of research in psychology, 1971–76, Part 1*. Popular Publication.
Pareek, U. (1981). *A survey of research in psychology, 1971–76, Part 2*. Popular Publication.
Pillay, S. R. (2017). Cracking the fortress: Can we really decolonize psychology?. *South African Journal of Psychology*, *47*(2), 135–140.
Ramanathan, P., & Singh, P. (2021). 'Searching for roots': Exploring the idea of home in Tibetan refugee youth living in Delhi, India. *Psychology and Developing Societies*, *33*(2), 324–346.
Ramanathan, P., & Singh, P. (2024). 'Don't forget Tibet': Understanding the discursive construction of Tibetan national identity through the identity entrepreneurship of the Dalai Lama. *European Journal of Social Psychology*, *54*, 959–970. https://doi.org/10.1002/ejsp.3060
Sears, D. O. (1986). College sophomores in the laboratory: Influences of a narrow data base on social psychology's view of human nature. *Journal of Personality and Social Psychology*, *51*(3), 515.
Sen, A. K. (1980). Equality of what?. In S. M. McMurrin (Ed.), *The tanner lectures on human value* (pp. 195–220). University of Utah Press.
Shamanna, B. R. (2022). Implementation research for public health and preventive health care in India. In *Health psychology* (pp. 54–70). Routledge.
Sharma, S., & Jogdand, Y. (2024). The nature of caste prejudice: A new look at prejudice, social identity, and casteism in India. *CASTE/A Global Journal on Social Exclusion*, *5*(2), 73–96.

Singh, P. (Ed.). (2009). Justice and diversity [Special Issue]. *Psychology and Developing Societies, 21*(1).
Singh, P. (2021). Navigating India's rich diversity in social psychological research. *Nature Human Behaviour, 5*(9), 1116–1116.
Singh, P. (2024, July 21–26). Promoting social well-being in contemporary times. In S. Suchday (Chair), *Psychosocial aspects of well-being.* [Symposium]. *33rd International Congress of Psychology*, Prague, Czech Republic.
Singh, R. (2022, June). *Life and work of a social psychologist in India: 1945-present.* Source. https://ahduni.edu.in/site/assets/files/2663/life_and_work_of_a_social_psychologist_in_india_june_3-_2022.pdf
Sinha, D. (1981). Social psychology in India: A historical perspective. In J. Pandey (Ed.) *Perspectives on experimental social psychology in India* (pp. 3–17). Concept.
Sinha, D. (1998). Changing perspectives in social psychology in India: A journey towards indigenization. *Asian Journal of Social Psychology, 1*, 17–32.
Sinha, J. B. P. (1993). The bulk and the front of psychology in India. *Psychology and Developing Societies, 5*, 135–150.
Sinha, J. B. P. (1997). In search of my Brahman. In M. H. Bond (Ed.) *Working at the interface of cultures: Eighteen lives in social science* (pp. 77–84). Routledge.
Sodi, T., & Han, B. (2021). Psychology of uncertainty and vulnerabilities COVID-19 pandemic related. [Special Issue]. *Psychological Studies, 66*(3).
Sodi, T., Han, B., & Singh, P. (2021). Special issue on psychology of uncertainty and vulnerabilities: COVID-19 pandemic related crisis. *Psychological Studies*, 1–4.
Stephens, N. M., Markus, H. R., & Phillips, L. T. (2014). Social class culture cycles: How three gateway contexts shape selves and fuel inequality. *Annual Review of Psychology, 65*(1), 611–634.
Stern, R. W. (2003). *Changing India: Bourgeois revolution on the subcontinent.* Cambridge University Press.
Sundararajan, L., Hwang, K. K., & Yeh, K. H. (2020). *Global psychology from indigenous perspectives.* Springer International Publishing.
Tajfel, H., & Turner, J. C. (1979). An integrative theory of intergroup conflict. in W. G. Austin & S. Worchel (Eds.), *The social psychology of intergroup relations* (pp. 33–47). Brooks-Cole.
Thapa, K., & Kumar, R. (Eds.). (2015). Social exclusion and mental health [Special Issue]. *Psychology and Developing Societies, 27*(2).
Triandis, H. C. (1994). *Culture and social behavior* (xvi, 330). McGraw-Hill Book Company.
Tripathi, R. C. (Ed.). (2010). The poor in developing societies [Special Issue]. *Psychology and Developing Societies, 22*(2).
Tripathi, R. C. (Ed.). (2017). Psycho-social bases of sustainable development [Special Issue]. *Psychology and Developing Societies, 29*(2).
Tripathi, R. C., & Kumar, R. (Eds.). (2019). Collective victimhood and its consequences [Special Issue]. *Psychology and Developing Societies, 33*(1).
Tripathi, R. C., & Pande, N. (Eds.). (2022). Behaviour in scarce resource environments [Special Issue]. *Psychology and Developing Societies, 34*(1).
Tripathi, R. C., & Sinha, Y. (Eds.). (2014). *Psychology, development and social policy in India.* Springer India.
Tripathi, R. C., & Srivastava, R. (1981). Relative deprivation and intergroup attitudes. *European Journal of Social Psychology, 11*(3), 313–318.
Turner, J. C., Hogg, M. A., Oakes, P. J., Reicher, S. D., & Wetherell, M. S. (1987). Rediscovering the social group: A self-categorization theory. Basil Blackwell.
Uskul, A. K., Bernardo, A. B. I., Gonzalez, R., Kende, A., Laher, S., Lášticová, B., Saab, R., Salas, G., Singh, P., Zeinoun, P., Thalmayer, A. G., Norenzayan, A., Chao, M. M., Shoda, Y., & Cooper, M. L. (2024). *Challenges and opportunities*

for psychological research in the majority world [Manuscript submitted for publication].
Vahali, H. O. (2009). *Lives in exile: Exploring the inner world of Tibetan refugees*. Routledge.
Vygotsky, L. S. (1978). *Mind in society*. Harvard University Press.
Wei, K. K., Teo, H. H., Chan, H. C., & Tan, B. C. (2011). Conceptualizing and testing a social cognitive model of the digital divide. *Information Systems Research*, *22*(1), 170–187.
Yeh, K. H. (2020). Pioneer of Chinese indigenous psychology: Prof. Kuo-Shu Yang. In *Global psychology from indigenous perspectives: Visions inspired by KS Yang* (pp. 33–44).

Index

For Product Safety Concerns and Information please contact our EU representative GPSR@taylorandfrancis.com
Taylor & Francis Verlag GmbH, Kaufingerstraße 24, 80331 München, Germany

www.ingramcontent.com/pod-product-compliance
Lightning Source LLC
LaVergne TN
LVHW021121300926
849160LV00010B/803

* 9 7 8 1 0 3 2 6 0 9 6 4 5 *